Health & Society

Health & Society
Critical Perspectives

Edited by James Gillett, Gavin J. Andrews, and Mat Savelli

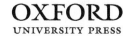
OXFORD
UNIVERSITY PRESS

OXFORD
UNIVERSITY PRESS

Oxford University Press is a department of the University of Oxford.
It furthers the University's objective of excellence in research, scholarship,
and education by publishing worldwide. Oxford is a registered trade mark of
Oxford University Press in the UK and in certain other countries.

Published in Canada by
Oxford University Press
8 Sampson Mews, Suite 204,
Don Mills, Ontario M3C 0H5 Canada

www.oupcanada.com

Library and Archives Canada Cataloguing in Publication

Health & society : critical perspectives / edited by James
Gillett, Gavin J. Andrews, and Mat Savelli.

Includes bibliographical references and index.
ISBN 978-0-19-901527-6 (paperback)

1. Health--Social aspects--Textbooks. I. Gillett, James,
1966-, author, editor II. Andrews, Gavin J., 1970-, author,
editor III. Savelli, Mat, 1982-, author, editor IV. Title: Health
and society.

RA418.H42 2016   613   C2016-900341-8

Cover image: © iStock/PM10
Chapter-opening photos: Chapter 1: Jose AS Reyes/Shutterstock.com; Chapter 2: Superjoseph/istock/Thinkstock; Chapter 3: Digital Vision/Thom
Northout/Thinkstock; Chapter 4: © MOHAMED NURELDIN ABDALLAH/Reuters/Corbis; Chapter 5: © Ed Kashi/VII/Corbis; Chapter 6: Kristoffer
TripplaarAlamy; Chapter 7: dpa picture alliance/Alamy; Chapter 8: BSIP SA/Alamy; Chapter 9: © T & L/BSIP/Corbis; Chapter 10: Bill Brooks/Alamy;
Chapter 11: Steve Hix/Fuse/Thinkstock; Chapter 12: © MIHAI ANDRITOIU / Alamy; Chapter 13: fivepointsix/Shutterstock; Chapter 14: Steven Scott
Taylor/Alamy.
Design graphic used throughout: Oleksandr Haisonok/Shutterstock.com

Printed and bound in Canada

2 3 4 — 19 18 17

Contents

Contributors

Gavin J. Andrews is a professor in the Department of Health, Aging, & Society at McMaster University. He was the inaugural chair of the department and currently serves as graduate chair. As a geographer, his research examines how place and space can influence a wide range of areas including health care, holistic medicine, aging, nursing, fitness, popular music, and phobias.

Jeffrey S. Denis is an assistant professor in the Department of Sociology at McMaster University. He studies the social psychology of racism and colonialism, antiracist and anticolonial activism, social inequalities in health, and social movements. He is the author of the forthcoming book Canada at the Crossroads: Boundaries, Bridges, and Laissez-Faire Racism in Indigenous-Settler Relations.

Joshua Evans is the human geography coordinator and an assistant professor in the Department of Human Geography at Athabasca University. His areas of interest include public health, hospital design, housing and homelessness, and urban policy.

Chelsea Gabel is an assistant professor in the Department of Health, Aging, & Society and the Indigenous Studies Program at McMaster University. Her research interests include Aboriginal health, health policy, and community-based participatory research.

Leigh-Anne Gillespie is a doctoral candidate in the Health Policy Ph.D. Program at McMaster University. Her research addresses aid agency policies and the ethical challenges of responding to humanitarian emergencies. Beyond this, her work as a research assistant at the McMaster Health Forum focuses on harm reduction interventions for people who use drugs.

James Gillett is an associate professor in the Department of Health, Aging, & Society and the Department of Sociology at McMaster University. His research focuses on individual approaches to health care and cultural understandings of health. He also studies health in relation to sport, animals, and media.

Amanda Grenier is an associate professor in the Department of Health, Aging, & Society at McMaster University, Gilbrea Chair in Aging and Mental Health, and the Director of the Gilbrea Centre for Studies in Aging. She is a social gerontologist with interests in the social constructs of aging, the relationship between public policy and the lived experience of older individuals, and social inequality. Her research draws on qualitative methods such as narrative and discourse analysis. She has published on frailty and late life transitions, and is currently finalizing a project on homelessness among older people.

Michel Grignon is an associate professor in the Department of Health, Aging, & Society and the Department of Economics at McMaster University. He is the director for the Centre for Health Economics and Policy Analysis and an Associate Scientist at the Institut de Recherche et Documentation en Économie de la Santé. His research focuses on the governance, finance, accessibility, and efficiency of health care systems.

Yvonne LeBlanc is an instructor in the Department of Health, Aging, & Society at McMaster University. She is a medical sociologist who has taught core sociology and sociology of health and illness courses at various universities in Ontario. Through qualitative inquiry, her research focuses on how people construct and negotiate health and illness, primarily through the intersections of health care, aging, and gender. She has used complementary and alternative medicine as a portal to understanding the mechanisms and processes that shape our understanding of how health and health care are experienced within contemporary society.

Anthony Lombardo is the executive director of the Canadian Association on Gerontology. He is an instructor in the Chang School of Gerontology at Ryerson University and has worked as a consultant in health research, health promotion, and grant development.

Raza Mirza holds a Ph.D. from the University of Toronto and has specialized in gerontology. He was previously a fellow of the Health Care, Technology and Place initiative of the Canadian Institutes of Health Research.

Elena Neiterman received her Ph.D. in sociology from McMaster University. Her research focuses on women's experiences of pregnancy and the postpartum period, midwifery and health professions, health care policy, and interdisciplinary study of the body. She is currently a lecturer at the School of Public Health and Health Systems at the University of Waterloo.

Dorothy Pawluch is an associate professor and former chair of the Department of Sociology at McMaster University. She currently serves as director of the university's Honours Social Psychology Program. Her research interests include the social construction of health knowledge, medicalization, constructions of deviance and social problems, health care professions, and complementary/alternative health care approaches. She is author of *The New Pediatrics: A Profession in Transition*, an exploration of pediatrics' move into the treatment of childhood deviance and behavioural problems. She has also written about the lived experiences of individuals diagnosed with HIV/AIDS.

Elizabeth Peter, RN, Ph.D. is an associate professor at the Lawrence S. Bloomberg Faculty of Nursing and a member of the Joint Centre for Bioethics and the Centre for Critical Qualitative Health Research, University of Toronto. Her scholarship reflects her interdisciplinary background in nursing, philosophy, and bioethics. Theoretically, she locates her work in feminist health care ethics, exploring the ethical dimensions of nursing work along with the ethical concerns that arise in home care. She is currently the chair of the Health Sciences Research Ethics Board, University of Toronto.

Mat Savelli is a postdoctoral fellow in the Department of Health, Aging, & Society at McMaster University. He obtained a D.Phil in the history of medicine from the University of Oxford and specializes in the historical and socio-cultural dimensions of mental health. He is currently researching the history of mental health care in Eastern Europe and the global advertising of psychopharmaceutical drugs.

Geraldine Voros is an associate professor in the Department of Health, Aging, & Society at McMaster University. She has designed and taught numerous courses on the subjects of health and aging and has received a number of accolades for her undergraduate teaching.

Foreword

Engaging with the Health Studies Scholarly Community ... Or, Why You Should Get Excited about This Book

Blake Poland and Pascale Lehoux

Books are powerful technologies. They open up the reader's mind. Their content can be shared endlessly with others. And the ideas they convey prompt new, more incisive inquiry. As such, books can be transformative.

While this book possesses the kind of power described above, it also performs something more important: it conveys what Karin Knorr Cetina (1999) calls an "epistemic culture" or a "culture of knowledge." An epistemic culture—in this case, critical health studies—brings forward what can be found "out there" that it deems as worth knowing. It defines the ways and purposes of knowing and makes explicit why one should care about that knowledge. Thus, the notion of "epistemic communities" as communities concerned with producing and disseminating knowledge is described by Haas (1992, p.3) as a "network of professionals with recognized expertise" who possess a "shared set of ... principled beliefs," "common practices," and a "conviction that human welfare will be enhanced as a consequence."

In this sense, critical health studies is also what Brown (2003) calls a "community of hope" or "community of promise," structured around the imagining and creation of a better future. It is productive insofar as it mobilizes opportunities for collaboration and change (Meyer & Molyneux-Hodgson, 2010). By carefully organizing the diverse yet interconnecting bodies of knowledge that contribute to the richness of health studies today, this book unlocks the door for readers to engage with a vibrant scholarly community.

The shared goal of this community is to examine health as a meaningful state of life, as opposed to a set of biomedical functions. To illustrate the many dimensions underlying the field, the book collects the thinking of scholars who draw on the social sciences to unpack (1) what constitutes health, illness, and care; (2) what ideologies underpin health and social care systems; (3) what health challenges individuals and communities face; and (4) the emerging dynamics that are shifting experiences of health.

Being Critical, Being Responsible

As readers will discover throughout the book, health studies scholars share a marked concern for criticality. This implies, among other things, being able to open up and engage in challenging conversations about established models of thinking and traditional authorities. Such conversations help students of health studies relate to, build on, reframe, or reject various knowledge claims. When interlaced within a single book, these conversations contribute to the shaping of a collective identity, which generates new forms of expertise and new ways of knowing.

By tackling the various cultural, political, social, and economic objects that are embedded in illness, health, and medicine, this book offers a solid introduction to the work of the health studies community. At the same time, its authors carefully set out the areas where complexity and puzzlement abound.

In principle, one may wish to see a point of articulation between what scholars define as "knowable" and what policy-makers or practitioners deem "useful to know." Yet, this book suggests that the relationship between knowledge and practice in health studies is not so straightforward. The knowledge–practice nexus reveals and deepens the moral foundations of research that critically explores what health, as a meaningful state of life, entails, and for whom. As academics who nurture a shared culture of knowing, health studies scholars seek ways to act responsibly when they develop new knowledge and put it into the public domain. This implies adopting a critical and reflexive posture that calls into question the power dynamics that are inherent in the relationship between those who decide and those for whom decisions are made.

Knowing Together

Each chapter in this book initiates a conversation that resonates with the other chapters that the book's editors have carefully assembled. Taken as a whole, these are epistemic conversations that have a far-reaching transformative potential because those who engage in them can be enriched, challenged, or even censured through the process. Epistemic conversations are, after all, conversations through which something is learned, even if the knowledge acquired may at times prove hard to stomach. Knowing the intricacies of health, illness, and medicine leaves no one undisturbed.

This book thus explains why health studies research is aspirational and shows how its researchers may articulate solidarity, humbleness, and creativity in their quest for knowledge. Scholarly practices are made up of, and structured by, the evolving disciplinary cultures prevailing in a given field. Mutual learning across disciplines is partly dependent on building shared knowledge and developing a common language, both of which enable the reinforcement of values and the modification or discarding of others.

More broadly, the book highlights the valuable contribution that the social and behavioural sciences make to understanding health, health care, and public health. While perspectives vary, the contributions of an explicitly "critical social science" perspective to understanding and explaining the nature and mechanisms of the individual, institutional, and societal conditions and forces that determine health include the following:

- "Social relations" are conceived as central to health. Health status, health-related behaviour, and professional and institutional practices are understood as being shaped by human social interaction and by cultural, organizational, political, and societal structures and processes.
- Problems are framed and addressed at multiple levels. Perspectives range from "micro" (individual/behavioural) to "meso" (groups, organizations) to "macro" (institutional/societal), often with reference to relationships across scale.
- Context is considered analytically important. Determinants, processes, and outcomes are viewed as contingent upon the circumstances and conditions in which they are located.
- Theory is employed as a key research resource. Theory is used to explain social processes that can only be inferred from observable phenomena (e.g., social class, power, racism, social learning) and to inform and link core assumptions, research questions, methodological design, data interpretation, and findings.
- Research methodology is aligned with the distinctive character of social/behavioural phenomena. A variety of qualitative, quantitative, and blended approaches, from varied disciplinary traditions, are designed to study phenomena that are mediated by human interpretation and meaning, and rooted in individual and social systems.
- A "critical" approach is taken to research and professional practice. Attention is directed to identifying underlying assumptions, the role of power in health and public health practices, and the political nature of knowledge and public discourse. (DLSPH, 2015)

A Vital and Timely Contribution

Critical Health Studies builds upon but also problematizes and distinguishes itself from mainstream dominant formulations. For the first time, this book (aimed at undergraduates beginning their involvement with health studies) brings together a range of disciplinary perspectives on what constitutes "critical health studies," at a time when health studies programs are proliferating. This is thus a timely and much-needed intervention in a rapidly expanding field.

The book attends to the social production of health and illness, as well as individual, institutional, and societal responses (health care systems, alternative and complementary medicine, social movements, health activism). A broad range of topics is covered, including social movements; social constructionism; ethics; healthism; social justice; globalization; transdisciplinarity; intersectionality; health inequity; One Health; neoliberalism; culture; political economy; iatrogenesis; the governance, funding, and regulation of health care systems; evidence-based medicine; epistemology and methods; social determinants of health; consumerism; and technology. It draws on a range of critical scholarship across the disciplines of health psychology, sociology, geography, economics, history, political science, and various fields of study (women's studies, Aboriginal studies, social movements, policy analysis, and so on). While there is some repetition of key concepts across chapters (e.g., culture, biomedicine, medicalization, political economy, professionalization) this is as it should be, given the centrality of these concepts and their interconnectedness. The use of a standard format of study questions, recommended readings, case studies of contemporary examples (with a decidedly Canadian and global health focus), chapter summaries, and chapter-specific reference lists conspire to make this a favourite for undergraduate learning. Overall, it is a superb introduction to critical health studies, and a valuable addition to any health studies program.

Books are powerful technologies because they contain and prompt crucial epistemic conversations that reflect, prolong, and may eventually modify cultures of knowing. Hence, what is there left to do when one has such a potent technology in hand? Discover the (critical) health studies scholarly community, share your understandings with others, and identify the key ideas upon which your own inquiries will draw.

References

Brown, N. 2003. "Hope against hype: Accountability in biopasts, presents and futures," *Science Studies*, 16(2): 3–21.

DLSPH (2015). The contribution of the social and behavioural sciences to public health. Toronto, ON: Dalla Lana School of Public Health. www.dlsph.utoronto.ca/discipline/social-and-behavioural-health-sciences.

Haas, P.M. 1992. "Epistemic Communities and International Policy Coordination," *International Organization*, 46(1): 1-35.

Knorr-Cetina, K. 1999. *Epistemic Cultures: How the Sciences Make Knowledge*. Cambridge, MA: Harvard University Press.

Meyer, M. and S. Molyneux-Hodgson. 2010. "The dynamics of epistemic communities." *Sociological Research Online*, 15(2): 14.

Acknowledgements

The editors would like to thank everyone who assisted in the production of the manuscript, especially the contributors. Completing the book was also made much, much easier through the input of two remarkable research assistants, Cristi Flood and Melissa Ricci. They were especially helpful in transforming disparate submissions into a coherent whole. Finally, we would like to thank the four anonymous reviewers whose feedback both highlighted the book's strengths and reshaped some important aspects of the text.

Part I

Introduction and Overview

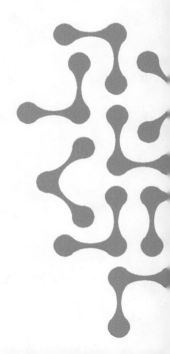

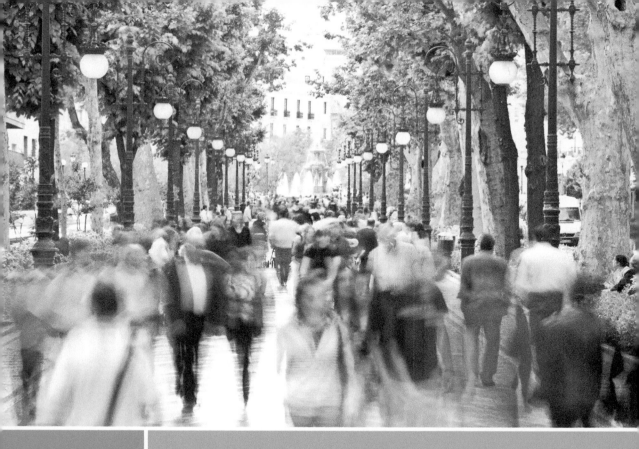

1

Introduction to Critical Health Studies

Gavin J. Andrews, James Gillett, and Geraldine Voros

LEARNING OBJECTIVES

In this chapter, students will learn

- what constitutes the field of critical health studies
- the nature of criticality
- the content of each chapter to come

Introduction

Critical health studies is a field of academic inquiry and teaching within which all of the following chapters comfortably sit. For many readers of this book, it also reflects the nature of the academic course they are currently taking, the degree program they are currently enrolled in, or the nature of their academic department.

This chapter is initially structured by two themes. The first, "health studies," describes the basic composition of the field. The second, "being critical," describes this specific approach and its priorities. A final section then walks readers through the remainder of book, summarizing the purpose and content of each remaining chapter.

Health Studies

Illness and medicine are important to people. This is unsurprising because the first is a negative life event and the second potentially relieves people from that event. Although we may not always be aware of it, these two concepts constitute much more than a biological process and a rational curative science. Through our experience of our own bodies, the numerous interactions we have had with doctors and nurses, our experiences with hospitals and clinics, and the ways in which illness and medicine are represented in the media, we are engaged with the breadth of the topic of health. **Health studies** picks up on this complexity, starting with the basic observation that the nature of illness, health, and medicine are all up for debate. Each has personal, collective, cultural, social, political, and economic dimensions that need to be accounted for.

As the name suggests, health studies is concerned with health (what else!). In this regard, reflecting the early ideas of the World Health Organization (WHO), health is considered as something particular in its own right, more than just the absence of disease (WHO, 1946). Indeed, health studies pays particular attention to the concept of "wellbeing," namely when individuals and groups are content, healthy, and in a good place in their lives. This entails having their basic needs fulfilled, with reasonable opportunities and capacities to meet these needs (Fleuret & Atkinson, 2007). **Wellbeing** is thus conceived by health studies researchers as a meaningful state of life. Most recently, researchers have been interested in it as an immediate experience and feeling that can arise in the moment (Andrews et al., 2014).

By contrast, the **health sciences**—a collection of disciplines that support and constitute medicine—are well established and well known. These can include:

- disciplines based around occupational categories such as nursing, occupational therapy, and pharmacy;
- disciplines based around medical categories and "basic sciences" (often about aspects of the body) including anaesthesiology, toxicology, genetics, immunology, and microbiology; and
- disciplines based around clinical specialties (types of services) including geriatrics, paediatrics, family practice, critical care, and mental health care.

"Health studies is composed predominantly of social science sub-disciplines, the most notable of these being health sociology (the study of the interactions and relationships between society and health—see Germov and Hornosty, 2011). Beyond this, health studies encompasses the following:

- Health geography (the study of how space and place affect and represent health and health care—see Gatrell & Elliott, 2009)
- Medical anthropology (the study of the bio-cultural and ecological aspects of health and health care—see Joralemon, 2009)
- Health psychology (the study of the cognitive and behavioural aspects of health and health care—see Ogden, 2012)
- Health economics (the study of different ways of allocating resources for health with different outcomes—see Palmer & Ho, 2007)

Indeed, by their very nature, these sub-disciplines help researchers address the aforementioned personal, collective, cultural, social, political, and economic dimensions of illness, health, and medicine.

However, the above list is far from exhaustive. Health studies also draws from, and is composed of, research from mainstream social science disciplines (including, for example, political science and religious studies), research from various humanities (including classics, history, philosophy, English, music, and other arts), and a range of contemporary interdisciplinary academic fields (including, for instance, women's studies, cultural studies, Aboriginal studies, social gerontology, and labour studies). And as if this picture were not complicated enough, the health sciences cannot be totally excluded from the field of health studies. There are scholars across a number of health science's constituent disciplines who produce critical research focused on health and society, including people working in public health, health services research, nursing research, or population health (Eakin et al., 1996).

Although the individual chapters to come outline their own focused areas of interest and inquiries, broadly speaking health studies asks the following questions:

- How are health and health care socially and culturally constructed (i.e., what constitutes health, illness, and health care to different people in different times and places)?
- What are the ideologies, principles, and powers underpinning health care and public health systems?
- What health challenges are facing individuals now? What will they face in the future? How do we experience these challenges?

Beyond this, the critical perspectives (as outlined in the next section) pose their own set of unique questions for health studies. These will be explored further on in the chapter.

Health studies research uses both **quantitative** research methods (including health records and statistics, census data, and survey questionnaires) and **qualitative** research methods (such as interviews, focus groups, observation techniques, and document analysis). It is, however, the latter group that is most popular. Data derived from qualitative research is well suited to answer the central questions of health studies, providing in-depth and person-sensitive perspectives (Bourgeault et al., 2013). Indeed, human circumstances are inherently complex, and a range of qualitative research methodologies is required to convey this complexity.

Health studies is not only diverse, it also an expanding field. This is reflected and supported by the increasing number of college- and university-based health studies programs and departments. Of course, these programs and departments are not all similar. Some are more scientific or bio medical in their approach, some are more humanistic, and some are combined with other subjects (such as gerontology, kinesiology, and cultural studies—see www.canadian-universities.net/Universities/Programs/Health_Studies.html).

Graduates of health studies programs enter a wide range of jobs, some going on take to specialist health professional qualifications (such as in public health, nursing, or medicine), others entering a variety of employment sectors (including health policy, health administration, health advocacy, health charities and NGOs, health IT, and health PR and advertising), Meanwhile, others join diverse private companies that produce health-related products and provide health-related services.

Being Critical

The hallmark of much of health studies is its "criticality," which distinguishes it from other forms of health research. Critical thinking has precedent, for example in the Marxist (radical) social science of the 1970s and 1980s, particularly in relation to its concern for social justice. However, critical research emerged strongly in the 1990s as something unique and broader (Blomley, 2006). Reflecting this development, in contemporary research we now see a critical approach adopted in most social sciences. These are known, for example, as "critical sociology," "critical geography," "and critical psychology." Across these disciplines, it is generally accepted that a number of core facets constitute and characterize a critical approach:

- **Challenging social and institutional norms, models of thinking, and power relationships.** Critical researchers do not simply accept that ideas, policies, services, and initiatives are appropriate simply because they are provided by those with power and authority. Instead, researchers should question them and be prepared to expose shortfalls, inequalities, and their consequences. Researchers might also question the fundamental ideas and concepts that are part of how power is exerted. Each will have relative merits, success or failures, and specific consequences.
- **Finding and questioning the ideas behind everyday social practices.** As Sayer (2009) notes, a critical approach goes beyond the consideration of practices—the things people do—to address the ideas and norms that inform these actions. Notably, critical research also develops and utilizes extensive bodies of thought as to why those ideas and norms are correct or incorrect and why they are held. So for example, as Sayer suggests, critical thinkers recognize that sexist practices are underpinned by ideas about women and men that feminism shows to be incorrect and entrenched.
- **Advocating alongside and on behalf of people and issues that are neglected or marginalized in mainstream policy, administration, and research.** It is observed that certain people—often the most vulnerable—"fall off the map" of policy, practice, and research. Critical researchers challenge the neglect of specific groups—such as disabled, LGBTQ, and Aboriginal peoples—and make a concerted effort to highlight the vulnerability, inequality, and oppression that that these groups experience.

- **Addressing pressing social and health issues that negatively affect individuals and populations.** It is argued that critical research should aim to alleviate mental and physical suffering, which is broadly a result of economic inequality, sexism, racism, homophobia, and other discriminatory beliefs and systems. It also aims to understand what constitutes human suffering, the extent to which this suffering is unacceptable, and what constitutes human flourishing. This interest brings health studies into proximity with broader social and welfare research.
- **Drawing on philosophy and social theory to inform research.** It is argued that this strategy can theoretically enhance research, make sense of empirical observations, and articulate some of the underlying meanings and processes involved. Typically, researchers engage with the work of specific continental philosophers. Beyond this, critical research involves a diversity of more general and often overlapping theoretical traditions that ebb and flow in popularity over time. For example, researchers may study issues within the framework of political economy, feminism, social constructivism, post-structuralism, post-colonialism, and/or post-humanism.[1] All of these theoretical perspectives can provide new ways of understanding the complex matters of health and illness.
- **Involving communities as partners in research, developing a "public" approach.** It is argued that much social science has to an extent "lost the plot," failing to directly engage with important public issues, debates, and agendas. However, scholars need not neglect this important potential aspect of their work; engaging with various "publics" can directly encourage social reform and change. This might, at times, involve direct action and an activist approach. As Wakefield (2007) suggests, there can be a real joy in working with others to change the world and make it a better place. Indeed, critical researchers might occupy a "third space" between academia and activism, continually and fluidly moving between the two (Blomley, 2007).
- **Thinking and acting "outside the box."** It has been said that criticality involves the production of new ideas and approaches, even those that might seem radical and unconventional, as they might better explain processes, tackle problems, and lead to positive change in the world (Parr, 2004). Such a bold approach requires courage on the part of researchers, as they must take risks with their scholarship.
- **Understanding how local situations and events are related to global scale processes.** The world is interconnected and interdependent. What happens in one place is connected to what happens in another. Hence, researchers need a global imagination. They also need to take responsibility for studying health issues in other non-Western places, realizing how Western values and systems have led to problems elsewhere. Specifically, global health involves critical consideration of (i) health phenomena of global significance, (ii) the local impacts of global health phenomena, and (iii) local health phenomena for which—from a moral perspective—international responsibility should be taken.
- **Expressing the aspirations of, and for, individuals and society.** It is argued that researchers need to articulate how they envision their ideal world and what this world entails. They need to be optimistic and provide a sense of a possible future, regardless of how unattainable it may seem (Blomley, 2008). In a world full of conflict, social problems, and health problems, academics need to address issues while still being a positive voice for change.

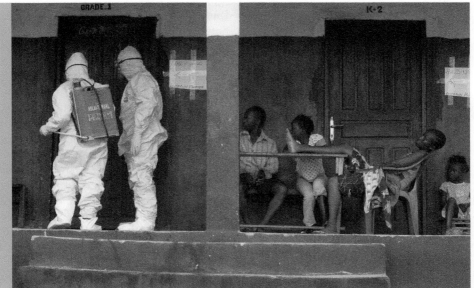

AP Photo/Jerome Delay/CP Images

One of the several aims of the critical perspective is to understand the relationship between local events and global processes. Some health scenarios, such as epidemics, can be linked to global processes relatively straightforwardly. What are some of the ways in which the West African Ebola virus outbreak, which started in 2014, can be critically considered both on a local and a global level?

- **Being humble and reflexive.** Kitchen and Hubbard (1999) note that the current divide between academia and "outside life" maintains academia's supposed "authority." It is thus suggested that researchers must situate their research in the same social and cultural world as the subjects and issues they study. Researchers must not think that they are higher or better than other people, that they are neutral, that their findings are objective, that they operate external to realities, or that they are impartial (Eakin et al., 1996). Rather, they must recognize the shortfalls of their own disciplines. Critical public health researchers, for example, recognize how public health involves the regulation and enforcement of behaviours (Eakin et al., 1996). Critical psychologists, meanwhile, acknowledge the shortfalls and damages of contemporary mental health care (Parker 1999), whereas critical geographers must come to grips with their own discipline's service to colonial, imperial, and nationalist projects (Smith & Desbiens, 1999).
- **Expressing solidarity.** As Blomley (2006) suggests, critical research must involve solidarity with people, particularly those who are oppressed and victimized. Researchers have an obligation to their fellow humans and to the world in general. As Castree (2000) argues, critical scholarship might be a liberal/left rallying point for anti-racist, anti-homophobic, feminist, and other politics, producing academic work (post-colonialist research, queer research, feminist research) that reflects broader public social movements.

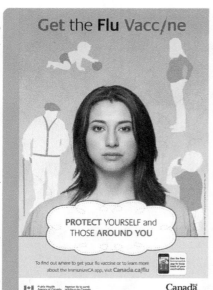

Analyzing public health campaigns from a critical perspective can provide valuable insights into how such campaigns affect individuals and communities. A critical researcher might ask of this poster, who is the target audience? Who are the people the poster identifies as being in need of protection?

- **Questioning the nature of "evidence."** It is noted how the idea of evidence-based health care (EBHC) has quickly become a global priority. However, the wide-ranging critique of EBHC highlights that, although it is appropriate that the best health care is provided in the best known ways, EBHC goes far beyond this objective, becoming a powerful movement in itself that espouses a dominant scientific worldview. EBHC selectively legitimizes and includes certain knowledge but degrades and excludes other—often qualitative—knowledge (Eakin et al., 1996). Moreover, it is argued that the EBHC movement is institutionally supported not only by medicine, but by the state and academia as well (Holmes et al., 2006). This is particularly troubling for critical researchers, many of whom believe that EBHC is uncritically accepted in academia as the "correct path." Critical health studies researchers argue that, in response, a critique is necessary for deconstructing this mode of thinking, and that resistance is ethically necessary given the powerful forces in play (Holmes et al., 2007).

CASE STUDY

Physicians and Gifts

Scholars from a variety of academic disciplines have analyzed a common practice within the pharmaceutical industry: the giving of gifts to physicians. On one end of the spectrum, this encompasses drug company representatives giving doctors branded pens or paying for lunch; in some cases, these gifts extend to free vacations and expensive office materials such as laptops. The practice of giving gifts is immensely controversial, prompting sociologists, anthropologists, and ethicists (among other social scientists) to take a critical approach to the subject.

Employing diverse methods and strategies, these researchers have made vitally important contributions to the debate over gifts. Social scientists have been studying gift giving for many decades, noting the very basic principle that gift giving increases the likelihood of a person being willing to reciprocate, whether through favours, consent, or gifts themselves (Mauss, 1954). Building upon this work, anthropologists have noted that gift giving is used by pharmaceutical reps for a variety of reasons including the establishment of trust, the creation of alliances, and building a sense of reciprocity (Oldani, 2004). Scholars have also demonstrated that gift giving appears to "work," as physicians who are more inclined to accept gifts are also more likely to prescribe expensive or inappropriate drugs (Spurling et al., 2010). Despite clear evidence of influence, most doctors see these gifts as harmless, believing that they are unlikely to shift their prescribing patterns. Yet, even small trinkets that might appear to be of little value (such as pens or coffee) seem to play an important role in changing physician behaviour around medication (Katz, Caplan, & Merz, 2010). In-depth studies of professional medical culture, meanwhile, indicate that many physicians may have very little individual choice when it comes to establishing gift-giving relationships with pharmaceutical companies; the "rules of the game" are structured in such a way so as to make such relationships almost unavoidable (Mather, 2005). These relationships are established very early in a physician's career and it is clear that the influence of industry on the profession has become normalized (Holloway, 2014).

In light of research that demonstrates that gift giving may give pharmaceutical companies inappropriate influence over physicians' prescribing, medical schools and professional associations have established guidelines to try and curtail this practice. In the spirit of critical social science, however, even these guidelines are now under scrutiny (Schnier et al., 2013).

Concerns and Criticisms

Critical research has itself been subject to criticisms of various kinds, which we must acknowledge rather than ignore:

- **The new conventional.** There are considerable differences of opinion on what constitutes critical research. On top of this, some are concerned that its growing popularity is weakening its radicalness and resolve (Parr, 2004). As Blomley (2006) notes, with so many academics undertaking critical scholarship, it has become quite ubiquitous and conventional.
- **A formulaic approach.** On a related note, some academics consider critical research to have become quite formulaic and predictable. As Blomley (2006) suggests, critical scholars conduct research through a process in which they often identify an oppressive relationship, find the ideology or social norm that creates it, reveal the experience of the oppressed, and conclude by noting less oppressive alternatives.
- **Over-theorizing the world.** As Gregory (2004) and Blomley (2007) note, there have been concerns that critical research has tended to over-theorize the world. Hence, empirical studies can become projects that illustrate researchers' own theories instead of pressing real-world problems and issues.
- **Naturalizing social situations.** There have been concerns that critical research essentializes and naturalizes social forces and human susceptibility to them (Sayer, 2009). Thus it can position phenomena—such as unequal power relationships and human suffering—as being almost inevitable. In turn, humans are consequently portrayed as powerless; their potential for coping, adaptation, and forcing changes is often hidden.

- **Lacking a movement.** As Cloke (2002) argues, critical research has never led to a consistent political movement or project with clear goals and regularly deployed approaches. Thus, critical research has been limited in its real-world impact and ability to force social and political change.
- **Academics make poor activists.** Finally there is a wide-ranging critique of the whole idea of academics as activists. As Blomley (2007) observes, academics have the luxury, time, and space to consider complex issues in depth, which might be their best contribution to society (rather than to politically organize others). Moreover, as Blomley (2008) suggests, critical academics are all too often comfortable middle class "champagne socialists" and "cocktail liberals" who merely talk radically and chat about revolution without actually acting. As such, political rallying and organizing may be beyond the scope of a critical researcher.

Research Tools

For students seeking to apply a critical health studies approach, there are a number of websites and academic journals that may prove useful. The following list is not exhaustive. These sources have been identified because they encourage researchers to carry out their work in the critical and flexible fashion outlined in this chapter.

- *Social Sciences & Medicine.* Elsevier Ltd.
- *Critical Public Health.* Taylor and Francis Group.
- *Critical Social Policy.* Sage Publications.
- *Health & Place.* Elsevier Ltd.
- *Journal of Medical Humanities.* Springer.
- *The Sociology of Health and Illness.* John Wiley & Sons Ltd.
- *Qualitative Health Research.* Sage Publications.
- *Social Theory and Health.* Palgrave MacMillan.
- *Health: An Interdisciplinary Journal for the Social Study of Health, Illness and Medicine.* Sage Publications.
- *BioSocieties.* Palgrave MacMillan.
- *Body & Society.* Sage Publications.
- *International Journal of Qualitative Studies on Health & Wellbeing.* Coaction Publishing.
- *Health and Social Care in the Community.* John Wiley & Sons Ltd.
- *Nursing Inquiry.* John Wiley & Sons Ltd.
- *Aporia.* www.oa.uottawa.ca/journals/aporia/about_aporia.jsp?lang=
- *Critical Approaches to Discourse Analysis across Disciplines.* http://cadaad.net
- *Revue Interdisciplinaire des Sciences de la Santé / Interdisciplinary Journal of Health Sciences.* www.riss-ijhs.ca

Moving Forward

Following this introduction, Chapter Two, "Disciplinarity in Health Studies" by Grenier et al. rounds off this first section of the book. Building on this chapter, it unpacks the notion of disciplines, what they are, and what makes them coherent. It then explains the ideas of multi-disciplinarity, inter-disciplinarity and trans-disciplinarity, and the insights that each approach provides for critical inquiry and understanding. Finally, it considers more generally the new understandings that can be gained, and the challenges that have to be overcome, in working across disciplinary boundaries.

The remainder—and bulk—of the book is then "issues led," taking the approaches outlined in the first two chapters and explaining aspects of health and health care. Section Two "Society, Health and Illness" commences with Chapter Three, "Health as a Social Construction" by Dorothy Pawluch. This chapter argues that social phenomena are not separate from society. There is no single overarching reality or "truth" that lies above and beyond us. Instead, all social phenomena develop in, and are relative to, their social contexts. The chapter explains this point with respect to health and health care, specifically engaging with ideas and debates around socialization, and biomedical objectivist versus social constructivist perspectives. Examples, such as various "contested illnesses," like fibromyalgia and irritable bowel syndrome, are used to examine these positions.

Chapter Four, "Cultures and Meanings of Health," by Raza Mirza, considers different ways of understanding and defining culture (collective, common ways of doing, being, and understanding) and articulates how culture shapes health, illness, care, and healing at different levels and in different ways. Attention is paid to what constitutes culture, specifically material objects, social relations, and ideas. Further, the chapter addresses types and scales of culture in society (such as ethnicities, religions, workplaces, and popular culture) and how they relate to health and health care. Finally, the role of culture in the popular, folk, and professional health sectors is explored, focusing on the concepts of illness and healing across cultures.

Chapter Five, "Social Intersectionality and Health," by James Gillett and Mat Savelli, explains how society is stratified and divided along structures of identity (for example, in terms of age, gender, ethnicity, class position, income, education level, disability, sexuality, and place of residence). The chapter explores how these social conditions and relations influence the experience of health and illness as well as health outcomes. Three structures of identity are examined individually before students are introduced to the theory of intersectionality.

Chapter Six, "Politics, Social Justice and Health," by Chelsea Gabel, is concerned with maximizing equality and rights with regard to health. It focuses on how this occurs through health education, advocacy and activism, and the ideologies and ideas underpinning them. The chapter also engages with movements that have arisen to improve health situations for individuals and specific populations.

Chapter Seven, "Globalization and Health," by Leigh-Anne Gillespie and James Gillett, poses the question: What is globalization? It then discusses the globalization processes through an examination of how countries, populations, and individuals are increasingly connected, integrated, and interdependent in a health context. Specific drivers of globalization such as market forces, technology, trade, law and regulation, and migration are explored. The chapter then addresses the impacts of global movements, global cultures and cultural politics, multiculturalism, international development, inequality, and environmental degradation. Finally, the specific concept of "global health" is deconstructed through the idea and example of One Health.

Section Three, "Health Care Paradigms, Systems, and Policies," commences with Chapter Eight, "Modern Biomedical Culture," by Elena Neiterman. This chapter explores the origins and development of biomedicine. It examines the key principles underpinning modern biomedical culture: scientific and rational analysis. The chapter demonstrates how biomedicine has a tendency to reject beliefs and practices based on anything else, favouring order and structure. The chapter addresses biomedicine's regulated structure and environment, its hierarchical power and knowledge base, its universal and generalizable aim, its mechanistic and technological character, and the involvement of ritual, identity, and symbolism. The chapter also considers, more broadly, the seeping of biomedical culture into contemporary culture: the "medicalization of society."

Chapter Nine, "Health Care Systems: Public and Private," by Michel Grignon, examines what health care systems do—construct and define illness and positive outcomes; allocate priorities and resources; and structure delivery of treatment. It also considers the nature of many normative aspects and concepts such as distribution, fairness, and risk minimization, and structural elements such as insurance. More generally, the chapter explores the historical basis, rationale, and development of publicly versus privately provided health care systems, with particular reference to Canada and the US.

Chapter Ten, "The Social Determinants of Health," by Anthony Lombardo, examines and contrasts the biomedical, behavioural, and socio-environmental models of health. In particular, this chapter highlights the growing acknowledgement that health and wellbeing are strongly rooted in communities and the environment, factors beyond the realm of medicine. The chapter pays particular attention to the relative impact of social "composition," such as one's affluence, class, and geographical location, on health. Further, it addresses the impact of the social context of health, that is, the resources available to people locally such as care facilities and social services. Finally, it addresses the impact of social capital and cohesion on health and welfare. The chapter concludes by considering the development of policies and programs initiated to identify and address the social determinants of health.

Chapter Eleven, "The Re-emergence of Other Healing Paradigms," by Yvonne LeBlanc, describes treatments and therapies that do not conform to the norms and practices of mainstream biomedicine. Historically, these have been considered as "traditional medicine" but are more recently described as "alternative," "complementary," or "non-conventional" medicine. The chapter explores key aspects of this wide-ranging and important phenomenon, including the classification of therapies, their historical evolution, the ideas that underpin them, and important aspects of their production, consumption, and integration with biomedicine.

Chapter Twelve, "Consumerism, Health, and Health Care" by Mat Savelli, describes the roots of consumerism in health and consumerist approaches to accessing and assessing health care. This chapter considers how advanced capitalism has created the informed and opinionated consumer of a wide range of health-related products and services. This has led to the evolution of the "expert patient"—people who actively track their health, possess in-depth knowledge about particular health issues, and expect certain things when they meet with medical professionals. Meanwhile, the health care system itself has become marketized: health care institutions are behaving more like corporations, using a variety of business tactics to embrace and manage their own market position. In particular, the example of medical tourism is used to showcase these trends in action.

Section Four, "Future Challenges and Directions," commences with Chapter Thirteen, "Technology," by Josh Evans. This chapter examines the increasing role of technology in how we experience, understand, and treat health and illness. In particular, the chapter argues that new technologies have expanded care beyond hospitals and helped to develop new services. Of particular concern is how technologies impact the form, experiences, and outcomes of people's interpersonal communications and relationships in health contexts. In this sense, technology can be inclusionary and liberating but also exclusionary and alienating. This chapter shows how technology can ultimately blur the lines between body and machine, human and non-human.

Chapter Fourteen, "Ethical Issues in Health and Health Care," by Elizabeth Peter, James Gillett, and Mat Savelli, introduces the concept of ethics and their application to health care. The bulk of the chapter focuses on some of the primary ethical challenges currently facing health care professionals and their patients. In particular, this chapter highlights how treatment decisions, access to care, physician shortages, medical error, end-of-life issues, and participation in medical research are important particularly when considering power inequalities and vulnerable populations.

In short, this book introduces students to the study of health from a critical social sciences approach. Using a combination of academic theory and real-life case studies, it demonstrates the complexity inherent in studying the concept of health in the contemporary world.

Chapter Summary

This chapter has introduced and described health studies as a multidisciplinary social science field of research which, in contrast to mainstream approaches in the health sciences, considers the social and cultural construction and aspects of health and health care, the ideologies and principles that underpin health and health care, and the health challenges facing individuals and populations. It introduced some of the key facets that constitute the field's critical approach, and walked readers through the book's remaining chapters and the subjects they address.

STUDY QUESTIONS

1. What are the key differences between health sciences and health studies?
2. What broad questions does health studies pose?
3. What are the key facets of a critical approach?

SUGGESTED READINGS

Blackwell, J. C., Smith, M. E., and Sorenson, J. S. (2008). *Culture of prejudice: Arguments in critical social science.* Toronto: University of Toronto Press.

Fay, B. (1987). *Critical social science: Liberation and its limits.* Ithaca, NY: Cornell University Press.

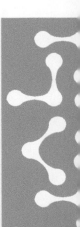

———. (1993). The elements of critical social science. In M. Hammersley (Ed.) *Social research: philosophy, politics and practice.* London: Sage.

WEB RESOURCES

What Is Critical Research? www.strath.ac.uk/aer/materials/1educationalresearchandenquiry/unit4/whatiscriticalresearch

Glossary of Social Sciences Terms: www.faculty.rsu.edu/users/f/felwell/www/glossary/Index.htm

Debates on health issues: http://healthydebate.ca

GLOSSARY

Critical health studies An approach to health that is characterized by "criticality." Critical health studies is interested in challenging and analyzing current conceptions of health and health care. This involves questioning social, political, and economic practices; current norms and ideologies; and practices that marginalize or negatively affect individuals or groups.

Health sciences The disciplines, typically scientific in nature, that work in conjunction with medicine. Examples include toxicology, genetics, occupational therapy, and pharmacy.

Health studies Addresses health, illness, and medicine through a social science, humanities, or interdisciplinary lens.

Qualitative Information that cannot be quantified (measured in numbers). Qualitative analysis utilizes interviews, observations, and other non-numerical data. Qualitative data addresses *how* something is rather than *how much* of it there is.

Quantitative Relating to numbers and measurable phenomena. Quantitative analysis deals with statistics, measurements, and other numerical data.

Wellbeing Being healthy and content with one's life, having one's basic needs met. More than just the absence of disease.

NOTES

1. For a definition of these social science terms, see the social sciences glossary in the Web Resources section at the end of this chapter.

REFERENCES

Andrews, G. J., Chen, S., & Myers, S. (2014). The "taking place" of health and wellbeing: towards non-representational theory. *Social Science & Medicine, 108,* 210–22.

Blomley, N. (2006). Uncritical critical geography? *Progress in Human Geography, 30*(1), 87–94.

———. (2007). Critical geography: anger and hope. *Progress in Human Geography, 31*(1), 53–65.

———. (2008). The spaces of critical geography. *Progress in Human Geography. 32*(2), 285–93.

Bourgeault, I., Dingwell, R., and de Viries R. (2010). *The SAGE handbook of qualitative methods in health research.* London: Sage

Castree, N. (2000). What kind of critical geography for what kind of politics? *Environment and Planning A, 32*(12), 2091–95.

Cloke, P. (2002). Deliver us from evil? Prospects for living ethically and acting politically in human geography. *Progress in Human Geography, 26*(5), 587–604.

Eakin, J., Robertson, A., Poland, B., Coburn, D., and Edwards, R. (1996). Towards a critical social science perspective on health promotion research. *Health Promotion International, 11*(2), 157–65.

Fleuret, S., and Atkinson, S. (2007). Wellbeing, health and geography: a critical review and research agenda. *New Zealand Geographer, 63*(2), 106–18.

Gatrell, A. C., and Elliott, S. J. (2009). *Geographies of health: an introduction.* Canada: John Wiley & Sons.

Germov, J. and Hornosty, J. (2011). *Second opinion: an introduction to health sociology* (Canadian Edition). Don Mills, ON: Oxford University Press

Gregory, D. (2004). *The Colonial Present: Afghanistan, Palestine, Iraq.* New Jersey: Blackwell Publications.

Holloway, K. (2014). Uneasy subjects: Medical students' conflicts over the pharmaceutical industry. *Social Science & Medicine, 114,* 113–20.

Holmes, D., Murray, S., Perron, A., and Rail, G. (2006). Entertaining Fascism? *International Journal of Evidence Based Health Care, 4,* 189–90.

Holmes, D., Gastaldo, D., and Perron, A. (2007). Paranoid investments in nursing: a schizoanalysis of the evidence-based discourse. *Nursing Philosophy, 8,* 85–91.

Joralemon, D. (2009). Exploring medical anthropology. Don Mills, ON: Pearson Education Canada.

Katz, D., Caplan, A. L., and Merz, J. F. (2010). All gifts large and small: toward an understanding of the ethics of pharmaceutical industry gift-giving. *The American Journal of Bioethics, 10*(10), 11–17.

Kitchin, R. M., and Hubbard, P. J. (1999). Research, action and "critical" geographies. *Area, 31*(3), 195–98.

Mather, C. (2005). The pipeline and the porcupine: alternate metaphors of the physician–industry relationship. *Social Science & Medicine, 60*(6), 1323–34.

Mauss, M. (1954). *The gift: forms and functions of exchange in archaic societies.* London: Cohen & West.

Ogden, J. (2012). *Health psychology: a textbook.* Maidenhead, UK: McGraw-Hill International.

Oldani, M. J. (2004). Thick prescriptions: toward an interpretation of pharmaceutical sales practices. *Medical Anthropology Quarterly, 18*(3), 325–56.

Palmer, G. and Ho, T. (2007). *Health economics: a critical and global analysis.* London: Palgrave Macmillan.

Parker, I. (1999). Critical Psychology: critical links. *Annual Review of Critical Psychology, 1*(1), 3–18.

Parr, H. (2004). Medical geography: critical medical and health geography? *Progress in Human Geography, 28*(2), 246–57.

Sayer, A. (2009). Who's afraid of critical social science? *Current Sociology, 57*(6), 767–86.

Shnier, A., Lexchin, J., Mintzes, B., Jutel, A., and Holloway, K. (2013). Too few, too weak: conflict of interest policies at Canadian medical schools. *PloS One, 8*(7), e68633.

Smith, N. and Desbiens, C. (1999). The International Critical Geography Group: forbidden optimism? *Environment and Planning D: Society and Space* 18, 379–82.

Spurling, G. K., Mansfield, P. R., Montgomery, B. D., Lexchin, J., Doust, J., Othman, N., and Vitry, A. I. (2010). Information from pharmaceutical companies and the quality, quantity, and cost of physicians' prescribing: a systematic review. *PLoS Medicine, 7*(10), e1000352.

Wakefield, S. E. (2007). Reflective action in the academy: exploring praxis in critical geography using a "food movement" case study. *Antipode, 39*(2), 331–54.

World Health Organization (1946). *The Constitution of the World Health Organization.* WHO Geneva.

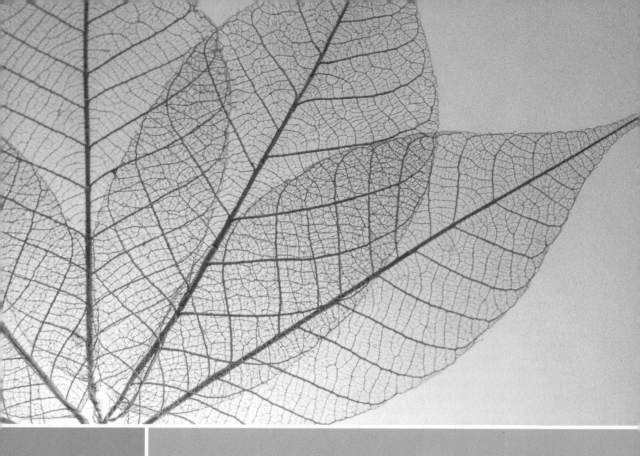

2

Disciplinarity in Health Studies

Amanda Grenier, Gavin J. Andrews, Mat Savelli, and James Gillett

LEARNING OBJECTIVES

In this chapter, students will learn

- the concept of disciplinarity
- how to work within and across disciplines in health studies
- to distinguish between the disciplines and fields that contribute to health studies

Introduction

Health and illness have social, political, cultural, and economic dimensions that extend beyond the biomedical perspective. The ideas we espouse as a society and our socio-cultural practices influence our definitions of health and our responses to illness. Thus, no singular theoretical perspective or methodology can fully capture the complexity of health. To address this complexity, critical health studies draws upon insights from a wide range of disciplines, conceptual fields of study, and professional domains to better understand health and illness. In doing so, these critical approaches seek to understand the meanings of health and illness across cultures and history. The aim is to scrutinize taken-for-granted knowledge and practices while exploring the ethical, political, and moral frameworks of health and illness. As the first chapter indicated, the field of health studies poses questions such as: What constitutes health? How do individuals and communities understand health and illness? How do political, economic, and medical ideologies impact these understandings of health and responses to illness? What are the underlying assumptions of decisions for funding health care? Are the decisions made about health and illness just, fair, and equitable? Do particular groups have better access than others? Critical health studies draws on a variety of approaches from across the social sciences (and other academic disciplines) in order to answer these questions and to better understand health and illness.

This chapter is an introduction to what is known as **disciplinarity**—the notion that different disciplines have unique ways of approaching a subject. For example, imagine a neighbourhood characterized by excessively high rates of obesity. In attempting to understand why this might be the case, experts from different disciplinary backgrounds would probably utilize very distinct approaches and tools as they try to answer the question.

- A geographer could map the physical environment, perhaps concluding that the high obesity rates are due to an abundance of fast-food restaurants and a lack of exercise facilities.
- A psychologist might interview local residents, determining that people are overeating to alleviate high rates of stress and depression.
- After conducting a neighbourhood-wide survey study, a sociologist could conclude that area residents typically work office jobs, meaning that they have few opportunities to burn off excess calories.

In this example, it is easy to see how each expert's disciplinary knowledge and methodological tools shaped their approach to understanding the neighbourhood's high levels of obesity. Each expert reached a separate conclusion regarding the primary cause of this complex phenomenon.

To understand the approach of critical health studies, it is important to have a strong grasp of the concept of academic disciplines, the boundaries that exist between them, and the ways that these can be crossed through collaborative research. This chapter is intended to introduce students to key approaches that have been taken in health studies. Emphasis will be placed on how we may draw on insights from (and move across) particular disciplines in order to produce complex understandings of the social, political, cultural, and economic dimensions of health and illness. The aim is not to find a definitive answer to any of the questions, or to identify a "fixed" approach, but to encourage students to develop an informed and open-minded stance. The approach taken in this chapter encourages students to think critically about how disciplinary knowledge and boundaries can ultimately influence our interpretations and decisions about health and illness.

By the end of the chapter, we hope that students can understand the concept of disciplinarity as it relates to the field of health studies. This background will provide the foundational knowledge required to appraise research and writing in health studies. The chapter unfolds as follows: first, it outlines what is meant by disciplinarity. This is followed by a review of key strands from the four most prevalent disciplinary approaches to critical health studies: sociology, psychology, geography, and ethics. Second, it distinguishes between multidisciplinary, interdisciplinary, and transdisciplinary work, and includes a discussion of the insights and challenges of studying health from various disciplinary perspectives. At the end of this section, we suggest that a collaborative approach to health studies that moves across disciplines can result in a more nuanced understanding of the issues at hand.

Disciplinary Approaches to Health Studies

As Mechanic (1995) has pointed out, societies are becoming increasingly stratified and diverse. Demographic change, shifting life trajectories, and new forms of knowledge have made health an increasingly complex matter. Moreover, as detailed elsewhere in this textbook, there is an increasing recognition that social issues and forces are central to both the causes and the remedies of health problems. Despite this understanding, health care interventions and systems are the products of a multitude of competing political beliefs. For all of these reasons, the complex matter of health is best debated and discussed from a range of academic disciplines and theoretical starting points.

The disciplines and perspectives represented in health studies vary greatly. In disciplinary terms, health studies is composed of contributions from the following:

- a number of social sciences (e.g., sociology, psychology, geography, political science, anthropology);
- several approaches from the humanities (e.g., English, history, the arts);
- wide-ranging empirically and/or conceptually based fields (e.g., cultural studies, women's studies, Aboriginal studies); and
- contributions from professional practice disciplines (e.g., nursing, social work, rehabilitation science).

Thus, the field of health studies is deeply rooted in "disciplinary knowledge." It must be stated, however, that the approach of a discipline can influence the way we understand a topic. Each discipline asks different questions, has its own ways of knowing, and uses varying analytical approaches. Take, for example, a researcher exploring young people's reasons for smoking cigarettes. If relying exclusively upon the methods and theories of psychology, she would likely uncover contributing factors related to the individual, such as a person's desire to rebel or appear more mature. By contrast, a researcher using a cultural studies approach might concentrate on the role of mass media in projecting an ideal of smoking as "cool." An anthropologist, meanwhile, might draw conclusions about youth social circles and the decision to take up smoking. In truth, all of these approaches may produce their own "correct" answers as to what prompts young people to smoke; their differing theoretical bases and methodological tools could account for their separate conclusions. Now we will further explore the constructions of knowledge in health studies and unpack the boundaries and approaches that are typical to each field.

Some Disciplinary Distinctions in Health Studies

Health studies is primarily concerned with the social study of health. Much of what is written and taught in health studies takes place through the lens of particular disciplines, such as sociology (see Nettleton, 2006; Bradbury, 2008; Nancarrow Clarke, 2008), psychology (see Brannon & Feist, 2009), geography (see Gatrell & Elliot, 2009; Brown, McLafferty, & Moon, 2010) and ethics (see Baykis, Hoffmaster, Sherwin, & Borgerson, 2012).

Sociology

In sociology, there is a long history of the study of institutions and the "subject." For example, a number of classic studies in sociology have focused on the power of institutions and institutional practices (see the works of Goffman, Foucault, and Bourdieu). As they demonstrate, institutions designed to protect and promote health (such as psychiatric hospitals and nursing homes) are also sites that empower some individuals (hospital staff) and disempower others (the patients). In general, sociologists focus on how social structures—especially those that are health related—shape the experiences of individuals who reside in them.

Health Psychology

Health psychology explores how people think and behave in relation to health and illness. Health psychologists perceive the mind and body as inherently linked. They develop psychological tools to understand why individuals may develop health problems and use these tools to help them avoid or manage illness. Key contributions in this field have examined the link between optimism and wellbeing (Scheier and Carver, 1985); daily stress and physical health (DeLongis et al., 1982; Antonovsky, 1979); and an individual's readiness to change health-related behaviours (Prochaska & DiClemente, 1986). By exploring the psychological mechanisms behind health-seeking (and health-harming) behaviours, these researchers have developed new strategies for the maintenance of health.

Geography

Geographers have focused on the ways in which space and place affect people's wellbeing. They have examined natural (Mitchell & Popham, 2008) and artificial environments (Morland & Evenson, 2009) and how these influence one's health. Further, geographers are interested in the connections between the environment and socio-cultural and political developments. Taking an interest in the spatial patterns of poor health, as well as the planning of health care services, health geographers have mapped the consequences of various geographical factors on health. Some issues they have addressed include people's proximity to health care facilities (Shannon & Dever, 1974) and sources of disease and poor health (Jones & Moon, 1987). They have also made vital contributions to discussions on globalization, migration (Bentham, 1988), and health inequalities (Curtis & Rees-Jones, 1998).

Ethics

The field of health care ethics addresses questions of morality in a variety of health-related contexts, including public health interventions (Childress et al. 2002), health care provision, and end-of-life care. Ethicists explore the moral dimensions of our attempts to maintain, improve, and manage health, casting a critical eye upon topics such as informed consent (Faden & Beauchamp, 1986), the right to die (Meisel, Cerminara, & Pope, 1989), reproduction (Overall, 1987), and the provider–client (or doctor–patient) relationship (Katz, 1984). Broader themes, such as national health care systems and global health, have also come under scrutiny. At its core, health ethics is concerned with issues such as equity, individual autonomy, and human dignity.

Conceptual Fields

A number of conceptually-based fields have greatly contributed to health studies. On the whole, the contributions from **conceptual fields** have drawn attention to the relationship between broader social structures and individual or local experiences, whether these are in the form of structural barriers, systemic inequities, and/or sustained disadvantages.

In cultural studies, for example, scholars have underscored the ways in which ethnicity and cultural identification inform understandings of health and illness (Spector, 1985; Kleinman, 1980). To gain a better understanding of the cultural studies approach, consider the public health movement through a cultural studies lens. The public health movement has drawn criticism from cultural studies theorists who argue that it enforces a particular moral order. When public health workers promote certain behaviours and value systems as "healthy," they marginalize beliefs and individuals who do not adhere to these criteria (Lupton, 1995).

Caring studies, another conceptual field, has long focused on questions of care across the life course. In particular, the field analyzes relations between formal and informal care; the relationship between health care and the state; family responsibilities; and women's care (see Armstrong & Scott-Dixon, 2008; Neysmith, 2001; Baines et al., 1998). Among others, issues in this field have ranged from those of **iatrogenic** effects of care (e.g., medicalization of child birth) (Cahill, 2001); the economic impacts of informal care (Waerness, 1984); and the emotional dynamics of mothering and eldercare (Chodorow, 1978).

Social gerontology, the social analysis of aging, draws attention to the social constructs and narrative experiences of objective classifications, such as frailty, dementia, and healthy aging (Kaufman, 1994; Kontos; 2004; Katz, 2005). Emerging fields, such as "cultural gerontology," have arisen through examining practices that relate to the body. Examining these practices and behaviours can help us develop new strands of inquiry around the body (Twigg & Martin, 2015).

In summary, conceptual fields have provided health studies with a number of important insights. This knowledge may not have been revealed through traditional disciplinary studies. As later sections of this chapter will demonstrate, combining disciplines allows for the production of many types of unique knowledge.

Professional Domains

Professional domains, such as nursing, social work, and rehabilitation science, have also contributed to the field of health studies. Although these contributions range from the macro (systems) level to the micro (individual) level, they are most visible at the meso level. As such, these contributions relate to organizational practices and the relationships between, for example, professionals and their clients. In this line of research, researchers have drawn attention to taken-for-granted assumptions and have raised awareness of alternative models and practices of care or healing (Arnold & Underman Boggs, 2011). Professional approaches have also spurred debate around the ethics of care. These debates question the ethical boundaries that guide professions (such as nursing and social work) as well as larger questions of justice and moral responsibility for health care (Tronto, 1993; Sevenhuijsen, 1998).

The starting point we use in this chapter is best described as a critical and transdisciplinary approach to health studies. This approach aligns with **critical perspectives** in the field of health studies (see Green & Labonte, 2008; Coppock & Hopton, 2000; Panitch & Leys, 2010) but places more emphasis on the idea that researchers and students can best understand health by moving across disciplines rather than working within one particular tradition. Each of the authors has a particular disciplinary background as a result of graduate training in social work/social policy (Grenier), health geography (Andrews), history of medicine (Savelli), and sociology (Gillett), as well as a practice of reaching across boundaries to conduct interdisciplinary and transdisciplinary work on health. Working within and across disciplinary boundaries is a reflection of our disciplinary training, our research, and our teaching experiences.

To reiterate, students should understand critical health studies as a flexible approach that borrows and adapts the theories and methods of various disciplines in the humanities, social sciences, and professional practice. In other words, there is no single or "correct" way to engage in critical health studies. Because health and health problems are inherently complex matters, they can best be understood by cutting across disciplinary boundaries. The next section of the chapter highlights several ways of working from more than one discipline.

CASE STUDY

Hearing the Voice

Although biomedical practitioners and lay people typically associate hearing voices with auditory hallucinations (one of the hallmarks of psychosis), for some individuals it is a regular component of their daily life. At Durham University in the UK, an interdisciplinary team of researchers have gathered together to explore this phenomenon beyond a strictly medical perspective. Through the Hearing the Voice project, these researchers are exploring people's lived experiences with voice hearing. In addition to trying to comprehend what the experience is actually like for individuals, they ask broader questions about how we interpret the phenomenon and the potential meanings of hearing voices.

The project may produce findings that could help inform therapeutic approaches within healthcare settings. However, the team's research methods draw upon a multitude of social science and humanities approaches. The research team includes experts in bioethics, geography, philosophy, history, theology, English and cultural studies, and the fine arts, alongside specialists in psychology and neuropsychiatry.

/continued

Such an interdisciplinary approach was deliberately chosen in light of the complexity of the subject. The research team frequently meets to exchange ideas, believing that the diversity of their disciplinary backgrounds can help to "guard against the development of reductionist accounts of voice-hearing." Project members regularly publish their findings for audiences within their specialized disciplines as well as for those more generally interested in the concept of hearing voices.

Source: Hearing the Voice: www.dur.ac.uk/hearingthevoice

Collaborative Approaches to Working across Disciplines

Recall that the concept of health cannot be defined in biomedical terms alone: culture, politics, economics, and other social factors all affect our understanding of what it means to be healthy (or ill). Thus, approaching health solely through one discipline cannot fully address its complexity. Increasingly, in both health care settings and the field of critical health studies, researchers are choosing to adopt critical perspectives that transcend individual disciplines.

In the first section, we focused on the contributions of different disciplinary traditions. In this section, we will discuss the practice of combining different fields to better understand a particular phenomenon. While the idea of drawing on different perspectives seems straightforward, there are some crucial distinctions to be made among multidisciplinary, interdisciplinary, and transdisciplinary analysis. While the differences between these terms are often blurred in practice, having a clear understanding of the distinctions between them is important. Understanding these terms allows individuals to make informed decisions regarding the theory and methods of their research projects and how their findings will be utilized.

All three approaches (i.e., multidisciplinary, interdisciplinary, and transdisciplinary) are similar in that they are processes of collaborative research that include knowledge from various disciplinary perspectives. Despite this similarity, however, these three collaborative approaches differ in their methods and processes; they generally produce very different results. We now review and outline these three approaches to highlight the differences among collaborative research strategies. We will consider the case study of older women and frailty through the lens of each type of collaborative approach to illustrate these differences.

Multidisciplinarity refers to a process of including many discrete disciplinary perspectives in one particular study. In a multidisciplinary approach, team members from many different fields work in parallel to understand a particular phenomenon or issue (Dyer, 2003). In this type of collaboration, representatives from various backgrounds apply their specific training and methodological traditions to the topic at hand. For example, a multidisciplinary team analyzing frailty among older women could include:

- a medical doctor studying the risk factors and best treatment of frailty;
- an occupational therapist focused on mobility changes;
- an anthropologist studying cultural variations in the meaning of aging;
- a sociologist studying the narratives or meanings associated with frailty; or
- a geographer studying the ways in which frailty may alter the older person's use of their home.

The result of multidisciplinary study is one with many, albeit disconnected, angles; the team works relatively independently to arrive at their own individual conclusions regarding different aspects of a project (Collin, 2009). While this is the most popular term used to denote a collaborative process of research, it is not necessarily the most common, nor is it considered the most effective. Each member of the research team contributes to the overall complexity of the study, but is relatively bound by the limits of his or her disciplinary knowledge (Dyer, 2003). Each contributor stays largely within the boundaries of his or her own field, using the methodological tools and theoretical assumptions traditionally associated with their discipline. As each member of the team acts as an independent specialist, there is often little communication between fields throughout the process. Maintaining these disciplinary boundaries can limit any new insights gained on a topic (see Rosenfeld, 1992). While multidisciplinary research may unearth several aspects of a phenomenon (such as frailty), the links between these aspects remain invisible.

Interdisciplinarity refers to a collaborative process by which researchers draw on their knowledge from various disciplines in order to understand a particular issue or topic. The prefix "inter" denotes a shared process and a is a synthesis of different disciplines coming together to integrate knowledge (Choi & Pak, 2006). In this process, the research tends to be conducted together within the guidelines of each disciplinary technique, with results

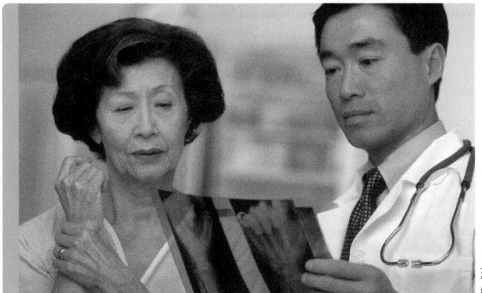

Flirt/Alamy

Frailty among older individuals can be considered through multiple interpretive lenses—and each interpretation of the concept of frailty can differently impact a study's findings, even if the studies use similar research methods. In a 2006 study by van Iersel and Rikkert, the researchers found that "the prevalence of frailty in a sample of 125 elderly people ranged from 33 per cent to 88 per cent, depending on the criteria used" (Bergman et al., 2006).

reported by each field (Rosenfield, 1992). For example, an interdisciplinary project examining the changing definitions of frailty might combine the long-term perspective gained from historical studies of aging (through historical research methods such as archival work) with a social policy approach. This approach could utilize questionnaires, interviews, and quantitative data. Combining these two fields might allow researchers to gauge the extent to which social programs, such as government welfare, have kept pace with changing conceptions of what it means to grow older. In our example, both the historian and the social policy expert might reach some common conclusions. In this sense, interdisciplinary approaches extend beyond simply sharing ideas between discrete disciplines. They produce knowledge that results from the overlap between these two approaches (Collin, 2009). Thus, this approach expands multidisciplinarity through collaborative communication, and allows for the solving of problems beyond the boundaries of each discipline (Dyer, 2003). Interdisciplinarity offers the potential for a greater integration of perspectives and viewpoints. Moving across perspectives, however, can be both a strength and a weakness. Interdisciplinary approaches involve productive collaboration and can yield novel insights. However, they may fail to retain the theoretical or methodological rigor that would be required for a similar piece of research rooted solely in one discipline. In other words, our example project might not be historically "pure" enough for historians, nor sufficiently policy-oriented to please the social policy world.

Transdisciplinarity moves across disciplines in order to understand a particular phenomenon or topic. Transdisciplinary research is considered to be a more comprehensive organization of research, promoting a shared, common conceptual framework (Rosenfield, 1992). Transdisciplinary approaches are often conceptual. They tend to involve multiple methods, and stretch across a number of fields to gain a more complete understanding of the phenomenon at hand. As such, transdisciplinary approaches are dependent upon effective communication among researchers to allow knowledge and skills to be shared across traditional boundaries, transcending the distinctions between disciplines (Dyer, 2003). In this sense, transdisciplinarity is a holistic approach that subordinates disciplines and looks at the dynamics of the project as a whole system (Choi & Pak, 2006). Individuals within such a research team focus on the overarching conceptual issues at hand and tend to work outside of the disciplines in which they were specifically trained. For example, a transdisciplinary study may be rooted in critical gerontology to challenge the dominant biomedical concept of "frailty." Frailty is a powerful social construction in health and social care, but it is also representative of a more complex socio-cultural construct of decline and impairment in later life. Although members of the research team analyzing the concept of frailty would all have been trained in specific fields (each possessing its own taken-for-granted knowledge and methodological tools), each researcher would be expected to work primarily in relation to the overarching framework.

In taking a transdisciplinary approach, the research team would move across various disciplines, practices, and sets of knowledge. They may look to the intersections between biomedical and socio-cultural interpretations, as well as the ways in which "frailty" is sustained and reinforced through professional practices. Studies could focus on any of the following:

• an individual's loss of physical strength, which is considered to signify frailty in the biomedical domain;

- ways in which acquiring impairment becomes a socio-cultural marker of decline;
- how older people structure stories about their experiences;
- the ways in which the concept of being "frail" may affect health-seeking behaviours.

Methods for such an exploration might include:

- an examination of the assessment instruments used in health and social care practice;
- observational studies focusing on the everyday life of elderly individuals in their homes and communities (e.g., using the bus or cooking meals);
- narrated accounts of their lives and experiences;
- photographs of older individuals depicting their strengths and vulnerabilities.

All of these approaches can help to challenge and problematize the construct of "frailty" (see Grenier, 2007; Grenier, 2012). From here, the analysis could outline how frailty, which takes place in relation to the bodies of older people through health and social care practices, can sustain powerful notions of decline and exclusion. The study could also tell us much about our perceptions of older people.

Transdisciplinary projects can also be linked to the critical project of "change." As methods become fully synthesized and theories broaden beyond disciplinary boundaries, new fields of inquiry may arise (Aboelela, 2007). Though the transdisciplinary process can lead to new understandings and richer conclusions, it requires flexibility and institutional support in order to be effective.

Insights and Challenges to Collaborative Research

While the above distinctions suggest that transdisciplinary approaches produce the most effective research results, each form of collaboration provides insights to understanding the complex matters of health. To varying degrees, all of these approaches provide for a more multi-faceted understanding of a specific phenomenon. A researcher rooted solely in one discipline would not be able to see, for example, the great diversity in how we conceptualize and understand frailty. Interdisciplinary and transdisciplinary approaches, in particular, provide researchers with greater flexibility in terms of theoretical and methodological starting points. As these researchers are not singularly tied to the primary tools or assumptions that guide a single field, they are freer to adapt their approach to meet the overall needs of the project or question at hand. This freedom is especially key when research data yield what appear to be inherent contradictions. For example, competing definitions of frailty might easily manifest themselves in discussions with health care providers, government officials, caregivers, and older adults themselves. Moreover, within these specific groups of people, one may encounter very different conceptions of frailty. A flexible approach, which allows researchers to move beyond the limits of any one particular field, could provide an opportunity to address these apparent contradictions.

While collaborative research provides opportunities to gain new insights, collaboration also involves its own set of challenges. Researching any particular phenomenon introduces complex dynamics that influence the research question, type of collaboration, and the research methods used. In taking a critical approach to health studies, researchers

| TABLE 2.1 | Multi-, Inter-, and Transdisciplinary Approaches to Health in Comparison | | |

Multidisciplinary	Interdisciplinary	Transdisciplinary
Involves several disciplines. Little interaction between researchers who work independently.	Involves several disciplines. Theories and methods from each discipline inform the others.	Involves several disciplines but researchers work beyond the limits of these fields.
Researchers have separate goals based on discipline.	Researchers share goals.	Researchers share goals and overarching framework.
Disciplinary boundaries remain in place.	Blurs boundaries between disciplines but disciplinary traditions largely maintained.	Transcends boundaries between disciplines. Little focus on disciplinary traditions.
Could be depicted by several totally separate circles.	Could be depicted by several partially overlapping circles.	Could be depicted by several overlapping circles, all encompassed within a large circle.

Source: Adapted from Choi & Pak (2006).

and students must consider issues such as power, structures that facilitate and block access to collaboration, and questions of what is possible within a particular context. This includes questions about what counts as "knowledge," and what is considered "valid" knowledge. Thus, while collaborative research frequently opens up methodological possibilities and new ways of forming knowledge, it remains a complex process characterized by negotiation.

Crossing Disciplinary Boundaries Outside of Academia

Recently, there has been an upswing in popular contributions to the discussion of health, which highlights the need to broaden our conceptualization and understanding of health and illness beyond academic and biomedical perspectives. These contributions (frequently artistic in form) aim to raise awareness regarding the limitations of the biomedical framework: they adopt, adapt, and transgress disciplinary perspectives in the hopes of enacting change outside of academic settings. These types of projects, including films, songs, websites, and plays, serve as important sources of knowledge for the public, disseminating novel ideas about health. At the same time, these projects are not totally divorced from traditional academic disciplines; they frequently use research-based approaches in their creation.

Through these new modes, one can document experience, challenge taken-for-granted assumptions and practices, and effect change. Most notably, there has been an increase in various research-based theatre initiatives as well as the use of photovoice methods and documentary film. Theatre groups, for example, have acted out their experiences of aging and age-related diagnoses, such as dementia. Two examples of research-based theatre are the

CASE STUDY

The Way I See It

The Way I See It is a photovoice project centred on the impact of housing on health, carried out by people living with HIV. These community researchers—individuals without academic research backgrounds who possess first-hand lived experience—spent two years using photography to explore and document how their lives and health were affected by housing. Ultimately, they demonstrated that individuals with HIV face specific barriers to accessing safe and affordable housing—a situation that profoundly affects their health. Beyond this, the project highlighted the concrete benefits of secure housing in the lives of people with HIV.

To publicize their findings, the community researchers engaged in a host of activities, ranging from academic conferences to public displays of their photos and events aimed at affected communities held during Homelessness Action Week. They also created postcards that could be used to lobby members of government to take action on HIV and housing. Some of the photos from the project continue to be displayed publicly at sites in Vancouver.

Facilitated by the British Columbia Centre for Excellence in HIV/AIDS, the Dr. Peter AIDS Foundation, and the McLaren Housing Society of British Columbia, *The Way I See It* was connected to a wider, overarching project on the broader experiences of people with HIV. The project provides a good example of how academic researchers can work with community members to transcend disciplines and open up new lines of inquiry and discussion.

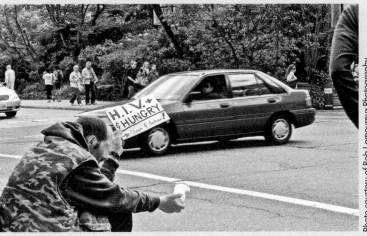

Photo courtesy of Rob Lamoureux Photography

Housing and homelessness is a critical issue in Canada; for example, Vancouver's count of homeless individuals increased 137 per cent between 2002 and 2010. This photo, taken by a participant of *The Way I See It* project named Rob, is entitled "Look Away." What do you think a project like this captures that other types of studies do not or cannot? Why can it be valuable for researchers in health studies fields to consider the lived experiences of the people they are studying?

Ages and Stages project in the UK, (www.keele.ac.uk/agesandstages), developed by researchers at Keele University and staff at the New Vic Theatre, and the play *I'm Still Here (Living with Dementia)*, developed by researchers Gail Mitchell and Christine Jonas-Simpson, and playwright Vrenia Ivonoffski (ACT II STUDIO, Ryerson University) in Toronto (see www. act2studio.ca). The first is a collaboration exploring the impact of theatre on ideas about aging. The second utilizes the perspectives of persons living with dementia and their family partners in care to explore individuals' journeys through dementia. Like many research-based artistic endeavours, it makes use of the arts' ability to connect with the audience on an emotional level. Through this connection, the project can explore issues fundamental to the illness experience, such as stigma and access to care.

Blogs, photovoice projects, and documentary films also share the experiences and stories of people's journeys through health and illness. These artistic endeavours can also be combined with approaches drawn from the social sciences. Take, for example, the *TimeSlips* project in the United States, an online resource that rethinks dementia through creative storytelling, "replacing the pressure to remember with the freedom to imagine" (www.timeslips. org). Such projects can be an effective way to disseminate information to audiences beyond of academic settings.

Further, consider the consumer/survivor movement within the world of mental health. Members of this movement have mental health–related issues, histories, and/or diagnoses; they take a critical approach to mainstream psychiatry and the mental health care field. These individuals have lent their knowledge and experience to a variety of projects seeking to critically address psychiatry and mental health care treatment more broadly. For example, many consumers/survivors have taken part in photovoice projects that aim to help marginalized individuals and communities communicate their stories and advocate for change (www. photovoice.org; www.photovoice.ca). Combining a person's own narrative with photography, photovoice projects have been used by mental health consumers/survivors to document their experiences with illness, stigma, and the health care system.

Chapter Summary

This chapter has highlighted the range of disciplines comprising critical health studies. It has shown the ways in which academics working across the social sciences, humanities, and conceptual fields have made important contributions to understandings of health. Moving beyond the contribution of these individual disciplines, this chapter has suggested that the complex matter of health is best understood by combining disciplinary approaches. Any singular approach drawing solely upon one discipline will likely fail to capture the nuances that inform a person's experiences of health and illness. Yet the ways in which researchers combine disciplinary methods and theories vary. Students have learned about three particular approaches: multidisciplinarity, interdisciplinarity, and transdisciplinarity, each of which has particular strengths and challenges. Finally, the chapter has highlighted the ways in which individuals and organizations outside of academia have adapted tools and ideas from cross-disciplinary critical studies of health to explore people's experience of health and illness. Through this type of exploration, they can advocate for change while contributing to the critical study of health and illness itself.

STUDY QUESTIONS

1. What are the key differences among multidisciplinary, transdisciplinary, and interdisciplinary research?
2. Why is it important to utilize collaborative research approaches when studying health?
3. What are the key challenges of conducting research across disciplines?
4. What benefits are produced from the collaboration between university researchers and community members and organizations?

SUGGESTED READINGS

Kessel, F., Rosenfeld, P.L., Anderson, N.B. (Eds) (2008). *Interdisciplinary Research: Case Studies from Health and Social Science.* Oxford, UK: Oxford University Press.

Mechanic, D. (1995). Emerging trends in the application of the social sciences to health and medicine. *Social Science and Medicine, 40*(11), 1491–96

Pohl, C. (2011). What is progress in transdisciplinary research? *Futures, 43*(6), 618–26.

WEB RESOURCES

ARJ: Disciplinarities. A music research blog: www.arj.no/2012/03/12/disciplinarities-2

Archives of the International Journal of the Creative Arts in Interdisciplinary Practice: www.ijcaip.com/archives.html

Amber Michelle Hill's TEDx Talk: Movement Uniting Cross-Disciplinary Work: www.youtube.com/watch?v=RMS9i4YIA0A

GLOSSARY

Conceptual fields A method of studying a subject by incorporating the views of multiple disciplines in a holistic way (e.g., women's studies, social gerontology).

Critical perspectives A way of studying a topic that addresses and analyzes the effects of institutional norms, models of thinking, power dynamics, and broader social influences on a given issue.

Disciplinarity The notion that different disciplines, or fields of study, have unique ways of addressing an issue.

Iatrogenic An illness or harm that is caused by medical examination or treatment. Iatrogenesis can be cultural, social, or clinical.

Interdisciplinarity An approach to an issue in which a researcher draws on his or her personal experience with and knowledge of different disciplines.

Multidisciplinarity An approach to an issue that uses the knowledge of various disciplines with little overlap or communication between them. In this approach, people with different areas of expertise work in parallel to reach discrete conclusions on a common issue.

Professional domains The knowledge and practice of specific trained professions (e.g., nursing, social work).

Transdisciplinarity An approach to an issue in which a researcher moves across various disciplines, looking at their intersections and how they relate to the overarching concept at hand. In such an approach, researchers tend to work beyond their usual disciplines.

REFERENCES

Aboelela, S. W., Larson, E., Bakken, S., Carrasquillo, O., Formicola, A., Glied, S. A., Haas, J., & Gebbie, K. M. (2007). Defining interdisciplinary research: Conclusions from a critical review of the literature. *Health Services Research, 42* (1p1): S45–46.

Adelson, N. (2005). The embodiment of inequity: Health disparities in Aboriginal Canada. *Canadian Journal of Public Health* 96(2): S45–S61.

Armstrong, P., Armstrong, H., & Scott-Dixon, K. (2008). *Critical to care: The invisible women in health services.* Toronto: University of Toronto Press.

Arnold, A. C. & Underman Boggs, K. (2011) *interpersonal relationships: Professional communication skills for nurses.* St Louis, MO: Elsevier.

Baines, C. L., Evans, P., & Neysmith, S. (1998) Women's caring: Work expanding, state contracting. in Baines, Evans and Neysmith (Eds), *Women's caring: Feminist perspectives in social welfare,* 2nd Edition. Toronto: Oxford University Press: 3–22.

Baylis, F., Downie, J., Hoffmaster, C. B., and Sherwin, S. (2004). *Health Care Ethics in Canada.* Cambridge University Press.

Bentham, G. (1988). Migration and morbidity: Implications for geographical studies of disease. *Social Science & Medicine,* 26(1): 49–54.

Bergman, Howard, Luigi Ferrucci, Jack Guralnik, David B. Hogan, Silvia Hummel, Sathya Karunananthan, & Christina Wolfson. Frailty: An emerging research and clinical paradigm—issues and controversies. *The Journals of Gerontology Series A: The Journal of Gerontology: Biological Sciences and The Journal of Gerontology: Medical Sciences* (2007) 62 (7): 731–37.

Birchenall, M. & Birchenall, P. (1998). *Sociology as applied to nursing and health care.* London: Bailliere Tindall.

Blaxter, M. (2010). *Health: Key concepts.* Cambridge: Polity Press.

Bradby, H. (2009). *Medical sociology: An introduction.* London: Sage.

Brannon, L. & Feist, J. (2010). *Health psychology: An introduction to behavior and health* (7th ed.). Belmont, CA: Cengage Learning.

Brown, T., McLafferty, S. & Moon, G. (2009). *Companion to health and medical geography.* Chichester: Wiley-Blackwell.

Bury, M. (2005). *Health and illness.* Cambridge: Polity Press.

Cahill, H. (2001). Male appropriation and medicalization of childbirth: An historical analysis. *Journal of Advanced Nursing,* 33(3): 334–42.

Chodorow, N. J. (1978). *The reproduction of mothering.* Berkeley: University of California Press.

Choi, B. C. & Pak, A. W. (2006). Multidisciplinarity, interdisciplinarity and transdisciplinarity in health research, services, education and policy: 1. Definitions, objectives, and evidence of effectiveness. *Clinical and Investigative Medicine,* 29(6): 351–64.

Collin, A. (2009). Multidisciplinary, interdisciplinary, and transdisciplinary collaboration: Implications for vocational psychology. *International Journal for Educational and Vocational Guidance,* 9(2): 101–110.

Curtis, S. & Rees Jones, I. (1998). Is there a place for geography in the analysis of health inequality? *Sociology of Health & Illness,* 20(5), 645–72.

De Haan, M., Dennhill, K., & Vasuthevan, S. (2005). *The health of southern Africa* (9th ed.). Cape Town: Juta & Co. Ltd.

DeLongis, A., Coyne, J. C., Dakof, G, Folkman S., Lazarus, R. S. (1982). Relationship of daily hassles, uplifts, and major life events to health status. *Health Psychology:* 119–36.

Dyer, J. A. (2003). Multidisciplinary, interdisciplinary, and transdisciplinary: Educational models and nursing education. *Nursing Education Perspectives,* 24(4): 186–88.

Gatrell, A. C. & Elliott, S. J. (2009). *Geographies of health: An introduction* (2nded.). Chichester: Wiley Blackwell.

Givens, P. & Reiss, M. (2002). *Human biology and health studies.* Delta Place: Nelson Thornes.

Jones, K. & Moon, G. (1987). *Health, disease and society: A critical medical geography.* New York, NY: Routledge.

Katz, J. (1984). *The silent world of doctor and patient.* New York: Free Press.

Katz, S. (2005). *Cultural aging: Life course, lifestyle, and senior worlds*. Broadview Press.

Kaufman S. R. (1994). The social construction of frailty: An anthropological perspective. *Journal of Aging Studies*, 8: 45–58.

Kleinman, A. (1980). *Patients and healers in the context of culture*. Berkeley: University of California Press.

Kontos, P. (2004). Ethnographic reflections on self-hood, embodiment and Alzheimer's disease. *Ageing and Society* 24(6): 829–49.

Lupton, D. (1995). *The imperative of health: public health and the regulated body*. London: Sage Publications.

Mechanic, D. (1994). *Inescapable decisions: The imperatives of health reform*. New Brunswick: Transaction Publishers.

Mitchell, R. & Popham, F. (2008). Effect of exposure to natural environment on health inequalities: An observational population study. *The Lancet*, 372(9650): 1655–60.

Moon, G. & Gillespie, R. (1995). *Society and health: An introduction to social science for health professionals*. London: Routledge.

Morland, K. B. & Evenson, K. R. (2009). Obesity prevalence and the local food environment. *Health & Place*, 15(2): 491–95.

Naidoo, J. & Wills, J. (2001). *Health Studies: An introduction*. Palgrave Macmillan Ltd.

Nancarrow Clark, J. (2008). *Health, illness and medicine in Canada* (5th ed.). Don Mills, ON: Oxford University Press.

Nettleton, S. (2006). *The sociology of health and illness*. Cambridge: Polity Press.

Neysmith S. (2001) "Caring and aging: Exposing the policy issues. In A. Westhues (Ed.) *Canadian Social Policy: Issues and Perspectives*. Waterloo: Wilfrid Laurier University Press: 397–412.

Overall, C. (1987). *Ethics and human reproduction: A feminist analysis*. London: Routledge.

Panitch, L. & Leys, C. (2010). *Morbid symptoms: Health under capitalism*. London: Merlin Books.

Parse, R. R. (1998). *The human becoming school of thought: A perspective for nurses and other health professionals*. London: SAGE Publications.

Phillips, D. R. (1990). *Health and health care in the Third World*. Essex: Longman Scientific & Technical.

Prochaska, J. O. and DiClemente, C. C. (1986). Toward a comprehensive model of change. In W. Miller and N. Heather (Eds), *Treating addictive behaviours: Processes of Change*. New York: Springer.

Rosenfield, P. L. (1992). The potential of transdisciplinary research for sustaining and extending linkages between the health and social sciences. *Social Science & Medicine*, 35(11): 1343–57.

Scheier, M. F. and Carver, C. S. (1985). Optimism, coping, and health: Assessment and implications of generalized outcome expectancies." *Health Psychology* 4(3): 219–47.

Segall, A. & Fries, C. J. (2011). *Pursuing health and wellness: Healthy societies, healthy people*. Don mills: Oxford University Press.

Sevenhuijsen, S. (1998). *Citizenship and the ethics of care: Feminist considerations on justice, Morality, and Politics*. London: Routledge.

Shannon, G. W., and Dever, G.E. (1974). *health care delivery: Spatial perspectives*. New York: McGraw-Hill.

Spector, R. (1985). *Cultural diversity in Health and illness*. Norwalk, CT: Appleton-Century-Croft.

Tronto, J. C. (1993). *Moral boundaries: A political argument for an ethic of care*. London: Routledge.

Twigg, J. and Martin, W. (2015). *Handbook of cultural anthropology*. London: routledge.

Waerness, K. (1984). The Rationality of caring. *Economic and Industrial Democracy* 5(2): 185–211.

Walters, K. L. and Simoni, J. M. (2002). Reconceptualizing Native women's health: An "Indigenist" stress-coping model. *American Journal of Public Health* 92(4): 520–24.

Part II

Society, Health, and Illness

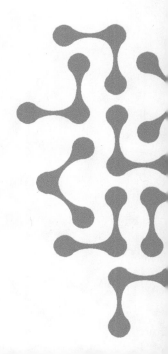

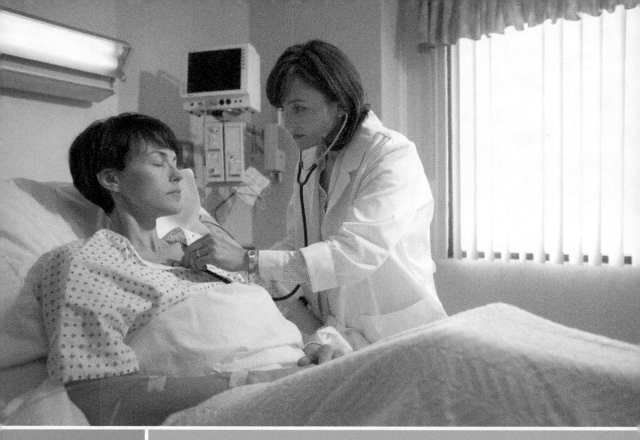

3

Health as a Social Construction

Dorothy Pawluch

LEARNING OBJECTIVES

In this chapter, students will learn

- the social bases of medical knowledge
- the social constructionist perspective of health studies
- processes of medicalization and demedicalization
- claims-making activity around contested illness
- lay constructions of health and illness

Introduction

We see some traits, like the colour of our eyes and hair, as simply a matter of difference. So why do we see the difference between an outgoing personality and an introverted personality as a health-related matter? We once understood homosexuality as a sin and then as mental illness; now we see it as only one among a range of a ways to express sexuality. How is it that the eating habits that doctors diagnose as anorexia or bulimia are seen by some of those who engage in these habits as simply a lifestyle choice? We previously considered forgetfulness as a normal part of the aging process, but now we are now inclined to see it as a sign of dementia or Alzheimer's disease. These are the kinds of issues that concern those who study health from a social constructionist perspective.

Social constructionism starts with the observation that nothing we think we know about the world, including health and illness, is either fixed or given. Though we may experience our world as an objective reality—something that exists apart from us and acts upon us—social constructionism holds that we are all engaged in interpreting, defining, giving meaning to, and making sense of the world around us (Berger & Luckmann, 1966; Hacking, 1999).

Does this mean, then, that there is no such thing as objective reality or "truth"? Is everything merely a question of interpretation? Constructionists are divided on this question. Some constructionists hold that objective reality does exist, but that our experience of it is mediated by the meanings we give that reality. In other words, there are multiple realities. These constructionists subscribe to a brand of constructionism known as *mild* or *contextual* constructionism. Other constructionists—often referred to as *radical* or *strict* constructionists—take what is best described as an agnostic stand. They argue that we cannot objectively say whether reality exists since we cannot know if anything is real beyond our own experiences. Ultimately, our interpretations and our sense of what is objectively real are all we really have. Either way, constructionists find common ground in exploring the social processes through which individuals create meaning. The concern then becomes to better understand *how* these interpretations and meanings are produced—how they are promoted, used, negotiated, and challenged—and the *consequences* in terms of how we behave.

There are few areas of study that have not been affected by the questions of social constructionism. Feminist scholars have looked at the binary construction of gender, exploring recent social movements that suggest gender is a continuum of possibilities beyond "male" and "female" (Lorber, 1996). Those who study race have moved beyond assuming that race is a natural biological category to investigate where the idea of race came from and how race is understood differently across time, space, and cultures. These researchers also explore why some groups have no concept of race at all (Maines & Kusnow, 2001). Those who study the human lifespan have turned their attention to the ever-fluctuating categories that have been constructed to carve up the trajectory of individuals over the course of their lives—childhood, tweens, adolescence, young adulthood, middle age, the young old, the middle old, and the very old (Holstein & Gubrium, 2000).

Applied to health, social constructionism problematizes the meaning of health and illness. Health is not treated as obvious or self-evident; illnesses are not treated as universal states in nature, waiting to be discovered. Social constructionists reject the "nature speaks" school of science. Instead, they treat health and illness as ideas whose meanings are constructed by social actors in and through their interactions with each other. These meanings or social constructs are as follows:

- *relative and socially contingent*: They arise in particular times, places, and social contexts.
- *defeasible*: They are constantly subject to contestation, challenge, and change. As Turner (2004, p. 37) writes, "... the classificatory paradigms of society, including medical classifications, become sites of political struggle and contest."
- *value judgements*: Social constructs of health make judgements about what is normal, good, acceptable and desirable.

Whether any particular condition is really a disease or whether particular understandings of health are right or wrong (and true or false) are not issues that generally concern constructionists. After all, according to strict constructionists, one cannot answer these questions without having some sort of privileged knowledge of what constitutes objective reality, what is "truly" a disease. For the contextual constructionists, the health-related opinions of social scientists are less relevant than those of social audiences; social actors make judgements that determine social practice and policies around health and illness. What happens as a consequence, in terms of our social practices and policies around health and illness, depends on these judgements. Our task, as social scientists, is to gain insight into how these processes play themselves out.

A useful way to learn more about the social constructivist perspective is to compare it to the social determinist approach (see Chapter Ten). The social determinist approach focuses primarily on the social factors that influence the health of populations. Social determinists take a realist position; health and illness exist "out there." People are either healthy or ill. The focus is on how health and disease are distributed, who stays healthy, who gets sick, and why. Social constructionism, on the other hand, raises questions of what counts as health and illness in the first place. From a constructionist point of view, health and illness are relative or subjective. In other words, they are a matter of definition. While social determinists ask what social factors lead to health or illness, social constructionists asks what social factors lead to our *understandings* of health or illness and why they are defined as such. "By studying how illness is socially constructed," Brown (1995, p. 267) has written, "we examine how social forces shape our understanding of, and actions towards, health, illness and healing."

The remainder of the chapter looks at four areas where social constructionism has made its greatest contributions to health studies.

The Social Construction of Medical Knowledge

The premise that health and illness are social constructions has led to a critical consideration of how medical knowledge is generated and used (Wright & Treacher, 1982). Eliot Freidson (1970) is largely responsible for pioneering this approach. His analysis focuses on the rise of the medical profession through the last part of the nineteenth and beginning of the twentieth centuries. Freidson argued that the medical profession had become dominant over other healing traditions because of the political process that eliminated competing methodologies. Scientific medicine was not necessarily more effective, but the profession had achieved a status that gave it a monopoly over the provision of health care services, making its practitioners the primary holders of medical knowledge. By virtue of their professional dominance, doctors became the final arbiters over health matters with the power to decide what constitutes health and who is sick.

However, Freidson stopped short of looking at the actual content of medical knowledge. He was not alone in this regard. In the past, social scientists generally did not concern themselves with the knowledge claims of medicine. Although the organization and practice of medicine were seen as being influenced by social factors that could be studied, medical knowledge itself was considered non-social—beyond social influence and therefore beyond social analysis. Medical knowledge was thus given an epistemologically privileged position.

Two developments within constructionism undermined this privilege. The first was a change in the social study of science, prompted by the publication of Thomas Kuhn's (1962) *The Structure of Scientific Revolutions*. This landmark book challenged the idea that science proceeds as a linear process of continual discovery. Kuhn suggested instead that the history of science consists of paradigm shifts. When a new **paradigm**, an explanatory framework, gains credibility it is adopted by the scientific community. In turn, the paradigm it replaces becomes obsolete. Kuhn's observations changed how scholars thought about science. Scientific knowledge was no longer viewed as reflecting social reality. While scientific "facts" were once "discovered," they were now perceived as social constructions. Attention turned to the social practices and contexts that produced those facts. Applied to medical science, the implication was that "[m]edical knowledge [and] medical practice [are] socially constructed. . . . Further, the objects of medical science are not what they appear to be; the stable realities of the human body and disease are in fact 'fabrications' or 'invention' rather than discoveries" (Bury, 1986, p. 137).

The second contribution to the theory of social constructionism is found in the writings of French social theorist Michel Foucault (1973; 1980). Foucault was centrally concerned with power. For Foucault, power is not something that rests with particular individuals, groups, or institutions. Rather, power is exerted through discourses or systems of language and knowledge. Discourses construct our realities and establish what is possible as far as how we feel, act, think, and relate to others and ourselves. **Medical discourse**, more specifically, structures our thinking about health and illness, what is normal or abnormal, and who has the expertise to define, diagnose, and treat disease. The key, however, is that these discourses are not naturally given. They are generated by particular societies and they can change. Each civilization, according to Foucault, defines its own diseases.

These two authors shifted our analyses of health and illness. Narratives of health and illness shifted away from "discovery" stories about medical knowledge to "constructed" stories. Discovery stories typically lay out uncritically the series of steps that led to a particular medical discovery; the discovery is shown as something that has always existed "out there." Contrarily, constructed stories highlight the social bases of medical "discoveries." Constructed stories highlight how social context—including prevailing cultural attitudes, social practices, and professional, corporate, and governmental interests—either facilitate or inhibit the success of certain *claims* about what exists "out there."

A good example of a socially constructed medical issue is found in Deborah Findlay's (1993) study of gynecological and obstetrical knowledge during the 1950s. Findlay's work is part of a large body of scholarship concerned with the ideological nature of medical knowledge about women and how this knowledge has been used as a tool of oppression against women (see Martin, 1987; Oakley, 1986; Verbrugge, 1976). Findlay analyzed medical textbooks and found that the ideas presented about women's physiology, pregnancy, and labour were infused with male-dominated cultural values. Particularly prominent was a pronatalist stance, an assumption that reproduction was the normal state for women and pregnancy was the *true* female condition. The textbooks valorized "pregnancy as a vocation" and proclaimed motherhood to be "one of the most important and serious jobs in the world" (Findlay, 1993, p. 131). There were also elements of classist attitudes implicit in the writing. Ideal mothers in these books were white, middle class mothers who concerned themselves with the bearing and raising of children. Findlay argues that the textbooks clearly reflected fears that the entry of women into the labour force in increasing numbers threatened the social order.

Some constructions of medical knowledge may serve a political agenda. Consider Thomas Szasz's (1981) analysis of the *drapetomania* and *dysaesthesia Aethiopis* labels. First described in the prestigious *New Orleans Medical and Surgical Journal* in 1851 by Samuel A. Cartwright, *drapetomania* referred to a disease characterized by an effort on the part of slaves to escape from their white masters. *Dysaesthesia Aethiopis* was its milder form or precursor, characterized by sulkiness and neglecting or refusing to work altogether. By problematizing and pathologizing these behaviours, the medical profession reinforced the practice of slavery, labelling those who acted to escape its injustices as "mentally ill." The medical profession, in this sense, served as an oppressor. Drawing out the political uses of these diagnoses and making the links to his broader critique of the mental illness label, Szasz (1981, p. 413) writes,

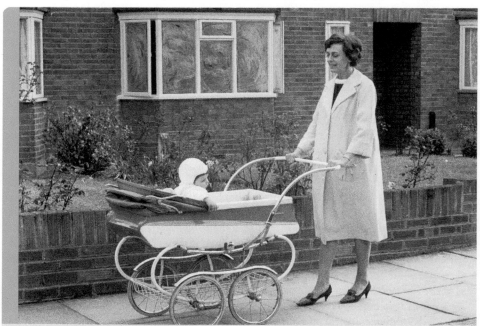

© Pictorial Press Ltd/Alamy

According to Deborah Findlay's (1993) study of gynecological and obstetrical knowledge in the 1950s, ideal mothers were depicted in textbooks as white, middle-class, and solely employed in raising their children. What implications could these assumptions potentially have had for how health in general would have been viewed? What do notions of ideal motherhood and maternal health look like today?

By substituting involuntary mental patients for Negro slaves, institutional psychiatrists for white slave owners, and the rhetoric of mental health for that of white supremacy, we may learn a fresh lesson about the changing verbal patterns man uses to justify exploiting and oppressing his fellow man, in the name of helping him.

Another example involves the case of ulcers. This example is particularly interesting as it shows how social factors can inhibit, not facilitate, the acceptance of a new knowledge claim. For decades, the common conception of ulcers was that they were caused by stress. When researchers began to claim that infection might actually be the culprit, the public resisted. According to Collyer's analysis (1996), the new theory about ulcers was not consistent with prevailing cultural attitudes about individual responsibility for body maintenance and a healthy lifestyle. People had become accustomed to thinking that there was no "quick fix" for ulcers and that stress management was the only cure. Collyer also describes the vested interests of the medical profession, which was not keen to have its well-established routines upset. Pharmaceutical firms, which saw no possibility for new profits in the treatment options connected to the infection theory of ulcers, were also reluctant to accept this new model. If ulcers could be treated simply with already available antibiotics, there was no incentive to support further research on the theory. Researchers who subscribed to the infection theory persisted in pressing their knowledge claims, becoming more strategic in how they did so. By the mid-1990s, Collyer observes, they were able to rally together a general consensus that the infection theory was correct, though there are still disagreements about mechanisms and other stomach-related conditions that may be involved.

There are many such analyses in the literature, demonstrating constructionists' continuing interests in the social forces shaping the content of medical knowledge.

Medicalization and Demedicalization

Another question that has drawn the attention of social constructionists is how various aspects of the human experience have moved into and out of the medical realm. **Medicalization** describes the process by which conditions and behaviours come to be defined as a medical problem (an illness, disease, syndrome, or disorder). Demedicalization refers to the opposite process, where conditions and behaviours once understood as medical problems are reconceptualized. Most of the research on the production of medical knowledge stresses the role of structural contexts and interests. The literature of medicalization and demedicalization, however, addresses human agency and the process of making claims.

Interest in medicalization originated with the work of Irving Zola (1972). He argued that the medical establishment was becoming a major institution of social control in society. The medical profession was claiming to be objective and morally neutral while making judgements about acceptable and unacceptable behaviours. Zola asserted that, under the guise of the objectivity and moral neutrality of science, medicine may act as an institution of social control. This process is "largely an insidious and often undramatic phenomenon accomplished by 'medicalizing' much of daily living, by making medicine and the labels 'healthy' and 'ill' relevant to an ever increasing part of human existence" (Zola, 1972, p. 487).

Zola's observations coincided with critiques emerging within medicine itself, more specifically regarding psychiatry's medicalization of mental illness. Psychiatrist Thomas Szasz

(1961; 1970), for example, wrote extensively about the medicalization of experiences he felt were essentially "problems in living" rather than illnesses. The writings of Ivan Illich (1976, p. 79), a philosopher and social critic, were also influential. Illich referred to the medicalization of life itself. From the unborn and newborn to the menopausal and old, the entire population is at risk: "Life is turned into a pilgrimage through check-ups and clinics, back to where it started."

The publication of Conrad and Schneider's (1980) book, *From Badness to Sickness: Deviance and Medicalization*, firmly established medicalization as a distinct area of study. Building on **labelling theory** and constructionist studies of social problems, Conrad and Schneider argued that behaviours that were once defined as immoral, sinful, or criminal were increasingly being given medical labels. These changes, they argued, represented paradigmatic shifts in understandings and responses to deviance, corresponding to broader changes in society. For example, the sin paradigm prevailed at a time when the Church was a dominant social institution. The sin paradigm gave way to a crime paradigm as secularism came to the fore; nation states and their criminal justice systems displaced religious authorities. Finally, perceptions have shifted to a disease paradigm with the rise of rationalism, science, and the increased power and prestige of the medical profession.

While these societal changes provided the context for redefinition, however, they do not *explain* the redefinitions. Medicalization does not happen without social actors doing something to bring about new understandings. Each and every case of medicalization, Conrad and Schneider insist, is the outcome of a successful claims-making effort. They included in their book accounts of such efforts for a number of conditions—alcoholism, homosexuality, hyperactivity in children, delinquency, mental illness, and opiate addiction.

Since the book's publication, medicalization literature has grown massively. Many studies are concerned with the medicalization of deviant behaviours and social problems such as homelessness, gambling, cult membership, child abuse, sexual compulsivity, transsexualism, post-traumatic stress disorder, and impairment among doctors (professional deviance), to name just a few (Billings and Urban, 1982; King, 1987; Loseke, 1995; Morrow 1982; Pfohl, 1977; Robbins and Anthony, 1982; Rossol, 2001; Scott, 1990; Snow et al., 1986). Other works address the medicalization of natural life processes, like aging (Estes and Binney, 1989; Fox, 1989; Kaufman et. al., 2004) and sleep (Williams et al., 2009). A number of cases relate specifically to women. While the redefinition of childbirth from a natural process to a medical event has long been an issue for feminist scholars, medicalization literature shows that the trend has moved well beyond childbirth. Medicine now pathologizes fear of childbirth, postnatal/postpartum depression and maternal anxiety, infertility, abortion, menstruation, sexual dysfunction, menopause, and sleep (Apple, 1995; Figert, 1996; Greil & McQuillan, 2010; Hislop & Arbor, 2003; Lee, 2003; 2006; McCrea, 1983; Tiefer, 2006). Women are particularly vulnerable to medicalization in a patriarchal society (Riessman, 1996).

Men are, of course, also subject to medicalization. Some conditions, such as andropause (male menopause), male sexual dysfunction (especially erectile dysfunction), baldness, male postnatal depression (Conrad, 2007; Kampf et al., 2013; Lee, 2004; Riska, 2003; Rosenfeld and Faircloth, 2006), show the pervasive trend of medicalization among all genders.

Children, too, have been particularly vulnerable to medicalization. Childhood misbehaviours such as naughtiness, mischievousness, and fidgetiness, for example, have been redefined as hyperactivity disorder, Attention Deficit Disorder (ADD) and Attention Deficit

Hyperactivity Disorder (ADHD) (Conrad 1975; 1996; Malacrida, 2003; Pawluch, 1996). But the list of medical labels available to apply to children, as well as the behaviours that we see as symptoms or disorders, continue to proliferate exponentially. One analyst has commented facetiously that we are determined to leave no child untreated (Frances, 2013).

The *Diagnostic and Statistical Manual of Mental Disorders* (DSM) has become a focal point for those interested in processes of medicalization. Published by the American Psychiatric Association (APA) and often described as "the bible of psychiatry," the DSM lists, classifies, and describes the symptoms for all recognized mental disorders. The DSM was published in its first edition in 1952. Its latest version, DSM-5, was released in 2013. Scholars have found it a useful document for tracking the medicalization (and demedicalization) of conditions. Analyzing contentious diagnoses (homosexuality, premenstrual syndrome, grief, temper tantrums, etc.) underscores the political nature of defining medical knowledge. Kirk and Kutchins (1992) have written about the origins of the DSM. The manual, they claim, presented itself as objective and scientific. This swayed professionals and the public into accepting its definitions as truth. However, controversy over the dramatic increase of symptoms and conditions included in the latest edition of the DSM has prompted even psychiatrists to question the manual and ask if psychiatry has gone too far (Frances, 2013).

A number of factors drive the medicalization process. Early studies emphasized the role of the medical profession. Medicalization was characterized as medical imperialism, an expression of professional dominance to expand its power (Freidson, 1970). That view is changing. Research has identified instances where the impetus for medicalization has come from lay groups, not medical doctors. Riessman (1983) has argued that women themselves have been proactive in seeking out medical labels for various aspects of their lives such as childbirth. They see themselves not as having been oppressed by this medicalization, but as benefitting from it. In the case of alcoholism, Alcoholics Anonymous played a central role in redefining alcoholism as a medical disorder. Medical professionals initially resisted the concept of alcoholism as a disease, but have since reconsidered (Schneider, 1978). The same process is seen in transsexualism (King, 1987), post-traumatic stress disorder (PTSD) (Scott, 1990), and Alzheimer's disease (Fox, 1989). Conrad and Potter (1999) have referred to these lay-driven campaigns as "bottom up" rather than "top down" medicalization.

The decline in the traditional dominance of the medical profession has led to other "engines of medicalization" (Conrad, 2005). Pharmaceutical companies have become major players in medicalization by taking a "pill for every ill" approach. These companies produce new drugs and promote their products both to physicians and the general public, thereby creating their own markets (Moynihan & Cassels, 2005). In several cases, including hyperkinesis, menopause, and erectile dysfunction, drugs were actually available to treat these conditions before an official diagnosis was recognized by the medical community. Accordingly, some analysts are now writing not about medicalization, but about pharmaceuticalization. Williams et al. (2009, p. 851) define pharmaceuticalization as "the transformation of human conditions, capacities or capabilities into pharmaceutical matters of treatment or enhancement."

The term *geneticization* (Lippman, 1991) has been coined to capture the impact of the growing interest in genetics on how we understand health and illness. This process is closely related to the Human Genome Project, which ran from 1984 to 2003 and mapped the complete human DNA code. Since then, genetics has become the new lens through which we try to make sense of complaints, difficulties, deviance, and social problems. Geneticization

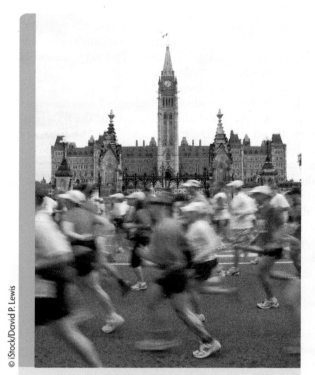

© iStock/David P. Lewis

Healthism refers to the emphasis on "correct" lifestyle choices as the route to health. Who are the main participants in popular events and fitness programs like marathon running? How do fitness activities like these affect the way we think about individual health?

has the potential to dramatically increase the range of individuals caught up in the medicalization net, since it targets not only those with problematized conditions, but also those simply genetically predisposed to conditions by virtue of carrying certain genes.

There is also the concept of healthicization. Healthicization refers to how the current emphasis on **healthism** (the idea of being proactive in health matters by making the right lifestyle choices) contributes to medicalization. Armstrong (1995) has argued that healthism, or what he calls "surveillance medicine," brings everyone into its network of visibility. Armstrong points out that since even the healthy are at risk of becoming ill, healthism problematizes normality itself. Lowenberg and Davis (1994) make the same point—that complementary and alternative therapies contribute to medicalization by expanding the traditional sphere of medical concerns. According to Lowenberg and Davis (1994, p. 581), medicine was once characterized by "a narrow, largely technical focus on symptomatology and disease." With the expanding presence of complementary and alternative medicine, the field of medicine has "a broadened domain including such health salient [sic] foci as nutrition, psychological and spiritual well-being, interpersonal relations and influences emanating from the environment." They highlight in particular the blossoming of multiple varieties of health and fitness programs to assist in stress reduction, biofeedback, smoking cessation, weight loss, and similar preventive lifestyle changes. In short, the pathogenic realm has expanded significantly.

The consequences of medicalization, as well as their "engines," are also increasingly of interest. Medicalization can be a double-edged sword. Medical labels are generally better and less punitive than criminal labels. But, as those who are on the receiving end of mental illness labels will attest, they are not necessarily less stigmatizing. Medical labels evoke sympathetic responses on the part of others, absolve us of responsibility for our actions, and may exempt us from our normal duties. But they also have the effect of turning individuals into victims and objects of pity. Using mental illness once again as an example, Rosenhan (1973) has

CASE STUDY

Medicalizing Introspection and Shyness

Over recent decades, health scientists and clinicians have been paying more attention to shyness, timidity, and introversion. Those who exhibit these temperaments are often diagnosed with social phobia, social anxiety disorder, and avoidant personality disorder (Lane, 2007; Scott, 2006). Consider the following case study of Jack, a 28-year-old male member of the Royal Australian Air Force who was diagnosed with social anxiety disorder:

> I reckon I was OK until high school. It was there that I started to get really anxious if I had to do a presentation to the class. I'd worry about it for days and the night before I couldn't sleep. When it came to the presentation, I'd be sweating, blushing, my mouth would go dry . . . it was like torture. It felt like everyone in the class was laughing at me. Other social situations were really difficult too. Going to parties, chatting up girls . . . I just couldn't do it. I'd stick close to one or two mates, let them do the talking, and just tag along. I've been pretty much the same ever since. (Australian Department of Veterans' Affairs, n.d.)

In her book, *Quiet: The Power of Introverts in a World that Can't Stop Talking*, Susan Cain (2012) explores the consequences of these trends. Introversion, she argues, along with sensitivity, seriousness, and shyness, is being defined as a second-hand personality trait, somewhere between a disappointment and a psychopathology. Our culture increasingly values assertiveness, promoting what Cain calls "the extrovert ideal." Those who are more cerebral and quiet are often told that they are "in their heads" too much: introverts may internalize an image of themselves as deficient, flawed, or sick in some way. Many of them will seek treatments for their "affliction," doing the best they can to pass in the world as extroverts.

But Cain argues that our cultural preference for extroversion also has consequences at a societal level. In our families, schools, and workplaces, we do not create spaces for introverts. Accordingly, we lose the potential contributions that introverts, as thinkers and individuals who reflect deeply, stand to make. In the process, we impoverish ourselves as a society. Rosa Parks, Gandhi and Eleanor Roosevelt, Cain points out, were all introverts.

(See Susan Cain's TED talk at www.ted.com/talks/susan_cain_the_power_of_introverts)

described psychiatric labels as sticky; once they are applied, they become the lens through which others will always view us.

At the societal level, medicalization has the effect of individualizing problems (Conrad & Schneider, 1980, p. 250). Since disease is understood as occurring within individuals, the solution or treatment is directed to individuals (and sometimes against their will). By conceptualizing childhood misbehaviours as sickness, for example, we are not considering the broader social forces that may be generating these misbehaviours. The *medical* label of ADHD does not, for example, take into account issues with the educational system, changing family structures, the effects of media, and other factors related to inattention among children.

Finally, medicalization depoliticizes behaviours. To illustrate this effect, Conrad and Schneider (1980) give the example of political dissidents in the former Soviet Union who were declared insane and committed to mental hospitals. The hospitals were not any more effective than prisons in containing the dissidents, but the psychiatric label neutralized the dissidents' message. Criticisms of the Soviet political and economic system became nothing more than a symptom of mental illness—the ramblings of the mad. Conrad and Schneider conclude that medicalizing behaviours stops us from considering the possibility that the behaviours may be deliberate, an "intentional repudiation of exiting political arrangements" (1980: 251).

Demedicalization

Medicalization, however, is a two-way street (Conrad, 1992, p. 224). If successful claims-making can result in "normal" conditions becoming medical problems, it can also lead to "diseases" being redefined as normal. Compared to medicalization, demedicalization has received relatively less attention. This may be a result of the intensive medicalization that has occurred over the past decades. But there have been notable exceptions—and signs that demedicalization may actually be increasing as well.

The classic example of demedicalization is homosexuality. An extensive campaign from the 1970s succeeded in having homosexuality removed from the DSM (see Bayer, 1981; Conrad & Schnieder, 1980; Spector, 1977). There has been considerable claims-making activity on the part of the disability-rights movement as well, redefining those with "handicaps" or the "disabled" as "differently abled." This type of language is framed as empowering, as opposed to debilitating. Within the larger disability movement there are specific groups, like the hearing impaired, who have promoted a "deaf culture" view of themselves. Deaf culture is a term meant to describe, in morally neutral terms, the quality that makes members of the community different. The community does not view their qualities as a pathology, but the only vocabulary that hearing culture has available to describe it underscores a deficiency—the inability to hear (Reagan, 1995). There are similar movements among the blind (McCreath, 2011).

There are many more recent examples of claims-making aimed at depathologizing or normalizing conditions, including the following:

- *The mad movement* frames those who are labelled as mentally ill as different but also gifted. The movement goes beyond the psychiatric survivors/consumers movement, which is largely about the legal and medical rights of those with mental illness. The mad movement challenges, in a more fundamental, way the very definition of mental illness as undesirable and a disease. The Icarus Project (www.theicarusproject.net), a site that promotes this alternative understanding of mental illness, describes itself as envisioning "a new culture and language that resonates with our actual experiences of 'mental illness' rather than trying to fit our lives into a conventional framework. We believe these experiences are mad gifts needing cultivation and care, rather than diseases or disorders." The movement urges those labelled as mentally ill to embrace their madness: if society allows mad individuals to act on their gifts, "the intertwined threads of madness, creativity, and collaboration can inspire hope and transformation in an oppressive and damaged world." (See also Farber, 2012; Glaser, 2008; LeFrancois et al., 2013.)

- *The asexuality movement* includes those who do not experience sexual attraction or desire. In a culture that understands sexual urges as ubiquitous and essential to being human, the lack of such urges has been constructed as a medical problem. Asexuality is defined as either a psychological issue, such as sexual aversion disorder or hyposexual desire disorder, or a bodily dysfunction that requires medical intervention. Asexuals encounter stigma from both the straight and LGBTQ populations, in spite of any shared experiences with marginalization. The asexuality movement primarily seeks to have asexuality legitimized as a biological or innate characteristic—a thing that actually exists—but also to have this state understood as just as natural and "normal" as sexuality (Pagan-Westfall, 2004; Scherrer, 2008).
- *The neurodiversity movement* holds that autism, Asperger syndrome, and other autism spectrum disorders are not pathologies but simply the results of normal variations in the human genome. This movement, like many of the others discussed here, insists that those who may not be neurotypical ("normal") should be recognized as a social category on par with gender, race, ethnicity, and sexuality. The neurodiversity movement frames applied behaviour analysis (ABA), a common treatment for autistic children, as a form of genocide, aimed at eliminating those who are not neurotypical from the world. In Canada, Michelle Dawson, an autistic woman, used this argument before the Supreme Court to successfully block government funding of ABA programs for children (Armstrong, 2010; Orsini, 2009).

What factors are promoting this increase in demedicalization? Some have suggested that the internet is responsible, but internet technologies really represent only more efficient ways of coming together to share and make sense of experiences. This new, efficient avenue of correspondence does not account for society's increasing contestation of medical knowledge. Ballard and Elston (2005, p. 239) offer an argument to explain this phenomenon. They argue that if medicalization was linked to modernity (the rise of science and the medical profession), then demedicalization is linked to society's move from modernity to postmodernity. With growing scepticism of "experts," we should expect to see more challenges to medical constructions of life's experiences. This is especially relevant to those who feel oppressed by these constructions. Recent social trends appear to validate this theory.

Contested Illnesses

Social constructionists have recently become interested in **contested illnesses** (Brown, 2007; Brown, Morello-Frosch, & Zavetovski, 2011; Moss & Teghtsoonian, 2008). Contested illnesses are "conditions in which sufferers and their advocates struggle to have medically unexplained symptoms recognized in orthodox biomedical terms, despite resistance from medical researchers, practitioners, and institutions" (Barker, 2010, p.153). As Barker points out, there has been a notable increase in the number of contested illnesses in recent decades. Such illnesses include chronic fatigue syndrome or myalgic encephalomyelitis (ME), fibromyalgia, irritable bowel syndrome, multiple chemical sensitivity disorder, environmental disease, sick building syndrome, Gulf War syndrome, post-traumatic stress disorder, urologic chronic pelvic pain, endometriosis, temporomandibular joint dysfunction (TMJ), tension headaches, seasonal affective disorder, and repetitive strain injury (RSI). Some of the most interesting recent work explores activism around gluten-related problems, food intolerances, and allergies (Copelton & Valle, 2009; Moore, 2014; Nettleton et al., 2010).

Those who suffer from these conditions generally experience serious distress. Symptoms can include pain, fatigue, sleep disturbances, and depression. Sufferers feel debilitated and unable to carry on with their lives as usual. They report that their quality of life is significantly compromised. Yet, physicians tend to be reluctant to deal with these conditions because of the uncertainly that surrounds them. Their symptoms can be vague, they are difficult to diagnose, their causes are unknown, and they are complicated to manage or treat. Since they are conditions that have not been officially recognized as diseases, many physicians are skeptical about whether they are even "real." Refusing to validate the experiences of those living with contested illnesses only increases sufferers' distress. Diagnoses give people permission to be ill and to take on the "**sick role**"; they are excused from many social expectations until

CASE STUDY

Endometriosis as Contested Illness

Doctors believe that endometriosis is linked to the presence of uterine tissue outside of the uterus, usually somewhere in the pelvic cavity. Many women who suffer from endometriosis, though not all, experience pain and problems with fertility. According to Whalen (2007, p. 957), the enigmatic nature of the condition causes much conflict. The medical community is divided over this issue, and endometriosis patients are often at odds with medical practitioners. Similar to other groups living with contested illnesses, women with endometriosis frequently encounter physicians who know little about the condition, minimize their distress, and dismiss their pain as an exaggerated account of "normal" menstruation.

This delegitimization, Whalen (2007) argues, explains why women with endometriosis have come together to create their own communities and patient support groups. But local groups are linked to a much larger virtual community called, tellingly, WITSENDO, which has members from over 60 different countries across the world. Endometriosis patient communities play a vital role for women with endometriosis, serving as sites of support, validation, and information sharing. But, more critically, Whalen argues, they open up a space for what she calls epistemic resistance. By this she means that the women who make up these communities also create their own body of knowledge about endometriosis—its patterns, symptoms, and manifestations, and effective ways to manage the condition. This body of knowledge, based on women's first-hand experiences, becomes the basis for challenging medical authority.

Many of these women see their experiential knowledge as better and more reliable than the knowledge of medical experts. They turn the tables on doctors. Doctors who discredit them are framed as misinformed, confused, or ignorant non-experts regarding the reality of endometriosis.

In essence, these groups make their own claims not only about endometriosis, but about who can speak knowledgably and credibly about the condition. They "collaboratively formulate and defend an understanding of what *counts* as 'good knowledge' in order to challenge medical authority and develop patient-centred knowledge claims" (Whalen, 2007, p. 959; emphasis in the original).

they are able to function at their normal level (Parsons, 1951). Refusing to acknowledge a person's illness prevents them from obtaining any relief that the sick role may offer.

Living with one of these contested illnesses, then, means coping not only with the symptoms but with medical uncertainty, public skepticism, and disparagement. Dumit (2006, p. 578) describes them as "illnesses you have to fight to get." In this sense, cases of contested illness offer an opportunity to explore the reverse side of the demedicalization process. Whereas demedicalization literature addresses efforts to resist disease labels, contested illness literature focuses on groups' efforts to have their experiences recognized as illness.

Researchers have investigated several facets of contested illness. One type of research addresses how individuals experience these illnesses. Such research typically focuses on the stigma and difficulties faced by those living with contested illnesses, especially in their encounters with physicians, employers, insurance companies, and the general public (Horton-Salway, 2004; Shriver & Waskul, 2006). Considerable attention has also been paid to these groups as health movements and to their collective efforts to have their conditions officially recognized (see Chapter Six). Emma Whalen's (2003; 2007; 2009a; 2009b) research on women with endometriosis illustrates many of the themes addressed in this literature. That many of these conditions are experienced mostly by women raises the question of whether they are modern-day labels for hysteria (Barker, 2010, p. 153).

Lay Constructions of Health and Illness

The chapter has focused thus far on themes having to do with the social construction of formal medical knowledge. But social constructionists have also looked at how individuals construct their health and illness at a more experiential level. At this level, the concern is less about "official" recognition for certain understandings and more about how individuals make sense of health and illness in the context of their own lives.

Among the first social scientists to write about the illness experience were Glaser and Strauss (1965; 1968; Strauss & Glaser, 1975), who challenged the then dominant understanding of the sick role as developed by Talcott Parsons (1951). The sick role refers to social expectations regarding how society should view sick people and how sick people should behave. According to Parsons, the sick role releases individuals from the normal demands and responsibilities in their lives. At the same time, though, the role comes with the expectation that individuals who are sick will seek out medical treatment and follow their doctor's recommendations. The concept of the sick role assumes the primacy of medical constructions of illness and the doctor–patient relationship. Doctors know best, and patients should be prepared to follow doctors' orders so that they can get well.

Glaser and Strauss, on the other hand, view individuals as active agents involved in making sense of their experiences in the context of their daily lives; this independence makes a clash of perspectives between doctor and patient inevitable. Their study of chronic illness, along with other studies through the 1960s (Davis, 1963; Goffman, 1963; Roth, 1963), shifted attention away from medical perspectives of illness towards individuals' subjective experiences.

A good example of how professional and lay perspectives can differ is the case of self-injury (Adler & Adler, 2007). Self-injury is an umbrella term that typically takes in behaviours such as self-cutting, burning, scratching, picking, and biting. The professional or "disease" view constructs these behaviours as symptoms of impulse control disorders such as borderline personality disorder, antisocial or histrionic personality disorder, or depression. Those who are not hospitalized are treated as outpatients. Many self-injurers, however, do not see themselves as lacking impulse control. On the contrary, they carefully plan their behaviour. From their point of view, self-injury can be a useful way of coping with anger, confusion, and frustration. In other words, they see self-cutting not as harmful, but as a helpful, therapeutic, and even health-enhancing practice. One self-injurer who had stopped the practice for a while and then decided to start again explained, "I think I wanted to have that feeling again, that release that I could only get from doing that, that calming sensation" (Adler & Adler, 2007, p. 554).

The 1980s witnessed a number of key conceptual advances in examining individuals' subjective experience with illness. Through his analysis of interviews with people living with rheumatoid arthritis, Bury (1982) developed the notion of a chronic illness as a biographical disruption. A biographical disruption is an experience that leads to a fundamental rethinking of one's life and self-concept. Similarly, Charmaz (1983) wrote about the social isolation that severely debilitating chronic illnesses can generate. In the face of these disruptions and threats to self, individuals often respond imaginatively and find ways to give their suffering meaning. Williams (1984) coined the term "narrative reconstruction" to capture the strategies that individuals employ in responding to illness. They construct narratives or stories that explain their diseased states. These stories "reconstitute and repair ruptures between body, self, and world by linking and interpreting different aspects of biography in order to realign present and past and self and society" (1984, p. 197).

Over the ensuing decades, there have been many more studies applying, refining, and extending these insights (Lawton, 2003 and Pierret, 2003 provide useful overviews). Some focus on specific diseases such as AIDS (Ciambrone, 2001; Weitz, 1991), Parkinson's disease (Nijhof, 1995), cancer (Frank, 2002), diabetes (Rajaram, 1997), and strokes (Pound et al., 1998). One's experience with illness varies according to age, stage of illness, or stage in the lifecycle, gender, race, class, and other aspects of individuals' social contexts.

Other studies focus on how individuals relate to the therapies or medications they are using. For example, Bell (2009) has looked at cancer patients and their constructions of chemotherapy. These perspectives may be counterintuitive from the perspective of the oncologists who treat them. Since patients define side effects as a sign that the therapy is working, those who experience no side effects often become anxious, while those with serious side effects may be reluctant to have their treatment doses reduced. A study of individuals with epilepsy (Conrad, 1985) showed that patients have a tendency to take their medication in ways other than how their doctors have prescribed them. This is defined as non-compliance from their doctors' perspective. For the patients themselves, however, playing with dosages represents an attempt to assert themselves over a condition that can make them feel as if they have little control. Studies such as these explain the tensions that often arise between individuals and their health care providers over disagreements in treatment plans.

Conrad and Barker (2010, S72) summarize the contributions of the social constructionist approach to the study of lay experiences in this way:

> This line of research brings to the fore aspects of illness that the tools of medicine are unable to reveal. A constructionist approach takes the subjective experience of illness seriously, examining the personal and social meanings of illness, and exploring how

illness is managed in the social contexts that sufferers inhabit. This research has given us a detailed and intimate view of the suffering that illness often represents, but it has also shown us that agency and resistance are key to the illness experience.

Chapter Summary

Health and illness are a central part of our everyday lives, but most of the time we do not question what these terms mean. Nor do we question why specific behaviours or conditions fall into one category or the other. We take these things for granted. For social scientists, the questions of who is healthy and who gets sick, why health care services are organized as they are, and who has access to these services are all important to ask. But all of these questions assume the existence of health and illness, and treat these terms unproblematically.

In this chapter we have looked at health and illness as social constructions. In other words, we have treated them as labels, meanings, or interpretations that are applied to certain behaviours and conditions. These labels come with certain consequences in terms of how we respond.

This chapter considered four main themes that have emerged from the social constructionist approach:

- The social construction of medical knowledge deals with the social bases of medical knowledge and how such knowledge is shaped by the social context within which it is produced.
- Medicalization covers the claims-making process involved in trying to have disease labels applied to deviant behaviours, conditions, or aspects of life traditionally viewed as normal. Demedicalization, on the other hand, covers efforts to have disease labels removed.
- The term contested illness refers to the claims-making activities of those who want their medically unexplained symptoms to be recognized in orthodox biomedical terms.
- Lay constructions of illness address how lay people construct and understand health and illness at an experiential level in the context of their own lives.

Each of these themes addresses some aspect of our constantly shifting conceptions of health and illness. Diseases of the past may not be viewed as disease today, diseases of the present may no longer be considered diseases, and other diseases await future "discovery." Health and illness, as social constructions, change because society changes. Human beings are continuously involved in the process of making sense of our experiences, ourselves, and the world around us.

STUDY QUESTIONS

1. What factors are necessary for a condition or process to become medicalized? Who is involved?
2. What are the key differences between medicalization and demedicalization? What do these differences say about society?

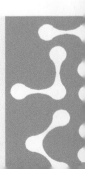

3. How can diseases or conditions be both "socially constructed" and "real" all at once?
4. What are the main differences between contested illnesses and those recognized by mainstream biomedicine?
5. What does social constructivism teach us about medicine and science more broadly?

SUGGESTED READINGS

Arksey, H. (1994). Expert and lay participation in the construction of medical knowledge. *Sociology of Health & Illness, 16*(4), 448–68.

Giles, D. (2006). Constructing identities in cyberspace: The case of eating disorders. *British Journal of Social Psychology, 45*(3), 463–77.

Scheff, T. (2009). *Being mentally ill: a sociological theory.* New Brunswick: AldineTransaction.

SUGGESTED WEB RESOURCES

Aimee Mullins, TED Talks: www.ted.com/speakers/aimee_mullins

The Icarus Project: Navigating the Space between Brilliance and Madness: www.theicarusproject.net

Selling Sickness (documentary film) (2004) Dir. Catherine Scott. Paradigm Pictures/Australian Film Finance Corporation Ltd: http://icarusfilms.com/new2005/sell.html

GLOSSARY

Contested illness An illness with inexplicable or uncertain medical symptoms. While patients experience the illness, it is unclear how or why. These illnesses may be source of contention between patients and medical practitioners (e.g., fibromyalgia).

Healthism The idea that, through making proper lifestyle choices, one can be proactive in maintaining one's health or becoming healthier. An emphasis on an individual's responsibility for their health.

Labelling theory The sociological concept that deviance is not an inherent quality but a label given by society. In this sense, something is not "other" until society perceives and claims it is so.

Medical discourse Society's conceptions of medical knowledge that influence our understanding of disease and its treatment (see Foucault, 1973; 1980). Medical discourse can vary between cultures.

Medicalization The process in which conditions and behaviours that were previously considered a normal part of life come to be understood as medical problems (e.g., the conceptualization of inattention and hyperactivity as ADHD).

Paradigm A widely accepted explanation or framework for understanding a given issue.

Sick role, the How society views sick people and how societies expect sick people should behave (see Talcott Parsons, 1951).

Social constructionism A theory that holds that knowledge, definitions, and social roles are not fixed or inherent but are a dynamic product of society. For example, gender roles are a social construct.

REFERENCES

Abraham, J. (2010). Pharmaceuticalization of society in context: Theoretical, empirical and health dimensions. *Sociology, 44*(4), 603–22.

Adler, P. & Adler, P. (2007). The demedicalization of self-injury: From psychopathology to social deviance. *Journal of Contemporary Ethnography, 36*(5), 537–70.

Apple, R. D. (2006). *Perfect motherhood: Science and childrearing in America.* New Brunswick, NJ: Rutgers University Press.

Armstrong, D. (1995). The rise of surveillance medicine. *Sociology of Health and Illness, 17*(3), 393–404.

Armstrong, T. (2010). *Neurodiversity: Discovering the extraordinary gifts of autism, ADHD, dyslexia and other brain differences.* Cambridge, MA: Da Capo Press.

Australian Department of Veterans' Affairs. (n.d.). Case study: Social anxiety disorder. Retrieved from http://at-ease.dva.gov.au/veterans/resources/case-studies/case-study-social-anxiety-disorder

Ballard, K. & Elston, M. A. (2005). Medicalisation: A multidimensional concept. *Social Theory and Health, 3,* 228–41.

Bayer, R. (1981). *Homosexuality and American psychiatry: The politics of diagnosis.* New York: Basic Books.

Barker, K. (2008). Electronic support groups, patient-consumers, and medicalization: The case of contested illness. *Journal of Health and Social Behavior, 49,* 20–36.

———. (2010). The social construction of illness: Medicalization and contested illness. In C. E. Bird, P. Conrad, A. M. Fremont, & S. Timmermans (Eds). *Handbook of Medical Sociology* (6th ed., pp. 147–62). Nashville, TN: Vanderbilt University Press.

Beck, U. (1992). *Risk society: Towards a new modernity.* New Delhi: Sage.

Becker, H. S. (1963). *Outsiders: Studies in the sociology of deviance.* New York: Free Press.

Bell, K. (2009). "If it almost kills you that means it's working!": Cultural models of chemotherapy expressed in a cancer support group. *Social Science and Medicine, 68*(1), 169–76.

Bell, S. E. & Figert, A. E. (2012). Medicalization and pharmaceuticalization at the intersections: Looking backward, sideways and forward. *Social Science and Medicine, 75,* 775–83.

Berger, P. & Luckmann, T. (1966). *The social construction of reality: A treatise in the sociology of knowledge.* New York: Anchor.

Billings, D. B. & Urban, T. (l982). The socio-medical construction of transsexualism: An interpretation and critique. *Social Problems, 29*(3), 266–82.

Brown, P. (1995). Naming and framing: The social construction of diagnosis and illness. *Journal of Health and Social Behavior, 35,* 34–52.

———. (2007). *Toxic exposures: Contested illnesses and the environmental health movement.* New York: Columbia University Press.

———, Morello-Frosch, R., & Zavestoski, S. (Eds). (2011). *Contested illnesses: citizens, science and health Social Movements.* Oakland, CA: University of California Press.

Bury, M. (1982). Chronic illness as biographical disruption. *Journal of Health and Illness, 4*(2), 167–82.

———. (1986). Social constructionism and the development of medical sociology. *Sociology of Health and Illness, 8,* 137–69.

Cain, S. (2012). *Quiet: The power of introverts in a world that can't stop talking.* New York: Crown Publishers.

Charmaz, K. (1983). Loss of self: A fundamental form of suffering in the chronically ill. *Sociology of Health and Illness, 5,* 168–95.

Ciambrone, D. (2001). Illness and other assaults on self: Women and HIV/AIDS. *Sociology of Health and Illness, 23*(4), 517–40.

Collyer, F. M. (1996). Understanding ulcers: Medical knowledge, social constructionism and Helicobacter Pylori. *Annual Review of Health Sciences, 6,* 1–39.

Conrad, P. (1975). The discovery of hyperkinesis: Notes on the medicalization of deviant behavior. *Social Problems, 23*(1), 12–21.

———. (1985). The meanings of medication: Another look at compliance. *Social Science and Medicine, 20,* 29–37.

———. (1992). Medicalization and social control. *Annual Review of Sociology, 18,* 209–32.

———. (2005). The shifting engines of medicalization. *Journal of Health and Social Behaviour, 46,* 3–14.

———. (2007). *The medicalization of society: On the transformation of human conditions into treatable disorders.* Baltimore, MD: Johns Hopkins University Press.

———— & Barker, K. (2010). The social construction of illness: Key insights and policy implications. *Journal of Health and Social Behavior, 51,* S67–S79.

———— & Potter, D. (2000). From hyperactive children to ADHD adults: Observations on the expansion of medical categories. *Social Problems, 47*(4), 559–82.

———— & Schneider, J.W. (1980). *Deviance and medicalization: From badness to sickness.* St. Louis: Mosby.

Copelton, D. A. & Valle, G. (2009). "You don't need a prescription to go gluten free": The scientific self-diagnosis of celiac disease. *Social Science and Medicine, 69,* 623–31.

Davis, F. (1963). *Passage through crisis: Polio victims and their families.* Indianapolis, IL: Bobbs-Merrill.

Dumit, J. (2006). Illnesses you have to fight to get: Facts as forces in uncertain, emergent illnesses. *Social Science and Medicine 62*(3), 577–90.

Estes, C. & Binney, E. (1989). The biomedicalization of aging: Dangers and dilemmas. *The Gerontologist, 29*(5), 587–96.

Ezzy, D. (2000). Illness narratives: Time, hope and HIV. *Social Science and Medicine, 50,* 605–17.

Farber, S. (2012). *The spiritual gift of Madness: The failure of psychiatry and the rise of the mad pride movement.* Rochester, VT: Inner Traditions.

Figert, A. E. (1996). *Women and the ownership of PMS: The structuring of a psychiatric diagnosis.* New York: Aldine de Gruyter.

Findlay, D. (1993). The good, the normal and the healthy: The social construction of medical knowledge about women. *The Canadian Journal of Sociology, 18*(2), 115–35.

Fox, P. (1989). From senility to Alzheimer's disease: The rise of the Alzheimer's disease movement. *Milbank Quarterly, 67,* 57–101.

Frances, A. (2013). *Saving normal: An insider's revolt against out-of-control psychiatric diagnosis: DSM-5, big pharma and the medicalization of ordinary life.* New York: William Morrow.

Frank, A. W. (2002). *At the will of the body: Reflections on illness.* Boston, MA: Houghton Mifflin.

Freidson, E. (1970). *Profession of medicine: A study of the sociology of applied knowledge.* New York: Harper and Row.

Foucault, M. (1973). *The birth of the clinic: An archaeology of medical perception.* London: Tavistock.

————. (1980). *Power/knowledge: Selected interviews and other writings.* Brighton: Harvester.

Giddens, A. (1990). *The consequences of modernity.* Stanford: Stanford University Press.

Glaser, G. (2008, May 10). "Mad Pride" Fights a Stigma. Retrieved from www.New Yorktimes.com/2008/05/11/fashion/11madpride.html

Glaser, A. & Strauss, B. (1965). *Awareness of dying.* Chicago, IL: Aldine.

————. (1968). *Time for dying.* Chicago, IL: Aldine.

Goffman, E. (1963). *Stigma.* Englewood Cliffs, NJ: Prentice Hall.

Greil, A. L. & McQuillan, J. (2010). Medicalization, intent, and ambiguity in the definition of infertility. *Medical Anthropology Quarterly, 24*(2), 137–56.

Hacking, I. (1999). *The social construction of what?* Cambridge, MA: Harvard University Press.

Hepworth, J. (1999). *The social construction of anorexia nervosa.* Thousand Oaks, CA: Sage.

Hislop, J. & Archer, S. (2003). Understanding women's sleep management: Beyond medicalization-healthicization? *Sociology of Health & Illness, 25*(7), 815–37.

Holstein, J. A. & Gubrium, J. F. (2000). *Constructing the life course.* Walnut Creek, CA: AltaMira.

Horton-Salway, M. (2004). The local production of knowledge: Disease labels, identities and category entitlements in ME support group talk. *Health, 8*(3), 351–71.

Illich, I. (1976). *Limits to medicine, medical nemesis: The expropriation of health.* London: Marion Boyars.

Jutel, A. (2009). Sociology of diagnosis: A preliminary review. *Sociology of Health and Illness, 31,* 278–99.

Kampf, A., Marshall, B. L. & Petersen, A. (2013). *Aging men, masculinities and modern medicine.* London: Routledge.

Kaufman, S. R., Shim, J. & Russ, A. J. (2004). Revisiting the biomedicalization of aging: Clinical trends and ethical challenges. *Gerontologist, 44*(6), 731–38.

Kirk, S. A. & Kutchins, H. (1992). *The selling of DSM: The rhetoric of science in psychiatry.* New York: Aldine de Gruyter.

King, D. (1987). Social constructionism and medical knowledge: The case of transsexualism. *Sociology of Health and Illness, 9*(4), 351–77.

Kuhn, T. S. (1962). *The structure of scientific revolutions.* Chicago, IL: University of Chicago Press.

Lane, C. (2007). *Shyness: How normal behavior became a sickness.* New Haven, CT: Yale University Press.

Lawton, J. (2003). Lay experiences of health and illness: Past research future agendas. *Sociology of Health and Illness, 25*(3), 23–40.

Lee, E. (2003). *Abortion, motherhood and mental health: Medicalizing reproduction in the United States and Great Britain.* New York: Aldine de Gruyter.

———. (2004). Pathologising fatherhood: The construction of post-natal depressions as "men's problem" in Britain. Retrieved from: www.kent.ac.uk/sspssr/research/papers/pathfather.pdf

———. (2006). Medicalizing motherhood. *Society 43*(6), 47–50.

LeFrancois, B. A., Menzies, R., & Reaume, G. (Eds). (2013). *Mad matters: A critical reader in Canadian mad studies.* Toronto, ON: Canadian Scholars' Press.

Lippman, A. (1992). Led (astray) by genetic maps: The cartography of the human genome and health care. *Social Science and Medicine, 35,* 1469–96.

Lorber, J. (1996). Beyond the binaries: Depolarizing the categories of sex, sexuality and gender. *Sociological Inquiry, 66*(2), 143–60.

Loseke, D. (1995). Writing rights: The "homeless mentally ill" and involuntary hospitalization. In J. Best (Ed.), *Images of Issues: Typifying Contemporary Social Problems* (2nd ed., pp. 261–86). New York: Aldine de Gruyter.

Lowenberg, J. S. & Davis, F. (1994). Beyond medicalization-demedicalization: The case of holistic medicine. *Sociology of Health and Illness, 16*(5), 579–99.

Maines, D. & Kusow, A. (2001). Somali migration to Canada and resistance to racialization. In D. Maines (Ed.), *The faultline of consciousness: A view of interactionism in sociology* (pp. 135–64). New York: Aldine de Gruyter.

Malacrida, C. (2003). *Cold comfort: Mothers, professionals and ADD.* Toronto, ON: University of Toronto Press.

Martin, E. (1987). *The woman in the body: A cultural analysis of reproduction.* Boston, MA: Beacon Press.

McCrea, F. B. (1983). The politics of menopause: The "discovery" of a deficiency disease. *Social Problems, 31,* 111–23.

McCreath, G. (2011). *The politics of blindness: From charity to parity.* Vancouver, BC: Granville Island Publishing.

Moore, L. R. (2014). "But we're not hypochondriacs": The changing shape of gluten-free dieting and the contested illness experience. *Social Science and Medicine, 105,* 76–83.

Morrow, C. K. (1982). Sick doctors: The social construction of professional deviance. *Social Problems, 30*(1), 92–108.

Moss, P. & Teghtsoonian, K. (Eds). 2008. *Contesting illness: Processes and practices.* Toronto, ON: University of Toronto Press.

Moynihan, R. & Cassels, A. (2005). *Selling sickness: How the world's biggest pharmaceutical companies are turning us all into patients.* New York: Nation Books.

Nettleton, S. (2006). "I just want permission to be ill": Towards a sociology of medically unexplained symptoms. *Social Science and Medicine 62,* 1167–78.

———, Woods, B., Burrows, R., & Kerr, A. (2010). Experiencing food allergy and food intolerance. *Sociology, 44,* 289–305.

Nijhof, G. (1995). Parkinson's disease as a problem of shame in public appearance. *Sociology of Health and Illness, 7,* 193–205.

Oakley, A. (1986). *The captured womb: A history of the medical care of pregnant women.* Oxford: Basil Blackwell.

Orsini, M. (2009). Contesting the autistic subject: Biological citizenship and the autism/autistic movements. In S. J. Murray & D. Holmes (Eds), *Critical Interventions in the Ethics of Healthcare: Challenging the Principle of Autonomy in Bioethics* (pp. 115–30). Surrey: Ashgate.

Pagan-Westfall, S. (2004). Glad to be asexual. *New Scientist, 184*(2469), 40–43.

Parsons, T. (1951). *The social system.* Glencoe, IL: Free Press.

Pawluch, D. (1996). *The new pediatrics: A profession in transition.* New York: Aldine de Gruyter.

Pfohl, S. (1977). The "discovery" of child abuse. *Social Problems, 24,* 310–23.

Phelan, J. C. (2005). Geneticization of deviant behavior and consequences for stigma: The case of mental illness. *Journal of Health and Social Behavior, 46,* 307–22.

Pierret, J. (2003). The illness experience: State of knowledge and perspectives for research. *Sociology of Health and Illness, 25*(3), 4–22.

Pound, P., Gompertz, P., & Ebrahim, S. (1998). Illness in the context of older age: The case of stroke. *Sociology of Health and Illness, 20,* 489–506.

Rajaram, S. S. (1997). Experience of hypoglycemia among insulin dependent diabetics and its impact on the family. *Sociology of Health & Illness, 19*(3), 281–96.

Reagan, T. (1995). A sociocultural understanding of deafness: American Sign Language and the culture of deaf people. *International Journal of Intercultural Relations, 19*(2), 239–51.

Riessman, C. K. (1983). Women and medicalization: A new perspective. *Social Policy, 14*, 3–18.

Riska, E. (2003). Gendering the medicalization thesis. *Advances in Gender Research, 7*, 59–87.

Robbins, T. & AnthoNew York, D. (1982). Deprogramming, brainwashing and the medicalization of deviant religious groups. *Social Problems, 29*(3), 283–97.

Rosenfeld, D. & Faircloth, C.A. (2006). *Medicalized masculinities*. Philadelphia: Temple University Press.

Rosenhan, D. L. (1973). On being sane in insane places. *Science, 179*(4070), 250–58.

Rossol, J. (2001). The medicalization of deviance as an interactive achievement: The construction of compulsive gambling. *Social Problems, 24*(3), 315–41.

Roth, J. (1963). *Timetables*. New York: Bobbs-Merrill.

Scherrer, K. (2008). Coming to an asexual identity: Negotiating identity, negotiating desire. *Sexualities, 11*(5), 621–41.

Schneider, J. W. (1978). Deviant drinking as disease: Alcoholism as a social accomplishment. *Social Problems, 25*(4), 361–72.

Scott, S. (2006). The medicalisation of shyness: From social misfits to social fitness. *Sociology of Health and Illness, 28*(2), 133–53.

Scott, W. J. (1990). PTSD in DSM-III: A case in the politics of diagnosis and disease. *Social Problems, 37*(3), 294–310.

Shriver, T. E. & Waskul, D. D. (2006). Managing the uncertainties of Gulf War illness: The challenges of living with contested illness. *Symbolic Interaction, 29*(4), 465–86.

Snow, D. A., Baker, S. G., Anderson, L., & Martin, M. (1986). The myth of pervasive mental illness among the homeless. *Social Problems, 33*(5), 407–23.

Spector, M. (1977). Legitimizing homosexuality. *Society, 14*(5), 52–56.

——— & Kitsuse, J. (1977). *Constructing social problems*. New York: Aldine de Gruyter.

Strauss, A. & Glaser, B. (Eds). (1975). *Chronic illness and the quality of life*. St. Louis: Mosby.

Szasz, T. A. (1961). *The myth of mental illness*. New York: Harper and Row.

———. (1970). *The manufacture of madness*. New York: Dell.

———. (1981). The sane slave: An historical note on the use of medical diagnosis as justificatory rhetoric. In G. P. Stone & H. A. Faberman (Eds), *Social Psychology through Symbolic Interactionism*, (2nd ed., pp. 405–13). New York: John Wiley.

Tiefer, L. (2006). Female sexual dysfunction: A case study of disease mongering and activist resistance. *PloS Medicine, 3*(4), e178.

Timimi, S. (2002). *Pathological child psychiatry and the medicalization of childhood*. London: Routledge.

——— & Taylor, E. (2004). In debate: ADHD is best understood as a cultural construct. *British Journal of Psychiatry, 184*, 8–9.

Turner, B. (2004). *The New Medical Sociology: Social Forms of health and Illness*. New York: W. W. Norton.

Verbrugge, M. (1976). Women and medicine in 19th century America. *Signs, 1*, 957–72.

Weitz, R. (1991). *Life with AIDS*. New Brunswick, NJ: Rutgers University Press.

Whelan, E. (2003). Putting pain to paper: Endometriosis and the documentation of suffering. *Health, 7*(4), 463–82.

Whalen, E. (2007). "No one agrees except for those of us who have it": Endometriosis patients as an epistemological community. *Sociology of Health and Illness, 29*(7), 957–82.

———. (2009a). Negotiating science and experience in medical knowledge: Gynaecologists on endometriosis. *Social Science and Medicine, 68*(8), 1489–97.

———. (2009b). *How classification works, or doesn't: The case of chronic pain*. Sage Handbook of Case-Based Methods (pp. 169–72). Thousand Oaks, CA: Sage.

Williams, G. (1984). The genesis of chronic illness: Narrative reconstruction. *Sociology of Health and Illness, 6*, 175–200.

Sleepiness. In S. Williams, J. Gabe & P. Davis (Eds), *Pharmaceuticals and Society*. Chichester: Wiley-Blackwell.

Wright, P. & Treacher, A. (Eds). (1982). *The problem of medical knowledge: Examining the social construction of medicine*. Edinburgh: Edinburgh University Press.

Zola, I. (1972). Medicine as an institution of social control. *Sociological Review, 20*(4), 487–504.

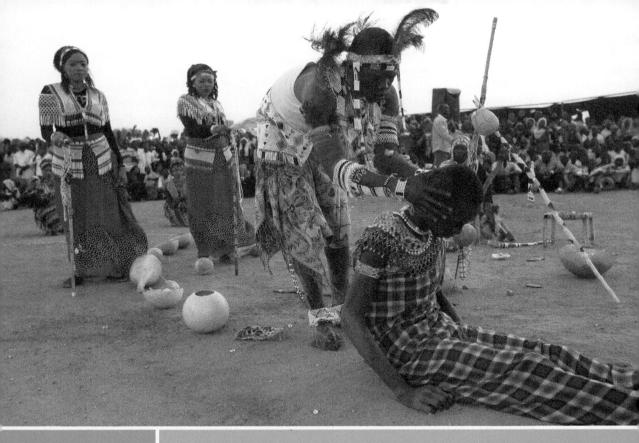

4

Cultures and Meanings of Health

Raza Mirza

LEARNING OBJECTIVES

In this chapter students will learn

- what is meant by culture and how it intersects with meanings of health
- why culture is a social determinant of health
- how material objects, social relations, and ideas shape and influence culture
- the relative importance of culture in relation to health care

Introduction

The concept of culture is difficult to unpack. This chapter articulates how culture—collective ways of doing, being, and understanding—shapes health, illness, care, and healing at different levels and in different ways. Specifically, attention is paid to the ways in which culture relates to health and health care. The role of cultures in the popular, folk, and professional health sectors is explored. More generally, the chapter analyzes the specificities and differences in illness and healing across cultures.

What Is Culture?

Almost two hundred conceptualizations and definitions of **culture** exist. Although the word *culture* is part of our everyday vocabulary, we do not have a universal understanding or interpretation of the term. More importantly, the terminology used to define culture is diverse. It depends on the context and who is using the term. The origins of the word *culture* can be traced back to agricultural contexts, where the term referred to the cultivation of crops and other harvestable goods (Williams, 1981). It was not until the eighteenth century that the term *culture* was extended to reflect a state of refinement or development that humans aspired to achieve (Williams, 1981). Based on this idea, those who were "cultured" had refinement in thought, beliefs, and actions (Williams, 1981). The effects of culture would allow one to evolve from a barbaric, uncivilized state to that of a civilized member of society. Ultimately, this individual would become a member of the cultural elite. This historical context of the term "culture" highlights the importance of group membership. The idea of culture as a developmental continuum remains embedded in our current conceptualizations of culture.

Historically, the concept of culture has been perceived and applied differentially based on the frame of reference. As such, defining the term is a complex process. Edward Tylor's (1871) definition of culture is one of the earliest. It defines culture from an anthropological perspective (see Table 4.1: Definitions of Culture). Critics of Taylor's definition say that it is too broad. It also assumes that one's capabilities are a result only of one's cultural upbringing; it ignores the role of biology in determining behaviour. However, what is important to note here is that this definition of culture suggests holistic elements of learning, sharing, and socializing that are necessary for culture to exist; this is consistent with our more modern definitions of culture.

Building on the idea that group membership is an important aspect of culture, famed American poet T.S. Eliot's (1948) *Notes on the Definition of Culture* argued that culture was inextricably linked to religion. His view was that culture could not develop outside of the context of religion, as people's religious beliefs determined their behaviour. From Eliot's perspective, group membership was dependent on a belief system such as Christianity or Christian ideology (1948). Eliot's work highlights again that not everyone has the same culture or is part of a culture sharing group. His belief was that the secularization of society would lead to a loss of religion and therefore a loss of culture. Again, what is important here is the belief that culture is an essential element of learning, sharing, and transmitting beliefs and behaviour.

One of the most cited definitions of culture comes from Kroeber and Kluckhohn (1952) (see Table 4.1). They reviewed the various ways (150 at the time) that the concept of culture had previously been defined, and ultimately devised their own definition.

TABLE 4.1		Definitions of Culture
Author	**Year**	**Definition of Culture**
Tylor	1871	"Culture is that complex whole which includes knowledge, belief, art, law, morals, custom, and any other capabilities and habits acquired by man as a member of society."
Linton	1945	"A culture is a configuration of learned behaviors and results of behavior whose component elements are shared and transmitted by the members of a particular society."
Eliot	1948	"Culture may even be described simply as that which makes life worth living. . . . It includes all the characteristic activities and interests of a people: Derby Day, Henley Regatta, Cowes, the twelfth of August, a cup final, the dog races, the pin table, the dart board, Wensleydale cheese, boiled cabbage cut into sections, beetroot in vinegar, nineteenth-century Gothic churches and the music of Elgar."
Parsons	1949	" . . . consisting in those patterns relative to behavior and the products of human action which may be inherited, that is, passed on from generation to generation independently of the biological genes."
Kroeber & Kluckhohn	1952	"Culture consists of patterns, explicit and implicit, of and for behavior acquired and transmitted by symbols, constituting the distinctive achievement of human groups, including their embodiment in artifacts; the essential core of culture consists of traditional (i.e., historically derived and selected) ideas and especially their attached values; culture systems may, on the one hand, be considered as products of action, on the other as conditioning elements of further action."
Hofstede	1994	"[Culture] is the collective programming of the mind which distinguishes the members of one group or category of people from another."
Ballard	2002	"Human cultures are cognitive structures; and since culture also provides a vehicle for communication, the phenomenon is best understood as the set of ideas, values and understandings which people deploy within a specific network of social relationships as a means of ordering their inter-personal interactions and hence to generate ties of reciprocity between themselves; in so doing it also provides the principal basis on which human beings give meaning and purpose to lives."
World Health Organization (WHO)	2004	"The learned, shared and transmitted values, beliefs, norms and lifetime practices of a particular group that guides thinking, decisions and actions in patterned ways."
Matsumoto	2006	"A shared system of socially transmitted behavior that describes, defines, and guides people's ways of life, communicated from one generation to the next."

In this table are a number of historical definitions and interpretations of culture. What is clear is that culture is whatever people perceive it to be. The term *culture* is often used in line with political or ideological agendas, and it is unlikely that there will ever be consensus in terms of what culture really is or means. The definitions of culture presented in Table 4.1 were selected to highlight that the concept of culture can represent multiple paradigmatic, political, and ideological standpoints. What we currently regard as "culture" could be best described as practices that are learned, shared, and transmitted, and that guide the behaviour and actions of members of a culture sharing group. With so many ways to look at and interpret the concept of culture, the utility of the term is often questioned. Critics argue that the notion of culture sharing groups creates bounded systems that are separate from the system at large. The notion hinges on the assumption that the realities and experiences of some people are separate and distinct from those of others. The elusiveness of the definition of culture does not mean that we should abandon our efforts to understand what culture is, but rather that we should shift our focus to one of the more enduring qualities of culture: culture is dynamic. In other words, as our notions of culture continue to change, so will our conception of the term.

From our review of the multiple ways that culture has been defined, we can say that definitions of culture share the following:

- notions of membership in a culture sharing group;
- elements of learning, sharing, and common beliefs and values that provide a frame of reference for members of the culture sharing group;
- a lens and world view for members of a culture sharing group to interpret and understand life, finding meaning in their experiences; and
- Transmission and maintenance of elements of culture among members of culture sharing groups or generations. Culture is transmitted through shared tangible and intangible elements such as symbols, objects, social relations, ideas, and knowledge. These elements may be understood only by members of a culture sharing group.

The term *culture* is often used interchangeably with the concepts of **race and ethnicity** (Ballard, 2002). Culture, race, and ethnicity all represent categorical differences among individuals, and these terms all suggest a transmission of some sort from one generation to another. But it can be argued that the concept of race differs from culture in that it is based on common assumed or imagined genetic characteristics (or biology) and ancestry. Ethnicity, on the other hand, is more about country or region of origin. While it is argued that culture is dynamic, and that the basis of culture is in social systems, race is assumed to be more about genetic lineage fixed through biology (Templeton, 1998). For example, the colour of our skin or our facial features are inherently genetic in nature and cannot be changed through social interactions. The differences between culture and ethnicity are more difficult to untangle. The term *ethnicity* is derived from the Greek word for foreign ("ethnos"), and loosely references the origin of birth of a group of individuals (Senior & Bhopal, 1994). For example, even if an individual is born in Canada but has ancestors from Latin America, it is the race of the individual's ancestors that determines ethnicity; in this case, the individual might still be considered Hispanic.

The terms *race*, *ethnicity*, and *culture* are all terms used to formulate an identity and group membership. Group membership is an important element of the concept of culture. Although we do not necessarily need to agree on a definition of culture, we do need to operationalize the term for our purposes, and differentiate it from other common terms such as *race* and *ethnicity*. In a broader sense, references to the concept of culture in this chapter will be made to help facilitate understandings of the experiences of members of a culture sharing group with respect to a larger collective of experiences. Emphasis will be placed on how culture is both a process and a state. The definition of culture that we will use is the one established by the World Health Organization (WHO) in 2004, which states that culture is "[t]he learned, shared and transmitted values, beliefs, norms and lifetime practices of a particular group that guides thinking, decisions and actions in patterned ways." The WHO's definition takes into account that culture produces identifiable patterns of behaviour among members of a culture sharing group within a social world.

Using culture as a tool, we can explore the experiences, perspectives, behaviours, lifestyle patterns, and social relations of groups. These experiences are not necessarily tied to biology, and as we will see in the next sections, culture can affect health and how we experience (and respond to) health and illness.

The Formation of Culture

Some aspects of culture are visible and some aspects are invisible. We often take for granted our interpretations of gestures, codes of behaviour, patterned ways of being, and the social relations we develop. For example, giving the "thumbs up" gesture, which is a common sign of approval in the North American context, is offensive in other places around the world. We were not born knowing that giving a "thumbs up" gesture was a sign of approval, of course, and therefore we must have learned this. In the previous section, we made the distinction between race and culture to highlight that culture is not embedded within our DNA. It is passed on—between generations—and is specific to a group. This leads to the question: How is "culture" formed?

One of the simpler ways that culture forms is between individuals who interact geographically. Returning to the example of the "thumbs up" gesture, the fact that it has different meanings in different places points to how practices are open to interpretation by different culture sharing groups. They are part of a cultural "language." Cultural traits such as behaviour, symbolism, communication, and interaction can be tangible or invisible. Culture is clearly quite complex.

There is great debate over what shapes a culture and its values, beliefs, and behaviours. It is undeniable that no single factor can explain the complexities of culture. One of the ways that anthropologists try to understand the culture of a group is by looking at the *organization* of cultural traits. Cultural traits are based on social interactions and communication. White (1975) envisioned culture as based on ideological, technological, and sociological subsystems. Building on this, Huxley's classification of structure was based on three factors: artifacts, social structures and relationships, and systems of belief (White, 1975; Huxley, 1955). Huxley, a biologist by training, hypothesized that these each of these components is interdependent—affected by and informed by the others.

The subsystem of artifacts gives us a better understanding of how members of a culture sharing group live. If you have ever been to a museum, you may have seen a display of ancient cultural artifacts such as primitive tools, eating utensils, musical instruments, or religious idols. This element of cultural traits is based on the visible, tangible material objects and even technologies that are part of a group's day-to-day living. Often included in the artifacts subsystem are the basic necessities that would allow members of a culture sharing group to protect themselves from others, feed themselves, and amuse themselves. Markov et al. (2008) suggest that the most important aspect of the artifacts subsystem of culture is the knowledge and techniques that coincide with the use of the objects. Knowing what a mortar and pestle is and how to use it to crush and prepare medicinal herbs, for example, illustrates the importance of shared knowledge. Without the information on how to use the apparatus, a mortar and pestle is just a bowl with a stick.

It is important to note that the transmission of information or patterns of behaviour can be linked back to social relations (Huxley, 1955). The structure and organization of a culture sharing group not only influences how individuals behave, but also regulates the role of the individual with respect to the larger cultural system. As Fellmann et al. (2007) point out, one's role, function, and expected behaviour within a culture sharing group is learned. Social relations are often maintained through intergenerational transmission of norms. An example of this is health related decision-making in traditional Chinese families. Strong intergenerational links suggest that "filial piety" or moral obligation may undergird the care relationship between adult children and their parents. According to Chinese tradition, the oldest adult male is the decision-maker for health and family matters. However, there is obvious influence from elders, including women, who can also assume the major role of decision-maker (Kolb, 2007).

The mobilization of care for parents by children in many families can be categorized as part of the belief systems of a culture. These systems can encompass almost anything that can be written, spoken, or communicated regarding beliefs, values, and morals. Literature, folklore, dietary preference, political thought, or even religious traditions would all be classified as elements of a culture's belief system. In any given situation, including times of health or illness, culture may govern what is considered beneficial and what is not. Take, for example, the Mediterranean diet. Olives are plentiful in certain areas of the world and are therefore a dietary staple. People in these areas have consumed a traditional "Mediterranean diet" for centuries, consisting of meals with high ratios of "good fats," wine, and fibre in the form of fruits, vegetables, and grains and a low intake of meats and dairy products. This diet is recognized by the United Nations as culturally meaningful (Trichopoulou & Lagiou, 1997), and is a good example of a cultural tradition. It touches on all three elements of culture we have previously discussed: members of this cultural group have the artifacts, such as farm equipment, necessary to cultivate such a diet; the social structure has helped to share this diet between generations; and members of the culture are aware of the health benefits of their food choices.

Often isolated by geography, culture sharing groups develop as a result of their exposure to a certain environment and modes of survival. This social organization can be based on age, gender, marital status, educational experience, or occupational rank. Cultural tools, modes of communication, family structure, and even food preferences are often such an inherent (and overlooked) aspect of everyday life that they we do not recognize them as elements of culture. Many cultural groups have similar characteristics but may not explicitly recognize these as cultural elements. Consider again the example of the "thumbs up" gesture. Many similar cultural groups share this gesture, but individuals may not immediately recognize it—regardless of its interpretation—as a characteristic of their own culture.

In the context of health, every culture may have its own understanding of the basic necessities for health. Each culture has a different understanding of the relationships among health care professionals, patients, and family members. Often, groups have common beliefs about preferences for medicines that are considered natural versus those that are not. As a result, culture can and does influence health. We will explore the implications for patient communication, patient behaviour, and approaches to health and illness in the next section.

Does Culture Affect Health?

The link between culture and health beliefs is not new, as Purnell and Paulanka (2003) highlight. Health services in North America are based on the principles of Western biomedicine, which may create discord between the health beliefs of some culture sharing groups and the context in which care is delivered. Based on the principles of Western biomedicine, North American health care uses prescription medicines to target and treat specific ailments. This system is based on values such as the patient's right to self-determination and autonomy. People whose values are based on other philosophies of medicine and health (e.g., Ayurvedic, traditional Chinese medicine) tend to have a strikingly different view of their bodies, health, illness, and treatment (Kong & Hsieh, 2011). For the Aboriginal community in Canada, traditional understandings of health are seen as inseparable from religion and spirituality (Robbins & Dewar, 2011). As such, health beliefs are often based on supernatural phenomena (i.e., invasion of the body by spirits) and health care is often delivered by a "medicine man" or shaman from the Aboriginal community.

In many First Nations cultures, like many other cultures, not only is the relationship between the patient and the health practitioner based on a shared understanding of health and illness, but there is also a common understanding of how to communicate issues of health. Patients often cite that communication issues have prevented them from receiving optimal care from practitioners (Efferth et al., 2007). In the North American context, health care professionals are encouraged to base communication with culturally diverse patients on a collaborative model, and to form a therapeutic partnership with the patient (and often their family) (Elwyn et al., 2014). However, in some cultures, patients will remain silent and passive, and defer all health care decisions to the health care professional (Leung et al., 2014). From a cultural perspective, such patients may understand their actions as appropriate and respectful. Without an understanding of the cultural basis for an individual's actions or behaviours, cultural cues are open to misinterpretation.

Not all members of a culture sharing group will draw on and prioritize the same elements of their culture. That is not to say that the health beliefs and modes of communication around health and illness are not often culturally grounded. Culture may influence philosophical assumptions about the nature of the body and the kinds of factors can cause illness. Individuals from culture sharing groups often learn about health, social relations with health care practitioners, and managing health and illness from previous generations. This information can come from within an individual's own family and more generally through interactions with other members of their cultural group. The effects of culture are vast. Members of a culture sharing group are often exposed to many diverse and sometimes conflicting views of health care, diagnoses, and treatment. As such, individuals may perceive that their beliefs are not valued and avoid the health care system completely, potentially resulting in serious health consequences.

Is Culture a Social Determinant of Health?

Our health decisions are influenced by our interactions with others, how we communicate, and how we understand health and illness. All of these are partially products of our culture; cultural factors clearly influence the health of group members in some way. The World Health Organization (WHO) has identified a number of non-medical factors that often impact (or determine) the health of individuals and societies (WHO, 2008). These factors are aptly dubbed the *social determinants of health*. In contrast to the medical determinants of health, social determinants can include the socio-economic status of a community, the built environment, and health-related behaviours of individuals. These factors may work together to make people healthy or unhealthy. A more expansive overview of the social determinants of health is presented in Chapter Ten; in this section we will provide a brief overview of how culturally grounded health rituals, traditions, and beliefs may contribute to some people being healthier than others.

From a social determinants of health perspective, culture and health are part of a larger interrelated group of factors that influence the wellbeing of an individual, a community, or society at large. The recognition that non-medical factors can often influence health underscores the fact that interventions based on a medical model of care (dominant in North America) may alienate or devalue other cultural conceptions of health, illness, and healing. As discussed earlier, cultural differences often manifest themselves as issues of communication within the health care system. As Knibb-Lamouche (2012) suggests, when a culture sharing

CASE STUDY

Culture, Health, and First Nations Peoples

Evidence of how social, economic, and environmental conditions have affected the health of members of Aboriginal communities in Canada can help contextualize the relationship between culture, health, and other social determinants of health.

The health beliefs of members of many Aboriginal communities can be classified as **holistic**, as not related simply to the mechanistic functioning (or dysfunction) of the body, but rather as part of a complex relationship between the mind, body, and soul (Ellerby et al., 2000). An important finding from research in Aboriginal communities is that many members of these culture sharing groups value and prioritize their cultural identity as fundamental to wellness (Ellerby et al., 2000). The issue of cultural identity is part of a larger narrative of loss for the Aboriginal community: the loss of land, language, and traditional health care practices weakened many facets of their culture as well as eroding control over community organization and resources.

The "Health of Canadians" report provided a snapshot of some of the issues faced by the Aboriginal community (Statistics Canada, 2012). These groups face disproportionally high rates of infant mortality and chronic illness such as cancer, cardiovascular diseases, and diabetes (Health Council of Canada, 2013). Male members of the Aboriginal community in Canada also experienced almost five-fold the rate of suicides when compared to male members of other non-Aboriginal groups (126 in every 100,000 versus 24 in every 100,000) (Statistics Canada, 2012).

group believes that the health care system does not respect their values and beliefs, the experiences of individual members may be negative. They may not comply with medication directives that do not fit their cultural frame of reference (Van Wieringen, 2002) and may choose to circumvent the professional health care sector altogether (Searight & Gafford, 2005). This phenomenon will be further discussed later in the chapter.

The experiences of the Aboriginal community in Canada are just one example of how culture is a social determinant of health. Canada is becoming an increasingly culturally diverse country; more and more cultures will come into contact with each other and may encounter the "dominant" culture in many ways. This is especially relevant in regards to the health care system. Greater attention must be paid to respecting and encouraging cultural competency among those who interact with members of various culture sharing groups. It will also be important to monitor population-level health activities that might create cultural inequalities.

Modern Medical Culture

As will be discussed at length in Chapter Eight, objectivity is an important element of the culture of modern medicine in the North American context. This section examines the meanings of objectivity within the context of health and illness, the techniques used by health care professionals to maintain objectivity, and the practices that help shape modern medical practice. Western societies, including Canada, continue to be characterized by increasing

Another report, "Improving the Health of Canadians" from 2004, further highlighted the interrelated nature of the determinants of health. The Aboriginal community has a strong spiritual connection to their land: the destruction and annexation of Aboriginal lands not only created a spiritual detachment, but also led to the pollution and contamination of Aboriginals' land and food supply (CIHI, 2004). The Aboriginal community has tried to maintain their food traditions, but cultivating, harvesting, and consuming food from contaminated land has had numerous negative health effects on the population. One study found unsafe levels of mercury in the diets of more than 50 percent of the population of one Aboriginal community (Chan et al., 1997). Elevated levels of pesticides and mercury have been found in the breast milk of mothers (Indian and Northern Affairs Canada, 2003).

Commentators on the poor health of the Aboriginal community in Canada often point to the impact of residential schooling. From 1892 to 1996, many Aboriginal youth were educated at federally run residential schools. Education in these schools was based on the controversial idea that residential schools would help assimilate and integrate the Aboriginal population into society by killing the "Indian in the Child" (Fournier & Crey, 2006). In many of these schools, Aboriginal youth were not permitted to speak in their own language or to practise their customs and rituals. Education in residential schools not only fractured the sense of community and ties between generations, but it created disconnect between members of families. This may have contributed to poor educational outcomes, income insecurity, and poor health (Fournier & Crey, 2006). The effects of the residential schools are still evident years later.

reliance on the biomedical model for addressing social, psychological, and biological problems. Modern medical culture relies on scientific rationalities (Wade & Halligan, 2004). This scientific emphasis suggests that "true" knowledge regarding health and illness can only be produced when science and medicine intersect.

As a result, the beliefs of modern medical culture have developed from the biomedical model of health and illness, Pasteur's (1880) germ theory, and a Cartesian mind–body dichotomy (Worboys, 2008; Mehta, 2011). At the very basis of modern medical culture is the assumption that illness results from an underlying pathological cause, and that addressing the pathological cause, usually through prescription pharmaceutical interventions initiated by a physician, produces a return to health (Mehta, 2011). By looking at health and illness from this perspective, commentators often argue that health, then, is simply the absence of disease. However, many agree that this is clearly not the case—recall the WHO description of health found in Chapter One. Modern medicine is materialistic in the sense that it prioritizes the treatment of cells, tissues, organs, bones, and muscles by health care professionals in order to restore health.

For modern medical culture, the acceptance of Pasteur's (1880) **germ theory** was crucial in establishing the scientific method as "truth," and this mentality is still evident in how modern medicine is practised (Worboys, 2008). With a greater focus on disease pathology and anatomy, the development of germ theory is particularly relevant for understanding the basis of modern medical culture. Germ theory successfully shifted the focus from healing

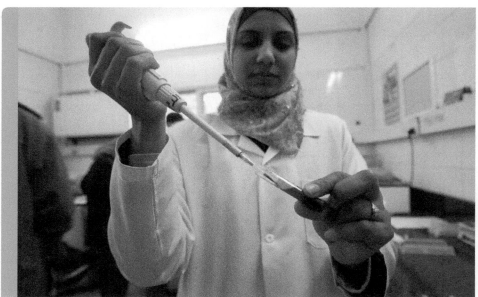

Photo by Abid Katib/Getty Images

Modern medical culture considers pathogens and bodily illnesses to be separate from the patients themselves. Diagnostic laboratory tests—which are not a part of all health paradigms—are often the definitive reason for a diagnosis in modern medical culture.

to disease, identifying invading pathological organisms as the cause of illness. In doing so, germ theory further substantiated the biological foundations of bodies. Soon after, vaccines and antibiotics entered the realm of medicine to help treat affected body parts. Today, modern medical culture remains grounded in current "best evidence," with a heavy reliance on advances in pharmacology and surgery to address issues of health, illness, and disease. In this regard, biomedical professionals are seen to be the gatekeepers of health.

Modern medical culture, by placing emphasis on the isolation (and treatment) of pathogens and body parts, sees physiological bodily illnesses as separate from the patients' psychological consciousness, and from social and cultural factors. The mind–body dichotomy that is prevalent in modern medical culture effectively isolates mental issues to the realm of the "non-physical," distinct from the "physical body." The physical body, in theory, is then reducible to the sum of its parts. Practitioners of Western medicine are those who are able to intervene on a biological level to restore order among the parts. This Cartesian model of the body, i.e., with mind and body as separate entities, manifests no embodied "energy forces," like intelligence, power, or self-movement (Mehta, 2011). The body is seen as a product of identifiable mechanical causality and subject to scientific analysis. To this day, Cartesian philosophy permeates the medical encounter in the Western world, expressing itself in the examination of the physical body and by de-emphasizing the lived experiences of the sick patient. Not surprisingly, medical training and modern medical culture are also grounded in objectifying the body and isolating the mechanical aspects of illness and poor health.

Modern medical culture takes a mechanistic view of the body and illness. It aims to isolate and suppress that which is causing problems in the body, such as toxins, viruses, or bacteria. While it cannot be ignored that science and rationality in Western medicine have allowed for the achievement of therapeutic triumphs, this success may come at the cost of neglecting important psychosocial and socio-cultural factors in the causation and treatment of disease. When symptoms are traced back to biological and pathogenic causes, illness is removed from the cultural context of the individual's life. Illness is thus reduced to a very clearly defined and isolated phenomenon, when in fact it might not be.

As a result, modern medical culture is concerned with causes more so than relationships. This can be seen in the study of anatomy (structure of the body) and physiology (functioning of the body) and in tools of diagnostic medicine that revolve around "that which can be seen." Whether through X-rays, observations through microscopes, or physical exams, the functions of organs in the body have been characterized by specialized observations—from the historical dissections of cadavers to the current reliance on molecular biology. These methods of observation have been an effective means to apply the scientific method in relation to the structure and function of the body.

However, the way in which people respond to illness is often not based on what would be considered "scientific rationalities." Our response to health and illness is just as important as the disease itself. Most people socialized within the North American context think of health and illness in relation to health care professionals. Modern medical culture has medicalized, or brought into the purview of the medical world, many issues and conditions that were previously not treated, diagnosed, or discussed as medical conditions (see Chapter Three for a more in-depth explanation). Issues are often medicalized when new modes of treatment are developed or we find a new way to define the issue (Conrad & Slodden, 2012).

As Chapter Three discussed, some conditions, such as anxiety and shyness, are now seen as mental health issues. Other diseases have also expanded as a result of new definitions.

Would you consider someone who is shy as suffering from a mental health issue? Would you think that this person requires treatment with antidepressants? According to the *Diagnostic and Statistical Manual of Mental Disorder* (DSM), traits associated with shyness may be indicative of a mental health issue called social anxiety disorder. Until the late 1970s, shyness was not associated with any disease state or medical condition. By the mid-1990s, however, shyness was one of the most commonly diagnosed mental health disorders in the United States; prescriptions for treating this "medicalized shyness" proliferated during this time (Lane, 2013).

The medicalization of many issues (previously seen as part of "normal" human variability) suggests that modern medical culture operates on the assumption that the biological imperative and modern medical advances are more influential on health (and quicker to respond) than environmental changes. From the perspective of sociologist Irving Zola (1973), modern medical culture's mechanistic approach to health and illness overestimates the importance of biological factors and medical technologies, and underestimates the role of non-medical factors related to social relations or culture. Zola (1973) introduced the concept of medicalization while arguing that defining human problems from a medical perspective meant that social problems would be addressed within the medical domain. The point is not that medicine as an institution is not useful or that medications and modern technologies do not save lives, but rather that reliance on medical expertise allows for greater social control over society. Medicine encroaches on or marginalizes other approaches to health and illness beyond the medical realm. This medical approach to help-seeking and illness-related behaviour minimizes the role of cultural and social values and beliefs that influence how individuals manage their health. Illnesses are consequently viewed only as biological issues within the body.

There is no doubt that the last century was full of medical milestones, and that pharmaceutical and technological innovation has improved our ability to address health problems. The development of modern medical culture has been grounded in the commitment to scientific inquiry, technological advances, and objectivity on the part of practitioners. Many aspects of the human experience that were previously seen as social issues are now increasingly referred to as medical problems. They are diagnosed by and treated by physicians, highlighting how modern medical culture is based on pathologizing, technological intervention, and the gatekeeper role of the health care professional.

Culture in the Professional Health Sector

Fictional characters in medical dramas are almost always running through the halls of a hospital to save yet another patient. These white coat–wearing heroes possess not only the knowledge that allows them to solve the mystery of illness and the power to cure and to comfort, but also the regulated ability to organize and deliver health care in society. Although the depictions of doctors and other medical professionals in medical dramas are often cited as highly inaccurate, there is great accuracy in the settings of these dramas.

Hospitals, teaching universities, and anatomy theatres are all venues for the transmission of medical knowledge. It is in these settings that esoteric medical knowledge is passed on to "qualified individuals" and becomes exclusive. Medical knowledge is thus controlled by teaching only hand-picked apprentices. It was the continuing disputes in the late 1800s over credentials that led to the recognition of doctors and "other organized healing professions" as distinct in the North American context (Kleinman, 1981). This facilitated the development of a professional health culture and sector. Before this point, nearly anyone could claim that they were a health care professional after a short period of training (Buerki & Vottero, 1996). Poorly coordinated medical education led to the perception that standards of practice were improper. There seemed to be little systematic theory, a small body of medical knowledge, and no such thing as professional culture or regulation. Freidson (1970) argues that law was used to define the practice of healing. Using political means and regulatory mechanisms created a distinction between health care professionals and non-healthcare professionals. As a result, patients who decided to seek help for an illness often had to choose between practitioners who were part of the **professional health sector** (i.e., doctors, nurses and pharmacists), and those in the non-professional health sector (i.e., chiropractors, naturopaths), sometimes characterized as "quacks" (Simpson, 2012).

Today, many of the practitioners who had been previously categorized as part of the non-professional health care sector have expanded their practice to become part of the changing landscape of health care professionals in North America. Culture in the professional health sector is based on values, norms, symbols, and language of various regulated health professions such as medicine, nursing, and pharmacy. Most importantly, the development of culture in the professional health sector is based on the inclusion of some as recognized health care professionals and the exclusion of others. For example, pharmacy culture is represented by symbols and events specific to being a pharmacist. Students who are accepted to pharmacy programs take an oath of professional ethics during their white coat ceremony, similar to that of medical students. This formal induction into the profession of pharmacy is an event that affirms the pharmacist's responsibility to the patient and his or her duty to the profession. Also, the mortar and pestle and the Bowl of Hygeia are symbols specific to pharmacy. They are used to differentiate the practice from other professions such as medicine and nursing (Stieb, 1970).

The culture of medical doctors, agreed upon by various commentators as the most dominant health profession (Buerki & Vottero, 1996), is often the model against which sociologists compare the cultures of other health care professions. In medical practice, symbols such as the white coat can represent "goodness," "purity," and a physical barrier between the doctor and the patient (Nash, 2014). The stethoscope and other diagnostic tools are symbols of the physician's intimate access to a patient's body (Rice, 2010). The clinical setting, arguably the institutionalized site of health and healing, is not only the domain of the health care professional, but also dictates the power dynamics of the relationship between those seeking health care and the professionals who provide it. This is true to such an extent that patients often experience elevated blood pressure and anxiety ("white coat syndrome") in their interactions with health care professionals in the clinical setting (Franklin et al., 2013). The social relationship between the patient and the health care professional is often characterized by the role the health care professional plays; the provider acts as a health advisor, legitimizes illness, serves as a gatekeeper to medical resources, and coordinates the patient's care.

Outside the realm of the clinic, patients access a range of explanatory frameworks for health and illness. These are based on social and cultural realities, often not associated with

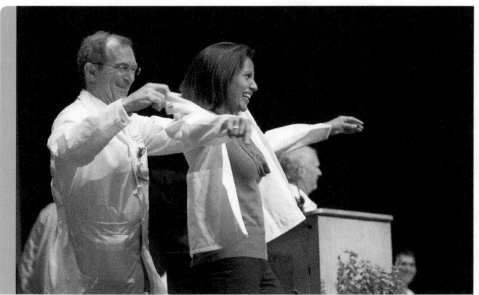

ZUMA Press, Inc/Alamy Stock Photo

The white coat ceremony has grown in prominence as a rite of passage in the culture of medical professions. This ceremony, which celebrates the transition of a student into the clinical realm, is symbolic of a person's entry into the professional health sector.

pathology or disease. As a result, there can be discord between the patient and the health care professional who is part of the professional health care sector. Consequently, patients may turn to alternative medical care (or practitioners from the folk health sector) as part of their decision to seek help.

Culture in the Popular Health Sector

Many people argue that North America is a facing an obesity epidemic, with fat, sugar consumption, and a lack of exercise to blame (Johnson et al., 2007). Although not everyone has reviewed the evidence, most people would at least agree that they have heard this statement, whether in a magazine, on television, or through social media. Culture in the **popular health sector**, often conceptualized as the informal health care system, includes lay information sharing. This sharing is similar to what happens on Facebook or through other social networks, such as one's family or community.

In the popular health sector, individuals are able to circumvent the professional health sector. Based on their understanding of health, illness, or their reliance on a "lay referral system," individuals can diagnose and treat their own symptoms. What is important here is that the perception of symptoms, or the sense that "something is wrong, or not normal," and how we experience health and illness are based largely on cultural factors. If the last time you suspected that you indeed had a cold, you looked up your symptoms online and decided you indeed had a cold (and not the flu), and that it was not serious enough to visit a health care professional, you managed your care as part of the popular health sector. You probably picked up some medication at a pharmacy (or decided to self-medicate with the healing powers of chicken soup), and then waited a few days to see if you felt better before seeing a doctor.

Not surprisingly, in North America the popular health sector is the largest of the three sectors that we will review (see Figure 4.1: The Professional, Popular and Folk Health Sectors). It is estimated that the majority of illnesses are managed informally as part of the popular health sector (CIHI, 2012).

Figure 4.1 provides an overview of the professional, popular, and folk health sectors that come together to form the health care system. The sectors in the health care system represent various points of entry and exit for individuals to respond to symptoms of poor health, to maintain their health, and to initiate and evaluate treatment options.

As studies suggest, symptom management is almost always the first course of action. Zola's (1973) model suggests that symptom management results from self-diagnosing and self-treating/medicating. This mode of help-seeking often involves how family members understand and assign meanings to actions such as seeing the doctor or deciding to use medications. Help seeking is also influenced by the degree to which these meanings are learned, modified, and transmitted between generations, if at all. This process happens within the context of the family and culture.

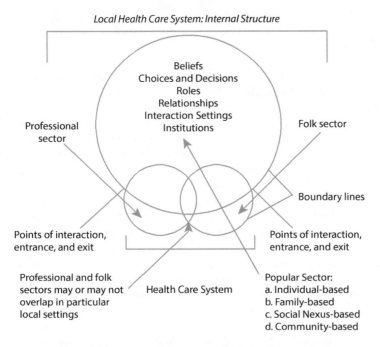

FIGURE 4.1   **The Professional, Popular, and Folk Health Sectors**

Source: Kleinman (1980), p. 50

When studying the origins of health behaviour, it is important to consider how the roles of familial health practices, intergenerational ties, acculturation, and culture influence the development of health-related beliefs. As Spector (1996) suggests, health-related practices or habits relate to early socialization and may be transmitted directly from parents to children. For example, families may rely on certain medicinal herbs, plants, or food (like chicken soup) to treat symptoms and illness. As Crespo et al. (2011) suggest, families have common history narratives that connect family members via certain rituals, rules and principles, and a collective memory of how to address issues of well being.

How we experience health and illness, and what we believe we should do in response to illness and disease, is influenced by culture. The conceptualization of what is a rational health action is in itself a social construct. While a health care professional may base her response on "clinical facts," a patient may base her mode of action on a divergent interpretive frame. The categorization of health sectors along the lines of professional, popular, and folk is often criticized for dividing the experiences of health and illness along the lines of "medical" and "non-medical." In the professional sector (objective, scientific, medical) the signs, symptoms and diagnoses are embedded within a system based on the scientific method. In the popular sector (subjective, unscientific, non-medical), realities of the patient's illness and disease are unique to that individual and are interpreted through a cultural and social lens.

CASE STUDY

Cleanses

In recent years, increasing numbers of Canadians have engaged in short-term dietary regimens, known as cleanses, hoping to lose weight or "detoxify." Although there are numerous types of cleanses, they all typically require individuals to limit themselves to very specific diets, eating precise amounts at particular times of day. For example, one famous cleanse calls for participants to adhere to a liquid-only diet for ten days: the only sources of permitted nourishment are tea and a mixture of lemonade, cayenne pepper, and maple syrup. In exchange for completing what many see as an extreme form of nutritional and sensory deprivation, many people believe that all of the toxins in their body have been "flushed out." As a result, these individuals report feeling lighter, happier, and more energetic.

The cleanse fad is a good example of the popular health sector in action. Despite the fact that many nutritionists and medical professionals reject the notion that these dietary regimens can produce health benefits—in fact, many warn that they may be dangerous to the individual—cleanses are still popularly conceived as a way to improve one's health. Although alternative health practitioners have long championed cleanses (millions of books have been sold on the subject), much of the information regarding cleanses is passed from person to person. Other forms of popular media carry celebrity testaments to the efficacy and benefits of cleansing. Thus, information about cleanses is largely transmitted outside the realm of biomedical discourse: physicians do not prescribe cleanses and popular belief in their benefits does not depend on conventional methods of biomedical research (such as **randomized controlled trials**). As a consequence, cleanses remain firmly rooted in the popular health sector.

It can be argued, based on our continued reliance on the popular health care sector, that neither the professional nor the popular framework for addressing health and illness are necessarily privileged or consistently prioritized. Rather, knowledge from health care providers can complement knowledge from family members, friends, and other lay referral systems. Often, when a chosen medical treatment does not work, the evaluation of the treatment takes place within the framework of the popular health sector. This process occurs regardless of whether the treatment was initiated and supervised by a health care professional or by a family member.

Culture in the Folk Health Sector

The complex web of cultural, structural, and social practices that individuals present in the clinical setting may conflict with the culture of the professional health sector. The popular health sector is often conceptualized as the bridge between the folk and professional health sectors, and the folk sector shares many overlapping features with both sectors. Similar to the professional health sector, health care within the context of the folk sector is administered by a practitioner (e.g., a shaman or a doctor of Ayurvedic medicine). The **folk health sector** is also linked to the popular sector through traditional healing practices that are often passed on between families and members of culture sharing groups. The folk sector is also known as complementary and alternative medical care (as opposed to the conventional medicine of the professional health sector; see Chapter Eleven). Herbalists, spiritual healers, and aromatherapists would currently all fall under this classification.

Kleinman (1980) popularized the systems approach to studying health care. This approach highlights how multiple systems of healing had previously existed before Western biomedicine flourished. In some form or another, this medical pluralism continues to exist in most places. In the typical "doctor visit" in North America, a patient usually first presents a set of symptoms (or complaints) to the physician. This social relationship between healer and patient is similar in the folk sector. In the professional health sector, the healer would now make a "systems inquiry" with the purpose of identifying the underlying systemic mechanisms for the disease or illness. At the end of the inquiry, there is a diagnosis, which usually isolates a cause. Finally, a treatment plan is discussed with the patient. This usually consists of prescription medication use, monitoring, and/or surgical interventions. These therapies are initiated to cure or eliminate the ailment and its associated symptoms.

In contrast, practitioners within the folk health sector operate with less specific objectives. They look to gather information, for instance, that could suggest a "pattern of disharmony." Within the context of traditional Chinese medicine (one example of a folk health system) this disharmony may be related to Yin and Yang or other imbalances that may be occurring (Jiang et al., 2012). Again, therapy aims to restore balance. It usually consists of the use of easily accessible medicinal herbs. Similar to the popular health sector, where individuals and groups rely primarily on one another for health advice, the patient and the healer in the folk sector share the same health beliefs, values, and assumptions about health and illness. The training of practitioners in the folk health sector is, for the most part, grounded in sacred or secular tradition. One other important feature of the culture of the folk health sector is that it is based on cultural congruence between the practitioner and the patient. As a result, there is a shared understanding of the meanings, interpretations, and significance of health and illness.

In the past, religious healers, families, friends, and neighbours were all "practitioners of folk health care." Healing practices were passed on from generation to generation, as they often still are within the popular health care sector (Kleinman, 1980). However, the scientific revolution of North America in the nineteenth century saw previously held ideas of health, illness, and treatment challenged by science. The formal regulation of health care practitioners and the intersection of science and medicine pushed the religious, cultural, and traditional aspects of medicine to the periphery of the health care system.

In some parts of the world there is no real distinction between the professional health sector and the folk health sector. Both sectors are very well integrated. With regard to traditional Chinese medicine, there is a common saying that before the proliferation of Western medicine in China, there was no division between the two systems; health care professionals would selectively access the appropriate resources to help the patient deal with their health issues. Whereas traditional systems of care such as Ayurveda (the traditional medical system in India) or traditional Chinese medicine might be based on the "laws of nature," an individual socialized in these systems of care may not be able to translate their understandings of health and illness within the context of Western medicine (Park et al., 2012). In a similar light, a doctor trained in Western medicine would not be equipped with the training to address issues such as an imbalance of Yin and Yang from this frame of reference. The tools (medications, diagnostic equipment), knowledge, and beliefs that are central tenets of medical care in North America may not translate cross-culturally, and vice versa.

The folk health care sector currently co-exists with the popular health care sector and the professional health sector in North America. All of these sectors help us recognize the varied options we have when maintaining our health or responding to episodes of illness. With continued globalization (see Chapter Seven), it will be necessary to foster medical systems and health sectors that acknowledge and incorporate varied cultural beliefs systems and previous health-related experiences within the context of medicine.

Fear and Illness across Cultures

Cultural beliefs about health and illness are often imbued with fear. How an individual understands and responds to their illness is often dependent on their culture. Life-altering and life-threatening diseases are no exception. In some cultures, even speaking the word "cancer" is considered taboo and uttering the word may lead to social consequences such as stigma and discrimination. These negative consequences result from the assumption that speaking of cancer (or, as it is often called, "that terrible disease") may promote the risk of developing cancer, that the afflicted individual somehow brought the disease upon themselves, or that a person who talks about their disease will die faster. Qualitative research on the experiences of patients with cancer reveals a common narrative in many cultures with regard to cancer disclosure: "We do not talk about cancer" (Ehiwe et al., 2012; Shang et al. 2014). As we have discussed, how members of a culture understand, interpret, and respond to an illness is based on social relations and culturally shared beliefs.

The cultural guidelines that may shape an individual's behaviour or worldviews also affect how individuals handle situations they perceive as "misfortune." For example, mental illnesses such as schizophrenia elicit great variation in responses between cultures (Abdullah & Brown, 2011). Beliefs around mental health issues, especially in African, Arabic, and South Asian culture, are often grounded in supernatural phenomena (Aghukwa, 2012). Collective values and beliefs often dissuade individuals from disclosing that they have mental health issues for fear of bringing shame to a family and stigma to the community. While new conditions are identified in the West on an almost yearly basis, it can be difficult to understand these experiences within the framework of another culture sharing group. Since understandings of health and illness are transmitted between generations and members of a culture sharing group, it can be difficult to "fit" a new illness into a culture's understanding. An example of this is the neglect of Alzheimer's disease in China: no concise terminology or language exists in China to explain how one is to understand Alzheimer's disease, and as such the diagnosis and treatment of this "variable condition" does not fit into the traditional system of cultural beliefs (Chiu et al., 2014). For example, trying to fit Alzheimer's disease into the context and classifications of culture and traditional Chinese medicine has led to the disease being labeled as stupidity, insanity, silliness, or lack of intelligence. Thus, the disease is treated as problematic and stigmatizing (Elliott et al., 1996, pp. 93; Chiu et al., 2014).

Attitudes and health beliefs are slow to change. Silence regarding illnesses such as cancer or Alzheimer's disease means that these illnesses may be misdiagnosed or their progress may be left unchecked. Despite the obvious flaws in these stigmatizing beliefs, members of culture sharing groups that deny, suppress, or shame various illnesses are less likely to participate in community-based interventions and screening programs, or to discuss these issues with health care providers. Although it is often assumed that cultural congruence between patient and provider promotes communication and understanding, a study by Mirza et al. (2014) found that patients often chose providers with similar cultural backgrounds to facilitate communication on certain subjects, but avoid talking about culturally taboo topics. They may feel that the health care providers from within their culture would look down upon them, discriminate against them, or shun them.

A similar fear of disclosure often exists in workplaces, another type of culture sharing group, where workers may be afraid to tell other members of the group that they are ill, or even to accept the fact that they are ill. A recent issue in workplace culture has seen sick employees "toughing it out" by coming to work even when they are ill, to avoid breaking their workplace's cultural code. Further, some employees may not disclose a mental health condition or life-altering disease for fear of stigma or termination (Morken et al., 2012). Employees are generally conscious of what a sick day costs a company. What is often not considered is the cost to the organization if the employee comes to work and infects others. Furthermore, employees who are often ill may fear reprisal from employers. They worry that the organization will be able to spread their work out among the other staff, or that their work will remain incomplete; either situation will degrade their standing as an employee.

On the whole, many people are very fearful about health and illness, especially when considering how to respond to these issues. Cultural transformations around long-held health beliefs of issues such as cancer and mental illness will be slow. Our meanings of illness may change as we are increasingly exposed to new perspectives.

Healing and Healers across Cultures

The meaning of health and illness is shaped by the context of cultural beliefs, norms, and values. The interrelationships among health, illness, healing, and those in a position to heal are complex and are often based on cultural frameworks of understanding. Healers are present in many cultures: religious healers, magicians, and practitioners could all be understood as part of both the popular and folk health sectors. Those skeptical of these healers often question why an individual would want to consult a traditional, spiritual, or religious healer. Critics contend that the practice of these ancient forms of medicine or healing requires "blind faith" and the acceptance of supernatural forces and cosmic influences. And while many of us will admit that we do not know how these forms of medicine work, or how these forms of healing are maintained across cultures, what we cannot deny is that they are perceived to work by the individuals who rely on them.

Traditional Chinese medicine (TCM) has undergone many of the changes that allopathic or Western medicine has undergone in the last 50 years, such as the establishment of regulated schools, a body of knowledge, and licensure. However, practitioners still consider the effects of the elements of earth, water, air, and fire on health (Lehmann, 2012). These metaphysical considerations are a fundamental part of TCM's approach to understanding the nature of the human being in relation to the world. The idea that *yin* and *yang* are forces, and are part of an intrinsic life force, *qi*, is important for understanding Traditional Chinese medicine. From the perspective of Chinese medicine theory, the Qi force within our bodies determines our state of health. It can be modified or depleted based on what we eat and whether we "abuse" our bodies (for example, with excessive alcohol consumption or smoking). How well *qi* is flowing within one's body is also critical to one's wellbeing (Xutian, 2012).

Some cultures believe that health issues such as alcohol-related liver damage, obesity, or infertility can be addressed by having a healer alter the state of mind of the afflicted person. This often takes the form of a trance or a magic spell. Even in North America, hypnotism for the treatment of smoking is gaining popularity (Hasan et al., 2014). Sorcerers, magicians, and shamans do not necessarily undergo formal training but may rather be "called" by spirits. Alternatively, they may succeed another healer, or may undergo a cycle of death–rebirth to establish themselves as healers. Winkelman (1990) suggests that these healers are found in all parts of the world, including the Aboriginal communities in North America. For example, illnesses in Aboriginal communities may be perceived to be a result of bodily invasion by foreign spirits or entities. As a result, traditional Aboriginal healers would use ointments, rituals, and prayer chants to remove the foreign element. In other cultures, sorcerers and magicians are cited as having expertise in the use of hallucinogenic plants. These practitioners are still relied upon, especially in African cultures, to cast or remove spells to address issues such as infertility (Winkelman, 1990).

While there is debate in the anthropological literature as to the origins of healers such as shamans and sorcerers, it is widely believed that this class of healers is often closely associated with religious beliefs (Winkelman, 1990). Religion often is reflective of cultural norms, views, and values. It provides guidelines for behaviour based on shared group beliefs. The culture of a religion may be based on a belief in God, superstitions, or ritualized social relations. An important religious belief across many cultures with regard to health and illness is that God or some other supernatural force is responsible for disability, disease, and even death (Islam & Campbell, 2014). A common theme in studies of patients with terminal or life-threatening illnesses is strong spirituality. These patients believe that that they will leave their fate in "God's Hands" (Meador, 2009). Islamic literature often associates illness and disease with "sins." Repenting for one's transgressions and making amends with God (Allah) can help individuals overcome their health issues (Ahmad et al., 2011).

Members of Muslim communities may turn to traditional healers such as Maulanas (priest-like spiritual leaders, Islamic scholars), and Hakeems (sometimes described as the equivalent of a medical doctor). These healers provide guidance and treatment in the case of ill health or disability. For these "custodians of religious culture," not questioning God's will is a major theme in response to episodes of poor health and illness. They generally suggest that an evil spirit (*jinn*) or a spell (*jaadu*) could be responsible (Ross, 2007). In such a case, healers may suggest making a charitable donation, as treatment protocols are embedded in superstitious beliefs. For example, in a study of children born with cleft lip and palate, some Muslim respondents believed that the child's disability could have been a result of the mother having held a knife or sharp object during an eclipse while pregnant (Ross, 2007).

Given the diversity of cultural explanations and interpretations of health and illness, it is surprising that many traditions of healing across cultures are grounded in similar principles and systems of care. Reliance on traditional healers across cultures remains strong in rural areas and developing countries. This is not only due to a shortage of health care providers from the professional sector, but also due to longstanding belief in the traditional modalities of care.

Research on Cultural Competency

With expanding cultural diversity in the Canadian population, the concept of **cultural competency** is increasingly relevant. Cultural competency ensures that health care professionals are able to provide appropriate care to individuals from a wide range of cultural backgrounds (Kleinman & Benson, 2006). There remains no universally accepted definition of cultural competency. The concept is broadly described by Betancourt (2002, p. 3), as "the ability of systems to provide care to patients with diverse values, beliefs and behaviors, including tailoring delivery to meet patients' social, cultural, and linguistic needs." Cultural competency is especially important with respect to communication between health care professionals and patients.

Language and cultural barriers create health disparities in many cultural groups within Canada. The idea that health care professionals can be trained in cultural competency, however, is contentious, and assumes a "one size fits all" approach to cultural groups and their health. For example, Chinese Canadians are now the second largest visible minority ethnic group in Canada, just behind the South Asian community (Statistics Canada, 2011), but this statistic actually masks the immense diversity within this group. On this basis, many people criticize cultural competency training programs as being based on the faulty assumption that there is a fixed culture that one can become proficient at understanding. Trying to understand "what people of a given ethnic group or culture will do" with regard to health and illness is problematic. With any culture sharing group, there is much intra-group diversity in members' interpretation of cultural norms, and also in their understanding of what constitutes a cultural issue.

As it stands, cultural competency training may create stereotypical views of patients and their adherence to cultural rituals, views, or practices, which may actually become barriers to health. Health care professionals may develop a prejudice or bias towards patients who belong to a culture sharing group. It is also problematic to assume that a family member or health care provider who shares the same ethnicity as a given patient also shares that patient's cultural identity and values. Health care professionals need to focus on understanding the culture of specific individual patients rather than assuming they can understand and predict the needs, motivations, and behaviour of a patient solely on the basis of their culture. Learning from the patient or their family members about the patient's preferences, values, and needs will likely yield a greater understanding and better quality of care than a cultural competency checklist.

In a health care system where providers pride themselves on providing high quality care to a very diverse population, cultural justifications of health care decisions may be too readily accepted at face value. The findings of Mirza et al. (2014) suggest that more focus needs to be on patients as individuals who interpret and shape their own ideas of "culture." The utility of cultural competency as it is currently taught in health care professional training programs needs considerable rethinking.

Chapter Summary

Culture is often described as one of the most complex words in the English language (Williams, 1981). The great range of understandings, meanings, and interpretations of what constitutes culture adds to the difficulties in operationalizing the term. Rather, there may be more value in understanding the common factors that constitute culture rather than trying to gain consensus on the precise definition of the term. Beliefs and norms around health and illness are often transmitted between generations. These norms are established as part of social relations through continued interactions with other members of a culture sharing group. Although culture may be shared among individuals, members of a culture sharing group are far from homogeneous and may prioritize and mobilize various aspects of culture to suit their own needs and goals. Furthermore, the boundaries around cultural guidelines, norms, activities, and shared behaviours are rather blurred and are not rigid or uniform. As a result, culture can be seen as dynamic and changing; the effects of a culture on its members are constantly in flux. As a determinant of health, looking at culture from the vantage point that some perspectives are prioritized, cultures can be arranged hierarchically, resulting in the emergence of a particular culture as dominant and others as subordinate. The subordination of cultural views and approaches to health may contribute to poor health outcomes.

The dominant biomedical culture in North America is based on objectivity and scientific rationality. As this is closely related to the professional health sector, other frameworks of understanding health and illness, such as the popular and folk health sectors, are pushed to the periphery of the health care system. This dichotomy has divided the health care system into two cultures: the professional sector, based on medical knowledge, and the popular and folk sectors, which are based on non-medical knowledge and beliefs. Often, disenchantment with the professional medical sector prevents members of some cultural groups from accessing its services. They may prefer to rely on their "own" healers for guidance and support in times of poor health and illness.

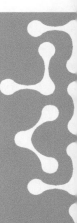

In some cases, the various cultures that make up the larger health and health care landscape are complementary and overlapping. At other times these are at odds with each other and are competing for patients. What is most important to note is that individuals have many different health care options to select from, and each provides a different way to address their issues. To best serve individuals from various cultures, it is necessary to strive to understand the unique needs of all patients from various culture sharing groups.

STUDY QUESTIONS

1. What are the main conceptual differences between culture, race, and ethnicity?
2. How did Pasteur's germ theory contribute to the process of medicalization?
3. Why is culture considered a determinant of health?
4. What similarities and differences exist between the cultures of the professional health sector, the popular health sector, and the folk health sector?
5. What are the benefits and drawbacks of cultural competency training in health care?

SUGGESTED READINGS

Horsburgh, M. (2006). The professional subcultures of students entering medicine, nursing and pharmacy programmes. *Journal of Interprofessional Care.* 20(4), 425–31.

Jahoda, G. (2012). Critical reflections on some recent definitions of culture. *Culture and Psychology,* *18*(3), 289–303.

Kleinman, A. & Benson, P. (2006). Anthropology in the clinic: The problem of cultural competency and how to fix it. *PLoS Medicine,* *3*(10), e294.

Meyer, V. (2003). Medicalized menopause, US style. *Health Care Women Int.,* *24*(9), 822–30.

SUGGESTED WEB RESOURCES

Health Council Canada. Making health care delivery culturally safe for Aboriginal people in urban centres: www.youtube.com/watch?v=a2tOddj6ypk

Singh, M. (2015, February 2). Blog: Why Cambodians Never Get "Depressed": www.npr.org/sections/goatsandsoda/2015/02/02/382905977/why-cambodians-never-get-depressed

GLOSSARY

Cultural competency The ability to work with, and for, individuals from a number of cultural groups. There is no widely accepted working definition of this phrase.

Culture This is widely defined, contested term. As culture is dynamic, there is no universal definition of the term. For the purposes of this text, *culture* is defined as the learned, shared, and transmitted behaviours that influence members of a given (culture sharing) group.

Folk health sector Encompasses healer-led medicine outside of the professionalized realm of biomedicine. Some examples include herbalists and spiritual healers.

Germ theory Louis Pasteur's germ theory identified pathological organisms as the source of illness; one of the key contributing factors to the evolution of biomedicine.

Holistic, holism Relating to the system as a whole. Holism refers to the notion that health and disease can be understood only by approaching the individual as a whole—the physical body, mental state, social factors, the environment, and so on.

Popular health sector Individuals' personal experiences with health or illness. The general population can consult one another, individually and as a group, to obtain health-related information, identify and diagnose their symptoms, or share their own health-related experiences.

Professional health sector Encompasses health care workers who have been licensed and regulated. Examples include nurses and doctors.

Race and ethnicity Contested terms. Some may use these terms to refer to genetic linkage and biological characteristics (e.g., skin and eye colour) but social scientists emphasize that these categories are socially constructed, with little true biological meaning.

Randomized controlled trials A research method that divides participants, at random, into two groups. Researchers will conduct some form of research on one group (for example, exposing them to a new drug) while the other group will be a "control" group (and therefore will not receive any new treatments or interventions). These trials are an intrinsic part of evidence-based medicine as they help determine the effect, if any, of a medical treatment.

REFERENCES

Abdullah, T. & Brown, T. (2011). Mental illness stigma and ethnocultural beliefs, values, and norms: An integrative review. *Clinical Psychology Review, 31*(6), 934–48.

Aghukwa, C. (2012). Care seeking and beliefs about the cause of mental illness among Nigerian psychiatric patients and their families. *Psychiatric Services, 63*(6), 616–18.

Ahmad, F., Muhammad, M., & Abdullah, A. (2011). Religion and spirituality in coping with advanced breast cancer: Perspectives from Malaysian Muslim women. *Journal of Religion and Health, 50*(1), 36–45.

Ballard, R. (2002). Race, culture and ethnicity. In M. Holborn (Ed.), *New Developments in Sociology.* Ormskirk: The Causeway Press.

Betancourt, J. R., Green, A. R., & Carillo, J. E. (2002). Cultural competence in health care. *Emerging frameworks and practical approaches.* New York: The Commonwealth Fund.

Buerki, R. A. & Vottero, L. D. (1996). The purposes of professions in society. In C. H. Knowlton & R. P. Penna, (Eds), *Pharmaceutical care.* London: Chapman & Hall.

Chan H. M., Berti P., Receveur O., & Kuhnlein H. (1997). Evaluation of the population distribution of dietary contaminant exposure in an Arctic population using Monte Carlo statistics. *Environmental Health Perspectives, 105*(3), 316–21.

Cheung, F. (2011). TCM: Made in China. *Nature, 480*(2), S82–S83.

Chiu, H., Sato, M., Kua, E., Lee, M., Yu, X., Ouyang, W., Yang, Y., & Sartorius, N. (2014). Renaming dementia: An East Asian perspective. *International Psychogeriatrics, 26*(6), 885–87.

Canadian Institute for Health Information (CIHI). (2004). *Improving the health of Canadians.* Ottawa.

——— (2012). *Drug expenditure in Canada, 1985–2012.* Ottawa.

Conrad, P. & Slodden C. (2013). The medicalization of mental disorder. In C. Aneshensel (Ed.), *Handbook of the sociology of mental health* (pp. 61–73). Dordrecht: Springer Science and Business Media.

Crespo, C., Kielpikowski, M., Pryor, J., & Jose, P. (2011). Family rituals in New Zealand families: Links to family cohesion and adolescents' well-being. *Journal of Family Psychology, 25*(2), 184–93.

Efferth, T., Li, P., Konkimalla, V., & Kaina, B. (2007). From traditional Chinese medicine to rational cancer therapy. *Trends in Molecular Medicine, 13*(8), 353–61.

Ehiwe, E., McGee, P., Filby, M., & Thompson, K. (2012). Black African migrants' perceptions of cancer: Are they different from those of other ethnicities, cultures and races? *Ethnicity and Inequalities in Health and Social Care, 5*(1), 5–11.

Eliot, T. S. (1948). *Notes towards the definition of culture.* London: Faber.

Ellerby, J. H., McKenzie, J., McKay, S., Gariepy, G., & Kaufert, J. (2000). Bioethics for Clinicians: 18. Aboriginal cultures. *CMAJ, 163*(7), 845–50.

Elliott, K. S., Di Minno, M., Lam, D., Tu, A. M. (1996) Working with Chinese families in the context dementia. In G. Yeo & D. Gallagher-Thompson (Eds), *Ethnicity & the dementias* (pp. 89–109). Washington, DC: Taylor & Francis.

Elwyn, G., Lloyd, A., Mav, C., Van der Weijden, T., Stiggelbout, A., Edwards, A., . . . & Epstein, R. (2014). Collaborative deliberation: A model for patient care. *Patient Education and Counseling, 97*(2), 158–64.

Fellmann, D., Getis, A., & Getis, J. (2007). *Human geography: Landscapes of human activities.* Columbus, OH: McGraw-Hill Education.

Fournier, S. & Crey E. (2006). Killing the Indian in the child: Four centuries of church-run schools. In R. C. Maaka & C. Anderson (Eds). *The Indigenous experience: Global perspectives.* Toronto, ON: Canadian Scholars' Press Inc.

Franklin, S., Thijs, L., Hansen, TW., O'Brien, E., & Staessen, J. (2013). White-coat hypertension new insights from recent studies. *Hypertension, 62*(6), 982–87.

Freidson, E. (1970). *Profession of medicine, a study of the sociology of applied knowledge.* New York: Harper & Row.

Hasan, F., Zagarins, S., Pischke, K., Saiyed, S., Bettancourt, A., Beal, L., Macys, D., Aurora, S., & McCleary, N. (2014). Hypnotherapy is more effective than nicotine replacement therapy for smoking cessation: Results of a randomized controlled trial. *Complementary Therapies in Medicine, 22*(1), 1–8.

Health Council of Canada (2013). Canada's most vulnerable: Improving health care for First Nations, Inuit and Métis seniors.

Hofstede, G. (1984). National cultures and corporate cultures. In L. A. Samovar & R. E. Porter (Eds). *Communication Between Cultures.* Belmont, CA: Wadsworth.

Hsieh, E. & Kong, H. (2012). The social meanings of traditional Chinese medicine: Elderly Chinese immigrants' health practice in the United States. *Journal of Immigrant and Minority Health, 14*(5), 841–49.

Huxley, J. S. (1955). Guest editorial: Evolution, cultural and biological. *Yearbook of Anthropology,* 2–25.

IMS Health Canada. (2005). *Canada Rx Report 2005.* Table 3: Retail prescriptions dispensed in Canada per capita by age.

———. (2008). *Canadian disease & therapeutic index.*

Indian and Northern Affairs Canada. (2003). *Human health—Canadian Arctic contaminants assessment report II.* Ottawa: Minister of Public Works and Government Services Canada.

Islam, F. & Campbell, R. A. (2014). "Satan has afflicted me!" Jinn-possession and mental illness in the Qur'an. *Journal of Religion and Health, 53*(1), 229–43.

Jiang, M., Zhang, C., Zheng, G., Guo, H., Li, L., Yang, J., . . . & Lu, A. (2012). Traditional Chinese medicine Zheng in the era of evidence-based medicine: A literature analysis. *Evidence-Based Complementary and Alternative Medicine.* doi:10.1155/2012/409568

Johnson, R. J., Segal, M. S., Sautin, Y., Nakagawa, T., Feig, D. I, Kang, D. H., . . . & Sánchez-Lozada, L. G. (2007). Potential role of sugar (fructose) in the epidemic of hypertension, obesity and the metabolic syndrome, diabetes, kidney disease, and cardiovascular disease. *American Journal of Clinical Nutrition, 86*(4), 899–906.

Kleinman, A. (1980). *Patients and healers in the context of culture: An exploration of the borderland between anthropology, medicine, and psychiatry.* Los Angeles, CA: University of California Press.

———. (1981). The meaning context of illness and care: Reflections on a central theme in the anthropology of medicine. In E. Mendelsohn & Y. Elkana (Eds), *Science and cultures, sociology of the sciences* (Vol. V, pp. 161–76). Dordrecht, Holland: D. Reidel Publishing Company.

——— & Benson, P. (2006). Anthropology in the clinic: the problem of cultural competency and how to fix it. *PLoS Med, 3*(10), e294.

Knibb-Lamouche, J. (2012). Culture as a social determinant of health: Examples from Native communities. In *Institute on medicine: Roundtable on the promotion of health equity and the elimination of health disparities.* Seattle: Institute of Medicine.

Kolb, F. (2007). *Protest and opportunities: The political outcomes of social movements.* Frankfurt: Campus Verlag.

Kroeber, A. L. & Kluckhohn, C. (1952). Culture: A critical review of concepts and definitions. *Harvard University Peabody Museum of American Archeology and Ethnology Papers, 47.*

Kreuter, M. W. & McClure, S. M. (2004). The role of culture in health communication. *Annual Review of Public Health, 25*(20), 1–17.

Lane, C. (2013). How shyness became an illness and other cautionary tales about the DSM. In M. Dellwing & M Harbusch (Eds), *Krankheitskonstruktionen und Krankheitstreiberei,* (1st ed., pp. 55–73). Wiesbaden: VS Verlag für Sozialwissenschaften.

Lehmann, H. (2012). A Westerner's question about traditional Chinese medicine: Are the Yinyang concept and the Wuxing concept of equal philosophical and medical rank? *Journal of Chinese Integrative Medicine, 10*(3), 237–48.

Leung, A., Bo, A., Hsiao, H., Wang, S., & Chi, I. (2014). Health literacy issues in the care of Chinese American immigrants with diabetes: A qualitative study. *British Medical Journal Open, 4,* 1–12

Linton, R. (1945). *The cultural background of personality.* New York: Appleton-Century-Crofts Inc.

Markov, K. R., Poryazov, S., Ivanova, K. R., Mitov, I., & Markova, V. (2008). Culture aspects of inforaction. *International Journal Information Technologies and Knowledge, 2*(4): 335–42.

Matsumoto, D. (2006). Culture and nonverbal behaviour. In V. Manusov & M. Patterson (Eds), *The SAGE handbook of nonverbal communication.* Thousand Oaks, CA: Sage Publications.

Meador, K.G. (2009). Clinical cases when patients say, "it's in God's hands." *Virtual Mentor, 11*(10), 750–54.

Mehta, N. (2011). Mind–body dualism: A critique from a health perspective. *Mens Sana Monographs, 9*(1), 202–09.

Minuchin, S. (1974). *Families and family therapy.* Cambridge, MA: Harvard University Press.

Mirza, R., Boon, H., Austin, Z., & Hsiung, P. C. (2014). Questioning the utility of "cultural competency" in caring for older Chinese patients. Unpublished manuscript.

Morken, T., Haukenes, I., & Magnussen, L. (2012). Attending work or not when sick—what makes the decision? A qualitative study among car mechanics. *BMC Public Health Open, 12*(813).

Nash, D. (2014). On the symbolism of the white coat. *Journal of Dental Education, 78*(12), 1589–92.

Nicolson, N. & McLaughlin, C. (1988). Social constructionism and medical sociology: The case of the vascular theory of multiple sclerosis. *Sociology of Health and Illness, 10*(1), 234–61.

Park, J., Beckman-Harned, S., Cho, G., Kim, D., & Hangon, K. (2012). The current acceptance, accessibility and recognition of Chinese and Ayurvedic medicine in the United States in the public, governmental, and industrial sectors. *Chinese Journal of Integrative Medicine, 18*(6), 405–08.

Parsons, T. (1949). *Essays in sociological theory.* Glencoe, IL.

Senior, P. A. & Bhopal R. (1994). Ethnicity as a variable in epidemiological research. *British Mediical Journal, 309,* 327–30.

Purnell, L. D. & Paulanka, B. J. (2003). Purnell's model for cultural competence. In L. D. Purnell & B. J. Paulanka (Eds), *Transcultural health care: A culturally competent approach.* Philadelphia: F.A. Davis Company.

Rice, T. (2010). The hallmark of a doctor: The stethoscope and the making of medical identity. *Journal of Material Culture, 15*(3), 287–301.

Robbins, J. A. & Dewar, J. (2011). Traditional Indigenous approaches to healing and the modern welfare of traditional knowledge, spirituality and lands: A critical reflection on practices and policies taken from the Canadian Indigenous example. *The International Indigenous Policy Journal, 2*(4). Retrieved from: http://ir.lib.uwo.ca/iipj/vol2/iss4/2

Ross, E. (2007). A tale of two systems: Beliefs and practices of South African Muslim and Hindu traditional healers regarding cleft lip and palate. *Cleft Palate Craniofacial Journal, 44*(6), 642–8.

Searight, H. R. & Gafford, J. (2005). Cultural diversity at the end of life: Issues and guidelines for family physicians. *American Family Physician, 71*(3), 515–22.

Shang, C., Beaver, K. & Campbell, M. (2014). Social cultural influences on breast cancer views and breast health practices among Chinese women in the United Kingdom. *Cancer Nursing.* ePub.

Simpson, J. (2012). The five eras of chiropractic & the future of chiropractic as seen through the eyes of a participant observer. *Chiropractic & Manual Therapies, 20*(1), 1–8

Spector, R. E. (1996). *Cultural diversity in health and illness* (4th ed.). Stamford, CT: Appleton and Lange.

Statistics Canada. (2011). *Immigration and ethno-cultural diversity in Canada. (Catalogue number 99-010-XWE2011001).* Retrieved from http://www5.statcan.gc.ca/access_acces/alternative_alternatif.action?t=99-010-XWE2011001&l=eng&loc=http://www12.statcan.gc.ca/nhs-enm/2011/as-sa/99-010-x/99-010-x2011001-eng.pdf

———. (2012). *First Nations & Inuit Health: Aboriginal Peoples Survey, 2012. Inuit health: Selected findings from the 2012 Aboriginal Peoples Survey (Catalogue Number: 89-653-X).* Retrieved from www.statcan.gc.ca/daily-quotidien/140826/dq140826b-eng.htm

Xutian, S., Cao, D., Wozniak, J., Junion, J., & Boisvert, J. (2012). Comprehension of the unique characteristics of traditional Chinese medicine. *American Journal of Chinese Medicine, 40*(2), 231–44.

Stieb, E. (1970). Edward Buckingham Shuttleworth 1842—1934. *Pharmacy in History; 12*(3), 91–116.

Templeton, A. R. (1998). Human races: A genetic and evolutionary perspective. *American Anthropologist, 100*(3), 632–50.

Trichopoulou, A. & Lagiou, P. (1997). Healthy traditional Mediterranean diet: An expression of culture, history, and lifestyle. *Nutrition Reviews, 55,* 383–89.

Tylor, E. B. (1871). *Primitive culture: Researches into the development of mythology, philosophy, religion, art, and custom.* London: John Murray.

Van Wieringen, J., Harmsmen, J., & Brujinzeels, M. (2002). Intercultural communication in general practice. *European Journal of Public Health, 12*(1), 63–8.

Wade, D. & Halligan, P. (2004). Do biomedical models of illness make for good healthcare systems? *British Medical Journal, 329,* 1398–1401.

White, L. (1975). *The concept of cultural systems: A key to understanding tribes and nations.* Columbia University Press: New York.

WHO. (2004). *A glossary of terms for community health care and services for older persons, by World Health Organization Centre for Health Development.* Retrieved from www.who.int/kobe_centre/ageing/ahp_vol5_glossary.pdf

———. (2008). *Commission on social determinants of health, closing the gap in a generation: health equity through action on the social determinants of health. Final report of the Commission on Social Determinants of Health.* Retrieved from www.who.int/social_determinants/thecommission/finalreport/en

Williams, R. (1981). Towards a sociology of culture. In *Culture.* Glasgow: Fontana.

Winkelman, M. J. (1990). Shamans and other "magico-religious" healers: A cross-cultural study of their origins, nature, and social transformations. *Ethos, 18*(3), 308–35.

Worboys, M. (2011). Practice and the Science of Medicine in the Nineteenth Century. *Isis, 102*(1), 109–15.

Zola, K. (1973). Pathways to the doctor: From person to patient. *Social Science and Medicine, 7,* 677–89.

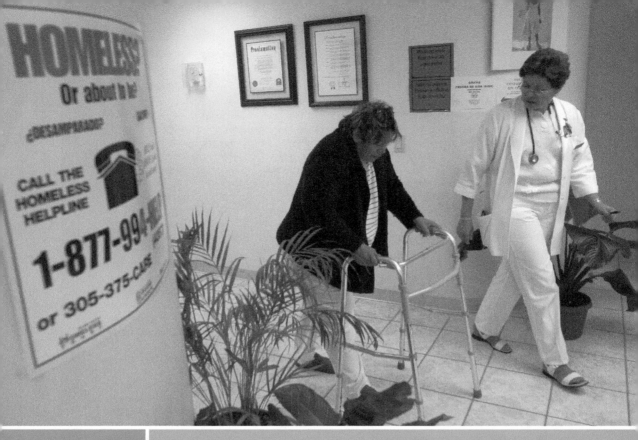

5

Identity, Intersectionality, and Health

James Gillett, Jeffrey S. Denis, and Mat Savelli

LEARNING OBJECTIVES

In this chapter, students will learn

- how social identity can affect one's health
- the role of social structures in forming identity
- about the concept of intersectionality and its relationship to health and illness

Social Identity and Health

Disparities in health across a society can be illustrated by what is often referred to as the "river story." This story serves as a parable to highlight the value of thinking about health in a broad social context. There are many versions of the story but it usually begins with a physician talking about what makes her profession challenging. She says being a physician is like standing on the bank of a river while a drowning person—a patient—floats by. The doctor jumps into the river, pulls the person out, and revives them. Just as she is done, two more people call for help in the river. Again, she goes into the river to save the drowning patients and as soon as they are safely on shore, more drowning patients appear, yelling for help. Reflecting on the story, the physician concludes that she spends so much of her day saving people from drowning in the river that she never has time to see who is pushing them from upstream.

This parable is used to demonstrate that health is influenced by "upstream" factors like the environment, social inequalities, poverty, sexism, and racism. Alongside such structural forces, certain lifestyle and behavioural patterns (like smoking, driving when fatigued, and drug use) can also contribute to ill health. In terms of producing health, the upstream contributors are just as significant as, if not more so than "downstream" factors. While downstream contributors, like health care services, are clearly important in promoting wellbeing, they generally come into play when people are already unwell. Upstream factors, on the other hand, play an even more important role in promoting wellbeing and preventing illness.

The river story can also provide an interesting perspective on the role of **social identity** in determining one's health. We see that people from different social backgrounds are more susceptible to the risks posed by upstream factors. Furthermore, when people from diverse backgrounds fall into the river, the way they respond and experience floating downstream varies according to their social identity.

In the social sciences the term *social identity* is used extensively; its meaning can be difficult to pin down. We all have a general sense of what it means: where one is from, our education and occupation, whether we are a man or a woman, our sexual identity, the ethnic heritage of our family, and even our passions and interests. This chapter utilizes the work of the sociologist Zygmunt Bauman (2000), who has written extensively on social identities in a globalized world. Without going into great detail, Bauman suggests that it makes sense to define social identify not as something fixed but rather as the product of **structures of identification**. How we develop our identity through these structures is seemingly contradictory. Our sense of self is built around structures that we all collectively encounter like gender, sexuality, class, and ethnicity. Yet our experience with these structures feels unique, individual, and different from anyone else's. This process of identification helps us understand how we are, ironically, bound together as a society through our desire to develop unique, individual identities.

In this chapter we discuss how structures of identification—or social identities—relate to health on two levels. On one level, as with the river story, societal structures regarding **gender**, **class**, race and sexuality pose health risks for individuals in unequal and complex ways. For instance, women are far more likely to experience domestic violence than men. This not only creates immediate physical harm but sets the basis for longer-term emotional and mental health problems. At another level, the way people experience and respond to health and illness also varies according to their social identity. For example, a gay man may respond to the mental trauma of domestic violence differently than a heterosexual woman. Finally, the chapter concludes by looking at the ways in which social identities intersect to create disparities in health as well as distinct conditions that shape the way people respond to illness. The chapter concentrates on three primary structures of identification: class, gender, and ethnicity.

Before beginning, it is important to understand the ways in which health status and health disparities can be measured. In general, social scientists and epidemiologists particularly rely on two concepts. The rate of **mortality**, or the number of deaths over a period of time across a specific population, is arguably the most commonly used measure of health or well being in a society. Childhood mortality is expressed as the number of deaths among children (under 12, for instance, or whatever definition of "child" is being used) over a period of time, usually a year. It is often expressed as a ratio of deaths per 1000 individuals. Pan et al. (2005), for instance, found that between 1979 and 2002, the annual childhood mortality rate declined significantly in Canada. However, the mortality rate among children due to suicide increased slightly. Through epidemiological studies like this one, we gain insight into the rate of change among a population; however, we are left to verify the reasons why fatal injuries have decreased but suicidality has increased.

A second common measure of health is **morbidity**. Put simply, morbidity is the prevalence and/or incidence of disease in a specific population. Keeping with the example of children, Emerson et al. (2006) studied the relationship between household income and health status in British children between the ages of 5 and 15. In this study, morbidity was defined as the prevalence of nine different types of diseases and illnesses (including injury) among 5- to 10-year-olds and 11- to 15-year-olds from households with a range of income levels. Co-morbidity describes cases in which people have more than one condition (asthma and an injury, for instance). Not surprisingly, the study found that the prevalence of morbidity and co-morbidity was higher among low-income households. Studies like this one make it possible to track the future incidence of a condition or disease in a population. Determining the prevalence of a specific type of morbidity makes it possible to evaluate whether an intervention is effective in preventing new occurrences of health problems in a specific population.

Social Class

Clearly, one's social class—a structure of identification—has a significant impact on health. The definition of social class is a highly debated topic in the social sciences. Most scholars would agree that the concept of social class helps us to understand the economic stratification of a society. In other words, social class—or socio-economic status (SES)—is a reflection or measure of each person's position in a society's economy. As the definition of social class can vary, so can the factors we consider when determining a person's social class. In the earlier study on the health of children, household income was used as a general measure of social class. To provide a more nuanced and comprehensive measure of social class, it is common to consider a person's education and occupation in addition to their income. Using such markers makes it possible to rank people in relation to their position in a market economy. This ranking according to social class is also referred to as the **social gradient**.

Social science research has shown evidence of a direct and complex relationship between health status and social class. Beginning in the 1970s, research demonstrated that health status and outcomes vary as a result of social inequalities associated with income, education, and occupation (Kitagawa & Hauser, 1973). In the United Kingdom, several large studies have raised greater awareness of the negative impact of social inequality on health and well being. The Black Report, published in 1980, was one of the first commissioned by a government to examine health disparities. While the study found that overall health had improved since the 1950s, there were increasing inequities in individual health status. It was initially thought that this was a result of ineffective health services. However, this inequality was actually a result of differences in social class or socio-economic status (Gray, 1982). The most privileged members of society fared much better across a range of health measures—morbidity and mortality—than those who were less privileged. Since the Black Report, similar reports (the Acheson Report in 1998; the Marmot Review in 2010) confirm the initial findings about the connection between social inequalities and health disparities.

One significant investigation of this kind is the Whitehall study of British civil servants. It began in the late 1960s and continues today, following both the initial and subsequent cohorts (Marmot et al., 1991; Heraclides et al., 2012). Across the hierarchy of the occupations in the civil service, those in higher positions have fared better in terms of both mortality and morbidity. The higher one's position in the civil service, in other words, the better one's health. The Whitehall studies demonstrate that differences in health are a product not only of income but also of social status and lifestyle behaviours. Subsequent studies began to look more closely at how factors like education and income affect health disparities. In Canada, for instance, Mustard and colleagues (1997) expanded on the Whitehall study by exploring the influence of education and income gradients on morbidity and mortality in Manitoba. The study found, predictably, a direct relationship between the social gradient and health. However, differences were greater among adults than children: the burden of the gradient increases over time, and income was more influential than education. In comparison to other developed nations, Canada is higher in health inequality given the degree of income inequality in the country.

As awareness of the social determinants of health has increased, scholars in developed countries have begun to explore more nuanced dimensions of these factors. The influence of socio-economic status on the health of children is a good example. In research on health inequalities, children occupy a unique position in that anything that affects them is cumulative. In other words, the effects of lower income on health may compound over the course of a person's life. Determining the level of influence of the social gradient is an important step in exploring the overall influence of inequalities on health. Across developed nations, research supports the claim that income and education differences are related to disparities in health. This connection is evident in Canada (Mustard et al., 1997), Germany (Reinhold & Jurges, 2012), and Australia (Khanam et al., 2009). Gradients in socio-economic status appear to have differential effects across the life course. To illustrate this point, Chen and colleagues (2006) argue that the effect of growing up in lower socio-economic circumstances is greater for adolescents than for younger children: age and the life course are important additional factors that affect the relationship between the social gradient and health.

Studies on health disparities across the life course have demonstrated the need for carefully timed interventions to decrease inequalities that lead to differences in mortality and morbidity. From the first studies in the 1970s, research on social class and health has identified policy and program interventions that could reduce the burden of the social gradient on the population. The mantra of reducing inequalities to improve overall health echoes across the last thirty years of research in this area. Strategies for addressing poverty through affordable housing, designing opportunities for education among lower-income citizens, and ensuring a fair wage are examples of initiatives intended to foster a fairer and healthier society.

Social class is one of the structures of identification that determines access to resources like income and education, thereby directly influencing a person's health over the course of their life. As an identity, social class can be very important to a person. It may be explicit in their society, like in Britain or India, where social position is publically and historically woven into a person's sense of self and the way they are treated. In the contemporary era, however, scholars argue that the significance of class status is becoming less central (Currie, 1992; Marshall et al., 2005). In countries like Canada or those in Northern Europe, social class tends to be more muted and in the background of self-identity. Despite this point, class is still significant when it comes to social inequalities and health disparities.

CASE STUDY

Class and Schizophrenia

For many years, researchers and health care workers have noted that rates of schizophrenia are far higher among individuals from lower-class backgrounds (Golderg & Morrison, 1963; Argyle, 1994). The exact reasons for this disparity, however, are the source of substantial debate, largely because the causes of schizophrenia are still unclear. On one hand, some theorists explain this phenomenon through what is called the social causation theory. Put simply, this model holds that individuals from lower-class backgrounds are more likely to receive a diagnosis of schizophrenia for a host of potential reasons. For example, these individuals tend to have limited access to health care resources, potentially resulting in complications during pregnancy and childbirth, many of which have been linked to the development of schizophrenia (Geddes & Lawrie, 1995; Hultman et al., 1999). Similarly, we know that working-class individuals generally have poorer health; mothers from lower-class backgrounds may thus be more likely to develop infections during pregnancy—another potential cause of schizophrenia (Sham et al., 1992).

Another theory holds that individuals from lower socio-economic statuses experience greater levels of stress (leading lives that are generally more insecure) and that this fact may be responsible for higher rates of schizophrenia (Gallagher, Jones, & Pardes, 2013). Other researchers (Kohn, 1972) have focused on variations in how individuals from different classes are socialized. They argue that individuals from neighbourhoods with lower SES are taught to be conformist and obedient rather than flexible and independent, leading to a general feeling that life is beyond their control. Evidence that could support this notion is that deficit schizophrenia (a variant of the disorder characterized by social withdrawal, blunted emotions, and difficulties in communication) is far more common among working-class individuals than those from the middle and upper classes (Gallagher et al., 2006).

Still another set of researchers reject the social causation theory, instead arguing that the correlation between lower SES and schizophrenia can best be understood as one of cause and effect: people with schizophrenia (regardless of their class background) find it difficult to obtain education and hold down steady jobs; as a result, they drift down the social gradient (Jones et al. 1993; Aro et al., 1995). In reality, all of these factors probably play some role in explaining why individuals from lower-class backgrounds tend to have higher rates of schizophrenia.

Race and Ethnicity

Like social class, race and ethnicity is a structure of identification that influences how we understand both ourselves and our health. The term *race* refers to the socially constructed categories that differentiate people based on cultural heritage (Smedley & Smedley, 2005). Racial categories, or ethnicities, can be a source of pride and collective identity among a community, as in the case of the Black Power movement in the late 1960s and the struggle for civil rights. Yet at the same time, racial categories can be used to discriminate when they are assigned specific meanings that disenfranchise ethnic communities on the basis of their cultural heritage. African Americans in the United States and the First Nations peoples of Canada provide examples of groups that have long suffered from systemic racism in North America (Regan, 2010; Alderman, 2010). The policies and practices that have historically supported racism against these groups (such the legacy of slavery and the residential school system) continue to differentiate people on the basis of racial categories. Through this process, these structures create inequalities and injustices that reverberate for all members of a society.

Research on the relationship between social identity and health extends beyond social class to examine race and ethnicity. In the United States, Nickens (1986) found differences in morbidity and mortality across different ethnicities. African Americans in particular fared worse compared to other ethnicities, especially in relation to Caucasian Americans. Seeking to understand health disparities and race, Dressler and colleagues (2005) examined four possible models that could account for the connection between health status and racial categorization: (1) genetic variation; (2) differences in lifestyle and behaviour; (3) level of psycho-social stress from life circumstances; and (4) social inequalities. Based on their extensive review, the authors argue that the social inequality model is the most plausible. The genetic variation model has no bearing on health disparities related to race.

In Canada, First Nations peoples experience a similar reality. In a study from 2005, Adelson examined the health of members of Aboriginal communities across Canada. On all measures of mortality, life expectancy, morbidity, and self-reported health status, Aboriginal individuals fared worse than other Canadians. The researchers also asked Aboriginal people what they perceived to be the most significant problems related to health and well-being. Participants mentioned broader social and political factors such as unemployment, substance abuse, suicide, and family violence. This study also highlights social inequities (related to race and ethnicity) as the primary factor that accounts for the drastic health disparities that First Nations peoples encounter. The kinds of inequities that exist in Canada have affected Aboriginal communities over a long period of time. Unless changes are made to address the underlying inequities, there will continue to be health disparities related to race and ethnicity.

The social inequities encountered by African Americans and First Nations peoples are compounded by their historical mistreatment within the medical system. For example, in the infamous Tuskegee experiment, researchers allowed rural African American men infected with syphilis to remain untreated in order to study the natural progression of the disease. Crucially, the researchers did not obtain the participants' consent for the experiment, nor were the men informed about the true nature of the study. Despite the existence of effective treatments for syphilis, these individuals were denied care. Such examples reflect what some believe to be a blatant disregard for and discrimination against racial minorities within medicine (Gamble, 1997). In Canada, the systemic barriers that Aboriginal people face in

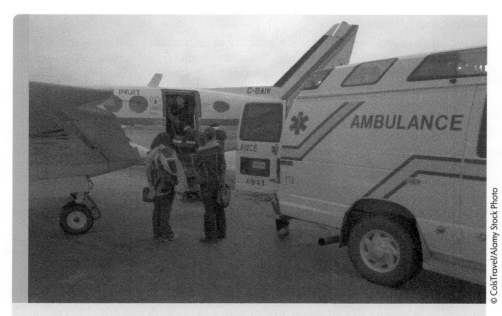

© ColsTravel/Alamy Stock Photo

The remoteness of many rural communities in Canada limits adequate health provision and can be a systematic barrier for certain populations (such as Inuit, First Nations, and Métis populations, who are disproportionately represented in remote communities). What are some potential ways to increase health care access for residents of remote communities?

accessing health care services, due to the structures in place within the reserve system or the remoteness of many communities, also limit health care provision (Brown & Fiske, 2001). On the whole, there are considerable ethnic and racial disparities in health care provision, and therefore health (Smedley et al., 2009).

As awareness of the social inequities facing racial minorities increases, a range of interesting initiatives hold promise for potentially decreasing health disparities. Kirmayer, Simpson, and Cargo (2003), for instance, argue that First Nations peoples' mental health can be improved by offering programs driven from within these communities, rather than imposed from outside. Concentrating on youth and community empowerment, these programs would address deeply entrenched inequities in health and health care services. Instead of simply concentrating on healing the individual—the approach favoured by dominant types of mental health care—these programs would aim at more collective forms of healing, targeting the broader community. Many First Nations communities are initiating their own programs and projects designed to combat the negative effects of racism and to alleviate its negative influence on health. As mentioned earlier, First Nations communities in Canada still experience health challenges at an alarming rate compared to the overall population. Health disparities across racial categories will continue, unfortunately, unless racially based systemic inequities are effectively addressed.

CASE STUDY

Race and Schizophrenia

The connections between health, race, and racism can be clearly seen when considering schizophrenia. For many decades in much of the Western world, black people have been far more likely to receive a diagnosis of schizophrenia than white people, even when controlling for other factors such as class and income (Fearon et al., 2006; Mukherjee et al., 1983; Strakowski et al., 1995). Why is it that psychiatrists and other physicians tend to overdiagnose schizophrenia in black individuals?

Researchers have advanced a wide range of theories to explain this phenomenon. As Krieger (1987) points out, psychiatrists, like many scientists, originally tried to explain health discrepancies between African Americans and Caucasians in terms of racial biology. They assumed that physiological differences in black individuals made them more prone to certain types of illnesses. This type of work relied upon racial stereotypes rather than any actual biological data.

It is clear that clinician bias continues to play a role in the overdiagnosis of schizophrenia in black individuals. As Trierweiler and colleagues (2000) note, psychiatrists are more likely to attribute paranoia and hallucinations (two common symptoms of schizophrenia) to African Americans than to other racial groups. Even when black individuals exhibit symptoms associated with other disorders (such as depression), they are still more likely to receive a schizophrenia diagnosis. Such notions have a long history in psychiatry; during the era of colonial expansion, many European psychiatrists argued that black populations in their African colonies were too "happy-go-lucky" to truly suffer from feelings of sadness and despair (Vaughn, 2013).

Historian and psychiatrist Jonathan Metzl's (2009) research on race and schizophrenia in the United States may provide another part of the answer. To begin, Metzl points to a long history of institutionalized racism in psychiatry, remarking upon diagnostic categories such as drapetomania, a diagnosis assigned to black slaves in the South who tried to escape their white masters. Metzl also notes that Caucasian anxieties about "black belligerence" during the civil rights movement helped spark a dramatic spike in the diagnosis of schizophrenia in African Americans. Coupled with pharmaceutical advertisements that reframed the illness as a "black disease," Metzl's work points to the fact that there are large, overarching structural issues that shape the way health care workers and society thinks about health, illness, and race.

Gender

Of the different structures of identification, gender is arguably the most evident and visible in our everyday lives. The identification of *male* or *female* is built into our environments, institutional structures (like the family), and most definitively into our sense of self (Wood, 2012). Conventionally, the gender order works as a binary dividing the world into either male or female. Masculinity and femininity each have their own associated meanings, and we understand gender in relation to these terms. These notions produce reproduce power differences and are often referred to as hegemonic (Connell & Messerschmidt, 2005). **Patriarchal** institutional structures emphasize male privilege and male domination, creating social relations that are oppressive to women and those men who do not embody or demonstrate traditionally dominant forms of masculinity.

HALF OF ALL CANADIAN WOMEN WILL EXPERIENCE AN INCIDENT OF PHYSICAL OR SEXUAL VIOLENCE.

Gender and health are intricately linked. This poster speaks to the fact that women are far more likely than men to suffer injury and death because of abusive relationships. How else does gender affect health?

This gender order creates the conditions for health disparities between men and women. One of the established trends in this research states that women live longer than men (lower mortality) but that they experience greater morbidity (Denton et al., 2004). This dilemma has sparked a number of interesting studies exploring differences between men and women, especially with regard to reported levels of illness. Denton and colleagues (2004) explored the factors that might help explain these differences, and put forward three possible sources: (1) psychological factors like stress and challenging life events; (2) health-related behaviours like exercise or smoking; and (3) social contextual factors like family structure, work, and age. In their findings they argue that "social structural and psychosocial determinants of health are generally more important for women and behavioural determinants are generally more important for men" (Denton et al., 2004, p. 2585). In other words, men may behave in ways that put their lives at risk either in the short term or the long term. Although these behaviours may be harmful, men will generally not develop illnesses as a result of these actions. Women, meanwhile, are better at taking care of themselves (and others) but, because of their life circumstances, are under pressures that can cause physical, mental, or emotional illnesses.

Annandale & Hunt (1990) argue that differences in morbidity are actually a result of our social understandings of masculinity and femininity. Rather than morbidity being a strictly sex-related biological phenomenon, it may have a social basis. In our society, higher rates of reported illness are generally associated with femininity. In such debates, it is instructive to take a multifactorial, non-reductionist approach, seeking value in the idea that phenomena like differences in morbidity among men and women are complex and the result of many intersecting forces combining together over time.

Regardless of why gender differences in health exist, scholars agree that one key way to redress them is by increasing gender equity. Unless men and women have similar access to resources, disparities in health outcomes will continue and arguably worsen. Further to this, despite improvements in gender equity, women continue to be subject to the negative and

CASE STUDY

Gendered Division of Mental Disorder

The gendered division of mental health diagnoses has intrigued commentators for quite some time. Why is it that women are more likely to receive some diagnoses including depression, anxiety disorders, eating disorders, and borderline personality disorder, whereas men experience higher rates of addiction, attention-deficit hyperactivity disorder (ADHD), antisocial personality disorder, and suicide (Rosenfeld et al. 2000; Kessler et al., 1994)? As ever, there are many potential explanations beyond biological difference.

Unsurprisingly, differences in socialization seem to contribute to the differential rates of mental disorder. Many theorists believe that typical female gender roles involve greater emotional awareness and openness in discussing vulnerability; these factors might account for the higher rate of depression and anxiety among women (Rosenfeld et al., 2000; Addis & Mahalik, 2003). Society's tendency to overtly sexualize women may also be a factor. Women are far more likely to experience sexual violence—an important contributory factor for the development of a range of disorders. Further, the pressure to maintain a particular body shape has been linked to the development of eating disorders (Mullen et al., 1993; Garner & Garfinkel, 1980). There is also the issue of gender bias in diagnosis. Some researchers have found that physicians are more likely to diagnose depression in women than in men, even when the same constellation of symptoms is present (Callahan et al., 1997; Stoppe et al., 1999).

Many of the risk-laden or harmful behaviours in which men are more likely to engage can also have a deleterious effect on their mental health. As teenagers and adults, males are more likely to abuse alcohol and illicit drugs—both of which can contribute to the development not only of addiction but of other mental disorders as well (Kessler et al., 1994). Men, perhaps because of gender role expectations, are also less likely to seek out assistance for emotional distress. Failing to engage in preventative or health-protective activities, such as psychotherapy, may explain why men have far higher rates of addiction and suicide (Komiya, Good & Sherrod, 2000; Delenardo & Terrion, 2014).

In the same way that a clinician's gender bias might increase the diagnostic rate of depression in women, theorists have speculated that gender expectations might be a reason that men are disproportionately diagnosed with certain types of personality disorders, namely antisocial and paranoid personality disorders (Rienzi & Scrams, 1991). Similarly, gender bias among teachers and parents might help explain why boys have historically been far more likely than girls to receive diagnoses of ADHD (Sciutto, Nolfi, & Bluhm, 2004). On the whole, it is clear that social conceptions of gender, beyond biological sex, play a vital role in the causation, reporting, and perception of mental illness.

harmful consequences of patriarchal forces that make them vulnerable to illness and harm. Raising awareness of issues like domestic violence and formulating programs and policies that seek to address the underlying causes of oppression are facets of a movement toward seeking gender equity to improve health for men and women (Bent-Goodley, 2007). Doyal (2000, p. 932) writes that "the only practicable strategy for reducing unfair and avoidable inequalities in health outcomes between men and women is to ensure that the two groups have equal access to those resources which they need to realize their potential for health." With regard to health, the challenge now is to articulate and put into place strategies that can overcome the deeply entrenched inequalities in the gender order. One approach that we examine in the next section is looking at the intersection between different structures of identification in order to better understand and reduce health disparities (Weber & Parra-Medina, 2003).

Intersectionality

In this chapter, the overall objective is to discuss the relationship between social identity and health outcomes along three structures of identification: gender, social class, and race. There are a number of other important structures related to identity that we are not able to address such as age, sexuality, illness, geography, and disability. Power relations that are embedded in the institutional structures of society create conditions whereby those with less access to resources are more vulnerable and at greater risk of illness, injury, and sickness. In addressing the consequences of social inequalities on health, scholars have begun to look more at the intersection between different structures of identification. Rather than studying the relationship between health and gender, or class, or race, research now tends to focus on the combined effect of intersecting social and power relations on health and health disparities. This perspective, known as **intersectionality**, developed from the theoretical work of important feminist scholars such as Kimberlé Crenshaw (1989) and Patricia Hill Collins (2000). It provides a useful and much needed way to think about how the many facets of a person's social identity relate to overarching power structures.

Taking an intersectional approach means attending carefully to unique health outcomes that result from the combination of different power relations and structures of identification. When examining health disparities, for instance, Kawachi and colleagues (2005) stress that the result is something greater than just combining data on race and class and adding them together. One cannot merely "add" the identities of "working class" and "Aboriginal" and assume that this produces a simple "doubling" of oppression. Rather, the interaction between the two social relations produces unique effects on the health of individuals and groups. Taking an intersectional approach to research allows for a more nuanced and detailed understanding of how and why health disparities arise. We can determine which strategies may be useful for addressing these disparities, both in specific contexts and more broadly across populations.

By examining multiple structures of identification together, one can witness the effects of this interaction. Rosenfield (2012) analyzes this issue directly in a study of gender, race, class, and mental health. In prior research, the assumption was that multiple forms of oppression—in this case, race, class, and gender—would usually compound one another and produce a "triple threat" with regards to mental health. While this is often the case, Rosenfield argues that there is a multiple, complex, and interactive effect across class, race, and gender that can create paradoxical or even contradictory results in terms of mental illness or one's ability to avoid illness. Studies taking an intersectional approach also do not privilege one category over another and tend to emphasize the importance of context, meaning, history, and experience in understanding health disparities (Hankivsky et al., 2008).

Chapter Summary

This chapter has explored the ways in which different facets of individuals' identities—notably social class, race, and gender—play an important role in shaping their health. It began by briefly exploring the concept of identity, noting that identity carries personal meaning but is also embedded in broader social structures. As a consequence, identity is important in shaping how we see ourselves and how others see and treat us. Depending on one's location, certain characteristics of identity are privileged while others are marginalized. In order to understand inequalities in health, it is fundamental to consider how individuals' identities structure their life experience; for example, they might face greater exposure to particular health risks or receive preferential care depending on their identity.

Social class, also known as socio-economic status, represents one very meaningful component of identity. Connected to a person's education, occupation, income, and family background (among other characteristics), class consistently produces substantial variability in health. In short, the lower one is on the social gradient, the more likely one will experience poor health. Within the framework of capitalism, class is an especially important driver of health inequalities. It can limit or promote a person's participation in a variety of activities such as job choices, educational opportunities, and overall lifestyles, all of which profoundly affects health.

Race and ethnicity represents another central element of an individual's identity. Race is a socially constructed category connected to a person's cultural heritage and physical appearance. Independent of any biological differences, race can have a profound effect on a person's health. It can structure their beliefs and behaviour around health while also influencing how they are treated by others. Within the context of North American society, where white identity is privileged, individuals from some racial communities (notably African Americans and First Nations peoples) experience much more illness and poor health.

Gender is another component of identity that greatly influences our daily life. Traditionally, gender has been divided into two primary categories—male and female—each associated with a variety of societal assumptions about what constitutes "proper" or "normal" behaviour. Unquestionably, this masculine–feminine binary deeply affects people's health far beyond the biological differences often associated with gender identity. In most places across the world, society is patriarchal: men with traditional masculine traits are at an advantage. Consequently, women, men whose behaviour deviates from this masculine norm, and individuals who identify outside the gender binary altogether all face greater barriers to good health.

Intersectionality is an important tool for seeking to understand how these and other components of identity affect health. Recognizing that identity interacts with overarching power structures, intersectionality examines the connections or intersecting points between various facets of identity, paying special attention to the issues of marginalization and privilege. Possessing certain combinations of identity traits (for example, being a working-class female or an Asian-American male) creates unique constellations that can significantly impact an individual's health. Intersectionality addresses the inseparable facets of human identity. Thus, it encourages us to dig deeper to understand the ways in which health inequalities are connected to a person's identity. If health equity is to be achieved, it will be necessary to understand the intersections between identity, power, and health outcomes.

STUDY QUESTIONS

1. How can we explain the relationship between the social gradient and health?
2. What are the main health differences between men and women? How can these be explained?
3. How might other facets of identity (such as sexuality or disability) affect health?
4. What are the connections between race, racism, and health status?
5. Why must we consider intersectionality when discussing identity and health?

SUGGESTED READINGS

Hankivsky, O. (Ed.). (2011). *Health inequities in Canada: Intersectional frameworks and practices.* Vancouver: UBC Press.

Harris, J. (2003). "All doors are closed to us": A social model analysis of the experiences of disabled refugees and asylum seekers in Britain. *Disability & Society, 18*(4), 395–410.

Haslam, S. A., Jetten, J., Postmes., & Haslam, C. (2009). Special issue: Social identity, health and well-being. *Applied Psychology, 58*(1).

Weber, L. & Peek, L. (Eds). (2012). *Displaced: Life in the Katrina diaspora.* Austin: University of Texas Press.

SUGGESTED WEB RESOURCES

Canadian Women's Health Network: Women and Mental Health: www.cwhn.ca/en/resources/mentalhealth

Peggy McIntosh's TEDx talk: How Studying Privilege Systems Can Strengthen Compassion: http://tedxtalks.ted.com/video/How-Studying-Privilege-Systems

Metzl, J. (2012, April 23). "Schizophrenia's Identity Crisis" Retrieved from www.youtube.com/watch?v=hzcIdCdPuUs

GLOSSARY

Class A component of one's identity, also known as socio-economic status. It is related to one's education, income, family background, and occupation.

Gender Unlike biological sex, gender has meaning beyond chromosomes; it involves complex social roles and expectations. Many societies divide gender along binary lines (men/women) but it should be noted that many individuals and societies recognize the existence of multiple gender identities.

Intersectionality The relationship between any and all of one's social identities. Posits that one's social identity is a result of the relationship between all of their various identities (gender, sexuality, race, class, etc.). None of these should be neglected.

Morbidity The prevalence and incidence of a disease in a given population.

Mortality The rate of deaths in a population over a period of time.

Patriarchal Relating to a patriarch, the male head of a society. In the context of this textbook, "patriarchal" refers to a male dominated society.

Social gradient Ranking in society based on socio-economic status and one's relative position in a market economy.

Social identity Our sense of self in relation to society as a whole and its broader social structures. While the definition of this term is not widely agreed upon, some components of social identity can include one's gender, race, and age.

Structures of identification Societal structures (e.g. gender, sexuality, class) that shape our individual experience and our identity, though our experiences are inherently different from anyone else.

REFERENCES

Acheson, D. (1998). *Inequalities in health: Report of an independent inquiry.* London: Stationery Office.

Addis, M. E. & Mahalik, J. R. (2003). Men, masculinity, and the contexts of help seeking. *American Psychologist, 58*(1), 5–14.

Adelson, N. (2005). The embodiment of inequity: Health disparities in Aboriginal Canada. *Canadian Journal of Public Health/Revue canadienne de santé publique,* S45–S61.

Alderman, D. H. (2010). Surrogation and the politics of remembering slavery in Savannah, Georgia (USA). *Journal of Historical Geography, 36*(1), 90–101.

Annandale, E. & Hunt, K. (1990). Masculinity, femininity and sex: An exploration of their relative contribution to explaining gender differences in health. *Sociology of Health & Illness, 12*(1), 24–46.

Annandale, E. & Hunt, K. (Eds). (2000). *Gender inequalities in health.* Philadelphia: Open University Press.

Argyle, M. (1994). *The psychology of social class.* London: Psychology Press.

Aro, S., Aro, H., Salinto, M., & Keskimäki, I. (1995). Educational level and hospital use in mental disorders: A population-based study. *Acta Psychiatrica Scandinavica, 91*(5), 305–12.

Bauman, Z. (2001). Identity in the globalizing world. *Social Anthropology, 9*(2), 121–29.

Bent-Goodley, T. B. (2007). Health disparities and violence against women: Why and how cultural and societal influences matter. *Trauma, Violence, & Abuse, 8*(2), 90–104.

Browne, A. J. & Fiske, J. A. (2001). First Nations women's encounters with mainstream health care services. *Western Journal of Nursing Research, 23*(2), 126–47.

Callahan, C. M., Kesterson, J. G., & Tierney, W. M. (1997). Association of symptoms of depression with diagnostic test charges among older adults. *Annals of Internal Medicine, 126*(6), 426–32.

Chen, E., Martin, A. D., & Matthews, K. A. (2006). Socioeconomic status and health: Do gradients differ within childhood and adolescence? *Social Science & Medicine, 62*(9), 2161–70.

Collins, P. H. (2000). Gender, black feminism, and black political economy. *The Annals of the American Academy of Political and Social Science, 568*(1), 41–53.

Connell, R. W. & Messerschmidt, J. W. (2005). Hegemonic masculinity rethinking the concept. *Gender & Society, 19*(6), 829–59.

Crenshaw, K. (1989). Demarginalizing the intersection of race and sex: A black feminist critique of antidiscrimination doctrine, feminist theory and antiracist politics. *University of Chicago Legal Forum, 140,* 139–87.

Currie, K. (1992). The Indian stratification debate: A discursive exposition of problems and issues in the analysis of class, caste and gender. *Dialectical Anthropology, 17*(2), 115–39.

Delenardo, S. & Terrion, J. L. (2014). Suck it up: Opinions and attitudes about mental illness stigma and help-seeking behaviour of male varsity football players. *Canadian Journal of Community Mental Health, 33*(3), 43–56.

Denton, M., Prus, S., & Walters, V. (2004). Gender differences in health: A Canadian study of the psychosocial, structural and behavioural determinants of health. *Social Science & Medicine, 58*(12), 2585–2600.

Doyal, L. (2000). Gender equity in health: Debates and dilemmas. *Social Science & Medicine, 51*(6), 931–39.

Dressler, W. W., Oths, K. S., & Gravlee, C. C. (2005). Race and ethnicity in public health research: Models to explain health disparities. *Annual Review of Anthropology, 34*, 231–52.

Emerson, E., Graham, H., & Hatton, C. (2006). Household income and health status in children and adolescents in Britain. *The European Journal of Public Health, 16*(4), 354–60.

Fearon, P., Kirkbride, J. B., Morgan, C., Dazzan, P., Morgan, K., Lloyd, T., & Murray, R. M. (2006). Incidence of schizophrenia and other psychoses in ethnic minority groups: Results from the MRC AESOP Study. *Psychological Medicine, 36*(11), 1541–50.

Frohlich, K. L., Ross, N., & Richmond, C. (2006). Health disparities in Canada today: Some evidence and a theoretical framework. *Health Policy, 79*(2), 132–43.

Gallagher, B. J., Jones, B. J., & Pardes, M. (2013). Stressful life events, social class and symptoms of schizophrenia. *Clinical Schizophrenia & Related Psychoses, 25*, 1–25. doi: 10.3371/CSRP.GAJO.112013

Gamble, V. N. (1997). Under the shadow of Tuskegee: African Americans and health care. *American Journal of Public Health, 87*(11), 1773–78.

Garner, D. M. & Garfinkel, P. E. (1980). Socio-cultural factors in the development of anorexia nervosa. *Psychological Medicine, 10*(4), 647–56.

Geddes, J. R. & Lawrie, S. M. (1995). Obstetric complications and schizophrenia: A meta-analysis. *The British Journal of Psychiatry, 167*(6), 786–93.

Goldberg, E. M. & Morrison, S. L. (1963). Schizophrenia and social class. *The British Journal of Psychiatry, 109*(463), 785–802.

Gray, A. M. (1982). Inequalities in health. The Black Report: A summary and comment. *International Journal of Health Services, 12*(3), 349–80.

Heraclides, A. M., Chandola, T., Witte, D. R., & Brunner, E. J. (2012). Work stress, obesity and the risk of Type 2 Diabetes: Gender-specific bidirectional effect in the Whitehall II Study. *Obesity, 20*(2), 428–33.

Hultman, C. M., Geddes, J., Sparén, P., Takei, N., Murray, R. M., & Cnattingius, S. (1999). Prenatal and perinatal risk factors for schizophrenia, affective psychosis, and reactive psychosis of early onset: Case-control study. *British Medical Journal, 318*(7181), 421–26.

Jones, P. B., Bebbington, P., Foerster, A., Lewis, S. W., Murray, R. M., Russell, A., . . . & Wilkins, S. (1993). Premorbid social underachievement in schizophrenia. Results from the Camberwell Collaborative Psychosis Study. *The British Journal of Psychiatry, 162*(1), 65–71.

Kawachi, I., Daniels, N., & Robinson, D. E. (2005). Health disparities by race and class: Why both matter. *Health Affairs, 24*(2), 343–52.

Kessler, R. C., McGonagle, K. A., Zhao, S., Nelson, C. B., Hughes, M., Eshleman, S., . . . & Kendler, K. S. (1994). Lifetime and 12-month prevalence of DSM-III-R psychiatric disorders in the United States: Results from the National Comorbidity Survey. *Archives of General Psychiatry, 51*(1), 8–19.

Khanam, R., Nghiem, H. S., & Connelly, L. B. (2009). Child health and the income gradient: Evidence from Australia. *Journal of Health Economics, 28*(4), 805–17.

Kirmayer, L., Simpson, C., & Cargo, M. (2003). Healing traditions: Culture, community and mental health promotion with Canadian Aboriginal peoples. *Australasian Psychiatry, 11*(s1), S15–S23.

Kitagawa, E. M. & Hauser, P. M. (1973). *Differential mortality in the United States: A study in socioeconomic epidemiology.* Cambridge, MA: Harvard University Press.

Kohn, M. L. (1972). Class, family, and schizophrenia: A reformulation. *Social Forces, 50*(3), 295–304.

Komiya, N., Good, G. E., & Sherrod, N. B. (2000). Emotional openness as a predictor of college students' attitudes toward seeking psychological help. *Journal of Counselling Psychology, 47*(1), 138.

Krieger, N. (1987). Shades of difference: theoretical underpinnings of the medical controversy on black/white differences in the United States, 1830–1870. *International Journal of Health Services, 17*(2), 259–78.

———, Chen, J. T., Waterman, P. D., Rehkopf, D. H., & Subramanian, S. V. (2003). Race/ethnicity, gender, and monitoring socioeconomic gradients in health: A comparison of area-based socio-economic measures—the public health disparities geocoding project. *American Journal of Public Health, 93*(10), 1655–71.

Macintyre, S., Hunt, K., & Sweeting, H. (1996). Gender differences in health: Are things really as simple as they seem? *Social Science & Medicine, 42*(4), 617–24.

Marmot, M. (2005). Social determinants of health inequalities. *The Lancet, 365*(9464), 1099–1104.

———, Allen, J., Goldblatt, P., Boyce, T., McNeish, D., Grady, M., & Geddes, I. (2010). *Fair society, healthy lives: Strategic review of health inequalities in England post 2010*. London: The Marmot Review.

——— & Bell, R. (2012). Fair society, healthy lives. *Public Health, 126*, S4–S10.

———, Friel, S., Bell, R., Houweling, T. A., & Taylor, S. (2008). Closing the gap in a generation: Health equity through action on the social determinants of health. *The Lancet, 372*(9650), 1661–69.

———, Stansfeld, S., Patel, C., North, F., Head, J., White, I., . . . & Smith, G. D. (1991). Health inequalities among British civil servants: The Whitehall II study. *The Lancet, 337*(8754), 1387–93.

Marshall, G., Newby, H., Rose, D., & Vogler, C. (2005). *Social class in modern Britain*. London: Routledge.

Metzl, J. (2009). *The protest psychosis: How schizophrenia became a black disease*. Boston, MA: Beacon Press.

Mukherjee, S., Shukla S., Woodle J., et al. (1983). Misdiagnosis of schizophrenia in bipolar patients: a multiethnic comparison. *American Journal of Psychiatry, 140*, 1471–74.

Mullen, P. E., Martin, J. L., Anderson, J. C., Romans, S. E., & Herbison, G. P. (1993). Childhood sexual abuse and mental health in adult life. *The British Journal of Psychiatry, 163*(6), 721–32.

Mustard, C. A., Derksen, S., Berthelot, J. M., Wolfson, M., & Roos, L. L. (1997). Age-specific education and income gradients in morbidity and mortality in a Canadian province. *Social Science & Medicine, 45*(3), 383–97.

Nickens, H. (1986). Health problems of minority groups: Public health's unfinished agenda. *Public Health Reports, 101*(3), 230.

Pan, S. Y., Ugnat, A. M., Semenciw, R., Desmeules, M., Mao, Y., & Macleod, M. (2006). Trends in childhood injury mortality in Canada, 1979–2002. *Injury Prevention, 12*(3), 155–60.

Regan, P. (2010). *Unsettling the settler within: Indian residential schools, truth telling, and reconciliation in Canada*. Vancouver: UBC Press.

Reinhold, S. & Jürges, H. (2012). Parental income and child health in Germany. *Health Economics, 21*(5), 562–79.

Rienzi, B. M. & Scrams, D. J. (1991). Gender stereotypes for paranoid, antisocial, compulsive, dependent, and histrionic personality disorders. *Psychological Reports, 69*(3), 976–78.

Rosenfeld, Sarah. 2012. Triple jeopardy? Mental health at the intersection of gender, race, and class. *Social Science and Medicine 74*(11), 1791–1801.

———, Vertefuille, J., & McAlpine, D. D. (2000). Gender stratification and mental health: An exploration of dimensions of the self. *Social Psychology Quarterly*, 208–23.

Sciutto, M. J., Nolfi, C. J., & Bluhm, C. (2004). Effects of child gender and symptom type on referrals for ADHD by elementary school teachers. *Journal of Emotional and Behavioral Disorders, 12*(4), 247–53.

Sham, P. C., O'Callaghan, E., Takei, N., Murray, G. K., Hare, E. H., & Murray, R. M. (1992). Schizophrenia following pre-natal exposure to influenza epidemics between 1939 and 1960. *The British Journal of Psychiatry, 160*(4), 461–66.

Smedley, A. & Smedley, B. D. (2005). Race as biology is fiction, racism as a social problem is real: Anthropological and historical perspectives on the social construction of race. *American Psychologist, 60*(1), 16.

Smedley, B. D., Stith, A. Y., & Nelson, A. R. (Eds). (2009). *Unequal treatment: confronting racial and ethnic disparities in health care*. Washington: National Academies Press.

Strakowski, S. M., Lonczak, H. S., Sax, K. W., West, S. A., Crist, A., Mehta, R., & Thienhaus, O. J. (1995). The effects of race on diagnosis and disposition from a psychiatric emergency service. *Journal of Clinical Psychiatry, 56*, 101–07.

Stoppe, G., Sandholzer, H., Huppertz, C., Duwe, H., & Staedt, J. (1999). Gender differences in the recognition of depression in old age. *Maturitas, 32*(3), 205–12.

Trierweiler, S. J., Neighbors, H. W., Munday, C., Thompson, E. E., Binion, V. J., & Gomez, J. P. (2000). Clinician attributions associated with the diagnosis of schizophrenia in African American and non-African American patients. *Journal of Consulting and Clinical Psychology, 68*(1), 171–5.

Vaughn, M. (2013). Suicide: A hidden history. In W. Kalusa & M. Vaughn (Eds), *Death, belief and politics in Central African history* (pp. 233–92). Lusaka: Lembani Trust.

Ward, E., Jemal, A., Cokkinides, V., Singh, G. K., Cardinez, C., Ghafoor, A., & Thun, M. (2004). Cancer disparities by race/ethnicity and socioeconomic status. *CA: A Cancer Journal for Clinicians, 54*(2), 78–93.

Weber, L. & Parra-Medina, D. (2003). Intersectionality and women's health: Charting a path to eliminating health disparities. *Advances in Gender Research 7*(a), 183–226.

Wood, J. (2012). *Gendered lives.* New York: Cengage Learning.

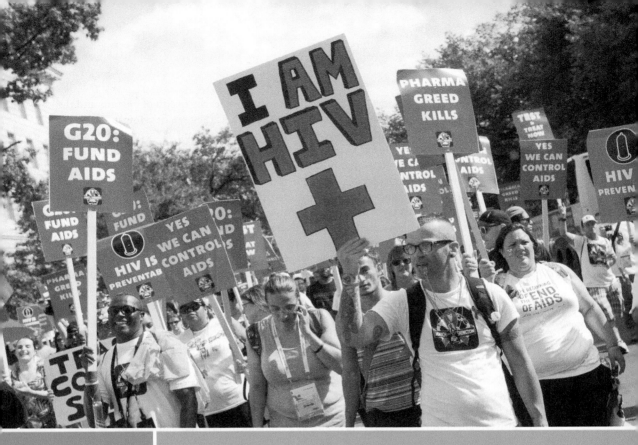

6

Politics, Social Justice, and Health

Chelsea Gabel

LEARNING OBJECTIVES

In this chapter, students will learn

- critical theories of social justice and their application to health
- the distinction between health advocacy and health activism
- important terms related to social movements and health
- the connections between broader social movements as they relate to health and illness

Introduction

As citizens, how do we balance the duty of the state to protect the health of citizens and the right of individuals to define and pursue their own health as they see fit? How much power should the state have over society? How can society control the state to ensure that the state always serves society's interests? One avenue is finding the will to organize. **Social movements** related to health are thus about mobilizing people for action. They form when individuals see or experience challenges around health. In light of these challenges, individuals and groups organize to alter the conditions, distribution of resources, attitudes, and laws that leave them disadvantaged. These movements are often centred around an issue, such as the movement for alternative medicine; a particular disease, such as finding a cure for breast cancer; or the health of a specific population, such as Aboriginal peoples. Ultimately, they are about citizens making choices about how to use their time, talents, and resources to make a difference. Movements gain momentum when they can convince the public that the cause is socially relevant. Gaining influence through shifting the mindsets of the wider public is challenging. In this chapter, students are asked to consider whether social movements really make a difference in achieving more social justice.

Social justice, in the context of health, refers to a situation in which all citizens share equal access to treatment and a fair allocation of resources regardless of their social status. Social justice, as it applies to health, has proven to be a top priority for Canadians; a lack of social justice would increase illness, disease, and mortality. Conversely, a just health care system would increase community democracy and foster healthier lives. The fight for social justice is often understood as one that is inherent to our fundamental rights and freedoms. The World Health Organization (1948, p.1) sees health as a fundamental right of citizenship:

> the employment of the highest attainable standard of health is one of the fundamental rights of every human being without distinction of race, religion, political belief, economics or social condition.

While a health care system born out of the principles of social justice can improve people's lives, many critics are concerned that the Canadian health system does not support social justice. This point is particularly relevant for women, refugees, and Aboriginal populations.

Many people question the assumptions we make about state control and health. For example, should the government have the right to limit access to alternative health care? Does the state possess the right to imperil our health in the name of economic development? Is it the government's responsibility to ensure that employers protect the health of their workers? Many of these debates centre around a broader question: should the government impose rules upon people when it comes to health or should it back off as much as possible? In this chapter, we will discuss these important questions with an emphasis on the proliferation of health advocacy, health activism, and health-related social movements. Bringing together the interdisciplinary study of health and illness with social movement theory, this chapter analyzes the goals and outcomes of political organizing around various health issues. It explores the goals, challenges, tactical strategies, and spirit of dissent of multiple social movements, with a focus on recent struggles in Canada.

CASE STUDY

Vaccination and the State

In 2014, the Ontario government made three more vaccines mandatory for schoolchildren, taking a hard stance against parents who failed to immunize their children. Students now had to be vaccinated against whooping cough, meningococcal disease, and chickenpox, in addition to six pre-existing required shots. These vaccines, part of the province's immunization schedule, are publicly funded. Unless parents apply for an exemption on religious or philosophical grounds, the province suspends students who have not been immunized.

Compulsory immunization laws are rare in Canada and only two other provinces (Manitoba and New Brunswick) have legislated vaccination policies for children entering school. Those in opposition to this policy feel that mandatory vaccination infringes on their constitutional rights. The so-called "Anti-Vaxx" movement gained substantial momentum after research, later revealed to by falsified, had linked the measles-mumps-rubella (MMR) vaccine to the development of autism spectrum disorders.

In the end, the debate juxtaposes the rights of the individual with the general public's right to health. The anti-vaccination movement is currently one of the most publicized health-related controversies in Canada.

Source: Born, Yiu, & Sullivan, 2014.

Theories on Social Justice

There are multiple meanings associated with the term *social justice*. It is a philosophical construct, as well as a political theory that dictates the shared obligations of the individual and society. In essence, social justice differs from the idea of individual justice as the latter applies only to obligations that exist between individuals. Also implicit in the concept of social justice is the notion that civil society is founded on the basis of a social contract. Through this contract we gain civil rights in return for accepting the obligation to honour the rights of others, giving up some of our own freedoms in the process.

Considerable disagreement persists among scholars over the definition of social justice. While there are many perspectives to consider, this section is primarily concerned with exploring how four dominant theories with very different perspectives apply to health.

The **libertarian** perspective on social justice supports the evolutionary yet impulsive creation of institutions. It opposes the creation of any institutions that challenge the distributive patterns of market order. Friedrich Hayek and Robert Nozick are two of the main proponents of the libertarian school of thought. For Hayek, judging individual outcomes based on conscious or deliberate actions is logical, but to apply this principle at a societal level is ineffective. Hayek's position is that market forces drive spontaneous, unexpected processes; we cannot causally link these phenomena to the decisions and actions of a central authority (Solimano,1998).

Similarly, Robert Nozick claims that social justice is an entitlement. He sees the distribution of resources as fair, so long as it is in agreement with three core principles:

1. Justice in acquisition—property may be acquired, as long as it is previously unowned. Theft, coercion, and fraud are unacceptable.
2. Justice in transfer—property may be transferred, as long as no theft, force, or fraud occurr in the transfer of said property.
3. Rectification—violations of the first two principles are to be rectified.

Nozick believes that individuals have a right to own property, which empowers them with the freedom to make decisions around what is theirs. Nozick argues for minimal state involvement and sees any state attempts to redistribute resources as unmerited. Additionally, Nozick does not see a need for the state to intervene in the lives of individuals who were born disadvantaged, like the poor or sick; rather, he states that individual charity should drive resource gifting for the disadvantaged. To Nozick, only two truths exist about resources: they are (1) preowned or (2) generated by individuals. They should not be seized by the state and redistributed for other purposes such as health care, poverty relief, or education (Solimano, 1998).

Classic utilitarians believe that the foundation of society is built around the mutual expectations and advantages of voluntary relationships. One of the more prominent utilitarians was John Stuart Mill. He argued that the delivery of societal goods should be for the "greatest net balance of satisfaction." This suggests that utility, that which is valued as good, should be shared accordingly to deliver the greatest good to the maximum number of people (Rescher, 1966). Society's organization should facilitate this delivery. This utilitarian perspective has been highlighted and reiterated as justification for numerous economic and social policies that benefit some groups over others. However, those who disagree with utilitarianism suggest that vulnerable populations are often affected at a greater rate than non-vulnerable populations. They may be further marginalized when they have to acquiesce for the good of those in privileged classes (Reamer, 2006).

The **Marxist** perspective differs sharply from the libertarian and utilitarian frameworks discussed above. The core of Marxist social justice is the right of subsistence. Subsistence rights are essential to sustain life (Peffer, 1990). The term refers to the right to things like nourishment, shelter, clothing, and medical care—the material essentials necessary to sustain life. There are three principles that underlie the Marxist perspective on social justice:

1. Rights to material resources—These should be positive and mutually beneficial. In other words, we as individuals benefit from a guaranteed minimum level of welfare. We also have an obligation to ensure basic living standards for others.
2. Individual duties to the natural rights of others—This position is also often championed by libertarians (an exception being the rigid guidelines around property rights that exclude ownership of any property that functions as a productive property).
3. Individuals should serve the common interest—Individuals may need to abandon interests that conflict with collective equity or aim to subvert social and economic equalities.

To summarize, these principles entail that individuals take on more than simply a moral burden for the basic well being of others. According to this theory, we have a commitment to promote human equality in all aspects of public and productive life.

John Rawls was one of the preeminent political philosophers of the twentieth century, and his concept of social justice is probably the most influential of the four theories discussed here. While most philosophers had dismissed the idea of the social contract by the start of the twentieth century, Rawls reinvented the concept through a "thought experiment," creating a theoretical account of the social contract. In essence, individuals would agree on how a just society is defined. He focused on elaborating the circumstances needed for a just social contract. Rawls argued that individuals would have to determine society's distribution of four primary goods: wealth and income, rights and liberties, opportunities for advancement, and self-respect. He believed that people would instinctively select tenets of social justice that benefited those in society who had no advantages. He criticized the utilitarian perspective as benefiting privileged classes of society. Rawls firmly believed in the idea that social values should be equally parcelled out, unless an imbalanced distribution would be fairer for society (1971). Rawls's original theory of social justice rested upon a few key principles:

1. Each person should have equal right to the most extensive system of personal liberties compatible with a system of total liberty for all.
2. Social and economic inequality should be arranged so that
    a) they benefit the least advantaged in society in the greatest way possible. (In other words, the least well off people are made as well off as possible—this could mean giving an unequal/greater amount to the people who are the least well off.);
    b) everyone in society has a fair and equal opportunity to obtain the social positions that permit them to make decisions about inequalities.

What does any of this have to do with health? Many people look to the state as a guarantor or provider of health and health care—these theories of social justice all address (in varying ways) health care as a human right. According to the libertarian perspective, the state should have as minimal a role as possible. It therefore envisions a very nominal social contract that rejects any claim of health care as a right. It assumes that individuals who desire a more fruitful array of services than those provided by the (minimalist) state will volunteer to join communities more reflective of their desires. Thus, the classic libertarian perspective opposes any positive right to health care.

Likewise, utilitarianism does not necessarily endorse health care as a basic human right. However, it does not rule out the possibility that health care may be universally offered if driven by social (i.e., government) policy. As long as a society determines that state-funded universal health care would be of maximum benefit to the majority of its members, it would be acceptable along utilitarian lines.

The Marxist perspective on social justice would argue that the health care system acts as a "mode of production" involving labour and collective ownership. Health care, if not provided unequivocally by the state, is commonly inferred as a recompense for labour. Therefore, the Marxist theory of social justice discussed previously concludes a universal positive entitlement to basic medical care (Peffer, 1990).

Finally, the **Rawlsian theory of social justice** provides for an entitlement to health care. In this theory, the right to health care rests upon two notions:

1. The difference principle—this idea posits that inequality within a just society can only exist if it is "of greatest benefit to the least advantaged members of society" (Rawls, 2001).
2. Fair equality of opportunity—society is obligated to provide "the general means necessary to underwrite fair equality of opportunity and our capacity to take advantage of our basic rights and liberties, and thus be normal and fully cooperating members of society over a complete life" (Rawls, 2001, p. 174).

Here, it becomes clear that Rawls considers the right to health care as fundamental in a free and equal society.

In conclusion, social justice is frequently in the background of debates around health care access and delivery in Canada and elsewhere. These theories are continually advanced and refined to help us think more critically about when health inequalities are just or unjust. They also help us to understand more clearly disparities in health care access and whether or not these are fair.

Health Advocacy and Activism

The previous section introduced students to the various theories of social justice and their application to health. This section discusses the politics of social justice by dissecting relationships between health activism and health advocacy and their role in challenging social injustice by using action that goes beyond the conventional or routine.

Health activism occurs when a marginalized group believes it is necessary to confront systemic inequities in the distribution of power and resources related to health. Such groups hope that, by illuminating power imbalances, distributions of privilege will be changed to give marginalized groups a greater say in health matters. The term *health activism* covers a wide spectrum of actions, each unique and specific to the type of change desired. Social movements have used health activism to accomplish broad, long-term goals. Geist-Martin, Berlin Ray, and Sharf (2003) state that health activism is born of an individual's desire for change that has broad social appeal; they cite actions such as lobbying, fundraising, and keeping health records as effective modes of health activism.

Additionally, health activism can be a mode of health citizenship, requiring citizens to become actively involved in individual and collective decision-making (Rimal, Ratzan, Arnston, & Freimut, 1997). For example, health consumer groups in the United Kingdom include patient groups centred on pain, illness, and loss. They are classified as voluntary organizations which seek to promote and represent the interests of patients with common experiences across a range of conditions such as heart disease, arthritis, cancer, and mental health (see Allsop, Jones, & Baggott, 2004).

Brown and Zavestoski (2004) differentiate between health activism and health advocacy. For them, health advocacy concentrates on education and functions within existing systems and the biomedical paradigm. Health advocacy is founded on experts within a system questioning existing principles and practices based on their knowledge and experience. They see health activism as a much more democratic process driven by the life experiences of lay people or celebrities. Jenny McCarthy's anti-vaccine campaign, for example, used personal narrative in an attempt to shift attitudes regarding vaccination policy. Both advocacy and activism attempt to change the status quo and alter research priorities. However, questions of conflict of interest and influence must always be considered in cases of activism: the rigour and scientific methods of advocacy are often absent from activism.

Health activism, according to Zoller (2005), can be viewed as a bottom-up social movement. Community organizers initiate grassroots campaigns to mobilize their fellow community members to effect change. In the campaign's initial state, the community organizers' grievances are typically localized, and similar communities or social groups may piggyback

CASE STUDY

Should Refugees Be Entitled to Canadian Health Care?

In 2012, Canada's federal government cut funding to refugee health care. Government ministers justified this decision on the basis that it would protect the immigration system from abuse. The Interim Federal Health (IFH) program had been designed to offer basic medical care for refugees who were waiting for their paperwork to be processed. Successful refugee claims would result in provincial health coverage, whereas unsuccessful claimants would be forced to exit Canada. The program, in place since 1957, has been the source of controversy.

Following cuts to the program, street demonstrations and legal challenges proliferated in protest. Refugee health experts and medical organizations from across Canada also registered their disapproval, arguing that this change would negatively impact refugees, spike medical costs, and affect Canada's international reputation.

Although the government remained firm in its decision, health advocacy did prompt some changes to the proposed legislation. The original draft revoked health care for all refugees, but subsequent revisions ensured that some refugees (most notably those whom the federal government invited) could continue to receive care. Additionally, many clinics and hospitals across the country took on the cost of refugee health care, with many physicians leading the charge against the changes. The Canadian Medical Association, for example, issued a statement indicating its firm opposition to the removal of the program, arguing that it violated basic medical ethics. Finally, some provinces have designed their own program to alleviate the damage caused by cuts.

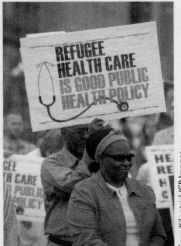

Following two years of demonstrations and legal challenges on the matter, the Federal Court ruled in July 2014 that the Canadian government's cuts to refugee health care constituted "cruel and unusual" treatment. However, only some of the cuts were reversed in the process.

Source: Adapted from Caudarella & Evans (2014)

on the movement. In turn, this broadens and further mobilizes the community's action. While top-down initiatives led by local elites also have the power to effect change, Zoller (2005) argues that this strategy has often worsened the condition of communities.

Understanding Social Movements

What is a social movement? The most extensive definition is offered by Castels (1996), who describes such movements as collective actions that transform the values and institutions of a society. Social movements challenge the boundaries between state and society, public and private. They bring the private into the realm of the public, and show how the private is political and how the state, too, is rife with "private" power relationships. The environmental movement would be an example of one such social movement. Social movements may also challenge dominant definitions of knowledge and science in the health field. In this way, movements aim to shift culture and knowledge, not just public policy (Orsini, 2008). Third, social movements are often said to engage in "repertoires of contention." That is, these movements may utilize radical strategies and tactics, sometimes tending towards the confrontational. Movements are often decentralized, democratic organizations or networks.

Smith (2014) attempts to close the gap between social movements and other representational vehicles such as interest and advocacy groups. First, she sees similarities in what they do. Interest groups arise from a sense of shared identity and use a variety of tactics to pursue their members' agendas. Social movements may engage in the narrow lobbying and representation often associated with interest groups. Second, she sees social movements as having purposive action while involving a network of actors and institutions. As such, interest groups, and indeed political parties, get bound up in these movements, becoming vehicles of representation of the identities and goals of social movements.

A final point in Smith's discussion urges us to avoid the trap of deifying social movements. Just as political parties come in all sorts of ideological colours, including racist and xenophobic ones, so too do social movements. Even in cases where an individual may identify with the values and goals of a social movement, it is worth bearing in mind that such movements, like political parties, makes decisions and choices that are open to critique.

Social change creates spaces for new identities and interests to form, and social movements aim to define and defend these identities and interests. Movements form vehicles to interact with the state, seeking to change state structures and policies; in turn, the state changes.

On the whole, social movements create a sense of shared identity for their members; naming, blaming, and claiming are three critical components of the preparatory phase of social movements.

- Naming identifies the problem. Some examples could include a sense of a lack of fulfillment, an individual psychological problem, or the patriarchal nuclear family. The naming process enables people to see that they share a problematic situation and fosters a sense of collective identity.
- The blaming phase sets out a series of relationships and begins to suggest who is to blame for the state of affairs. For example, patient groups may blame regulatory drug agencies for not approving new and potentially life-saving medications.

- Last, the claiming phase transitions from blaming someone or something to making claims for change to end whatever hurt or injustice has been identified. One example of this process would be a social movement pushing for the establishment of a government inquiry into inappropriate medical practices at a local hospital. Such an inquiry might lead to financial compensation for those who were injured by these harmful practices.

In developing identities and making claims of interest, social movements are working within the world they know. While social movements contest certain social relationships or ways of seeing the world, they may unconsciously treat others as natural, or even actively reinforce them as a way of trying to rally support and legitimacy. Idle No More is an example of a social movement that represents changing patterns of engagement among Indigenous peoples. Broadly speaking, its adherents aim to retain their culture and identities while reinforcing links among Indigenous people worldwide. Thus, Aboriginal communities have developed a sense of solidarity to fight what has impacted many of them. In the Canadian context, the Idle No More movement has drawn considerable attention to the vast health disparities between Aboriginal and non-Aboriginal peoples.

There tends to be a cyclical nature to social movements: we see periods of mobilization, where new organizations appear and new frameworks are created, and then periods of demobilization when these movements wind down. Mobilization appears to be tied to opportunity more than deprivation—a sense that successes are within reach. The social movement literature draws our attention to what are sometimes called political opportunity structures—features of the external political environment that affect the ability of movements to challenge authorities (Tarrow, 2005). Such elements of the political environment, like the accessibility of the political system, instability in political alignments, or having influential allies, incentivize people to undertake collective action. This can affect their odds of success or failure. Movements mobilize in reaction to a favourable political opportunity structure, but they also change that structure by altering policy and state institutions. They can also domesticate movements by drawing them in to routinized forms of interaction (i.e., the traditional way of doing things), sapping the movement's imagination and resources. New state institutions can also co-opt leaders of social movements into bureaucratic jobs. At the same time, however, these changes also link the social movement to the state. With a closer relationship to the state, social movements may receive a sympathetic hearing and get advanced information of upcoming social changes, enabling them to produce policy expertise and relevant research. In short, there are both advantages and disadvantages for health social movements developing closer ties to government.

Masson (2012) discusses the complex relationship between social movements and the state. She asks questions, for example, about how women's organizations affect government policy. Masson develops two theoretical arguments. The first is about scale and argues that opportunities for social movements are shaped in part by state structure. As such, social movements have to strategically tailor their strategies to these institutions, bearing in mind the distribution of responsibilities between national and regional levels. In the case of Canada, some responsibilities rest firmly with the federal government (such as defence), whereas many social responsibilities, such as education and health, are primarily provincial concerns. In hoping to alter many health care policies, it would thus make most sense to target provincial institutions, such as the ministry of health. Alternatively, one can contest this existing distribution of power and demand that decisions be taken elsewhere, perhaps by lobbying for the federal government to become more involved in matters traditionally left to the provinces. For example, consider Canadian health care. Provincial governments have the constitutional power to make health care decisions, yet the "Save Medicare" campaign tends to focus on national standards. This approach may be ineffective if there is not enough support for changing where the decision is taken, and individual provinces may start dismantling the system if the federal government is otherwise preoccupied.

Why do people bother forming specific (health) interest groups and movements? After all, political parties provide an obvious way to come together and represent specific interests though democratic institutions. With that in mind, why do those in power pay attention to social movements and allow them to have influence? Here are three key ideas:

1. Political parties may lack a clear mandate: Even when platforms detail what a party plans to do, they can never hit all of the key details; those details may be worth fighting over. Take, for example, Stephen Harper's Conservative government's decision to rescind Canada's support for the Kyoto Protocol—an international agreement that promotes health by binding governments to act on climate change. The government claimed to be in favour of an alternative climate change strategy but never explained the specific details of what this alternative plan might look like. With no clear plan, groups with a stake in climate change policies, ranging from environmentalist organizations to oil companies, attempted to influence the government's approach to this policy. Now take a field that is not as politically volatile as climate change, such as the issue of fertilizer run-off from farming activities. The resulting pollution of rural rivers and streams was not a hot issue in past federal and provincial elections, but governments must still create a policy on this issue. Political parties may approach this issue with different ideas about how active the government should be in environmental regulation and so forth. Without any sort of clear mandate on the issue, however, government officials are likely to listen to those groups with a direct interest in the matter to get a sense of the best course of action. In this instance, social movements would be ideally placed to try and influence policy on this matter.

2. Representation: Despite problems of accountability, social movements can claim to speak for certain interests. They demonstrate their dedication to these issues by maintaining a membership and mobilizing it through letter writing campaigns, demonstrations, and so on. Political parties, interested in winning votes, may need to be responsive to some demands. Thus, health social movements can help shift policy by encouraging political parties to develop specific stances on particular issues.

3. Expertise: Some groups have more knowledge about certain topics than the government does. In the case of new reproductive technologies, for instance, certain groups got a hearing with the government because they could claim expertise about the technical, legal, and scientific issues surrounding these technologies.

A Look at Health Social Movements

The previous section discussed the importance of social movements in general. This section defines these movements more specifically as they relate to health issues. For many years, a concerted and organized class of social movements has consistently challenged political and scientific authority. These are known as health social movements (HSMs) (Brown, 2011). The structural organization of HSMs is often bottom-up. They have been highly successful in effecting social change in areas ranging from improving the occupational health of workers in the Industrial Revolution to advocating for women's health through the modern-day feminist movement (Brown et al., 2004). Advances in AIDS research, funding, and treatment are direct results of HSM activists (Epstein, 1996). More recent HSM activity is reflected in the way medical research practices are carried out (Morgen, 2002).

HSMs also challenge the way we think about individual and collective identity. As Michael Orsini (2008, p. 480) points out,

> [w]hile some might assume that the primary challenge for some HSMs, especially those representing persons living with stigmatizing conditions, might be to mobilize supporters in the first place, one of the most interesting features of such movements has been their ability not only to do so but also to include interested people who are not actually affected by the condition or illness.

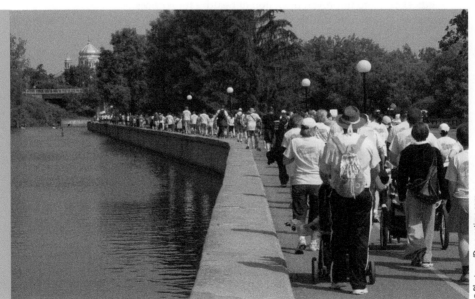

© Photawa/Dreamstime.com

The breast cancer movement, with its distinctive use of pink, has successfully become one of the most prominent and well-marketed social movements in health, having become sufficiently influential in its activism to involve people who do not have experience with breast cancer themselves. What can other movements learn from this one? What negative aspects are there to health care movements that have outgrown their grassroots origins?

The breast cancer movement is one such example, especially when we consider some of its more radical offshoots that focus their attention on the environmental causes of cancer. This particular group has the ability to mobilize women who are not living with breast cancer. It is also important to point out that in addition to the regular challenges those involved in movements encounter, many HSM activists also face the additional burden of being ill, which can hinder their ability to mobilize.

HSMs may contest social issues in different ways. For some HSMs, the main challenge is to move scientifically legitimate medical conditions, which are accepted within official circles, onto the political agenda (Brown et al., 2004). For example, if we look at asthma, activists do not need to spend a significant amount of time convincing others that it is a legitimate medical condition. Instead, asthma offers an opportunity to challenge wider environmental issues that disproportionately affect people living with asthma. A further example relates to high rates of diabetes among Canada's Aboriginal population. While no one would dispute the fact that diabetes is a legitimate chronic disease, there is a more concerted effort to address the reality that Aboriginal populations are more severely affected by diabetes.

Brown and his colleagues (2004) divide HSMs into three categories. These include:

1. **Health access movements**—as their name implies, these focus on equitable access to medical care and improved provision of health care services.
2. **Constituency-based health movements** focus on health inequalities among groups and may be based on structures of identification like race, ethnicity, or gender.
3. **Embodied health movements**—these focus on the experience of disease and illness, addressing etiology, diagnosis, treatment and prevention.

The authors acknowledge that the boundaries of these categories may blur and movements may fit into one or more of these categories. For example, they argue that environmental justice movements can be both embodied and constituency-based because they are established by people with an illness or fear of illness while still addressing inequality. Conceptually, it is difficult to determine the difference between these two categories because many embodied health movements (e.g., breast cancer, AIDS) are focused on inequalities among different people as they address diagnosis, treatment, and prevention. The differences between these three categories are further discussed below.

Health Access Movements

Health access movements seek to improve the accessibility, quality, and delivery of medical care (Zoller, 2005). These movements utilize activities such as labour campaigns and patient activism to enhance doctor–patient relations. Historically, medical care workers have used activism to force changes in care delivery. Health access movements can also consist of identity-based advocates, who aim to increase sensitivity in medicine while improving access for Indigenous populations and other similar groups. For example, Aboriginal peoples living in Canada experience their own particular challenges with health care and are linked with wider community-oriented advocacy and activism. The health care needs of Aboriginal communities, however, can often become lost in government bureaucracy. All permanent residents, including First Nations people living on reserves, are supposed to be provided with full access to health care services as per the Canada Health Act. However, many health care services are not available in First Nations communities, despite legal requirement—a problem highlighted by health access movements.

Constituency-Based Health Movements

Constituency-based health movements address health inequality and health inequity based on race, class, gender, ethnicity, or sexual differences (Brown, 2011). Constituency-based groups address unbalanced outcomes and unsound science, and try to identify any oversights by the scientific community. Examples would be the women's health movement, the gay and lesbian health movement, and the environmental justice movement. The women's health movement also contains elements of both health access social movements and embodied health movements. For example, the women's health movement aims to increase access to health services for women, a characteristic of health access social movements, but also challenges assumptions about psychiatric diagnoses for premenstrual symptoms, a characteristic of an embodied health movement. Brown and his colleagues (2004, p. 53) note that "by virtue of having a large categorical constituency, the women's health movement directly raises issues of sex differences and gender discrimination, and it represents a large population with specific interests, so that the constituency nature is significant."

Similarly, members of the environmental justice movement are normally concerned with their own health and/or their fear of illness. However, on a wider scale, they are also concerned with the health effects of polluting facilities and their impacts on marginalized populations. As a result, these organizations have similarities to both health access-based movements and constituency-based health movements (Brown, 2011).

Embodied Health Movements

More recently, scholars have called our attention to the development of HSMs focused on a specific illness or disease. Classified as embodied health movements, these groups bring together individuals who may share a common experience of illness and who, frequently, seek to create awareness and alter political and scientific policy regarding their condition. In doing so, these groups challenge dominant medical and scientific ideas about their condition. One famous example can be seen among early AIDS activist groups, where activists used the same organizational and political skills honed in the gay and lesbian rights movement to raise awareness of and create action on AIDS. Ultimately, these groups successfully influenced policymakers and played a central role in shifting scientific and medical thought around HIV treatment (Epstein, 1996).

Health as a Driver of Social Movements

Why is it necessary to pay attention to HSMs? Orsini (2008) argues that the attainment of health is becoming a dominant theme in politics because policy-makers are interested in reflecting the needs and desires of citizens. Some scholars view this popular concern with health as healthism, a contemporary ideology focused on the importance of health and wellness.

Health has always been a concern, of course, but why has it taken on such urgency today? There are many varied answers to this question. Sociologist Frank Furedi (2005) argues that there are four possible factors that account for our current focus on health:

1. *The imperative of medicalization.* In essence, the notion of medicalization means that problems we encounter in everyday life are reformulated as medical ones. Thus, medical labels are attached to everyday experiences that were previously understood as a normal part of life. As described in other chapters within this book, medicalizing seems to have accelerated in recent years.
2. *Illness is now as "normal" as health.* Early theories of medicalization viewed being healthy as the norm, with sickness being an outlier. Today, the scales have balanced: sickness and health are viewed as equal occurrences. Even healthy individuals are viewed as potentially ill. Illness is now a part of our collective identity.
3. *Health as a moral compass for human experience.* Natural, organic foods and medicines are explicitly viewed as morally superior to processed or genetically modified alternatives. Our cultural narrative emphasizes the importance of health in determining our livelihood.
4. *The politicization of health.* Politicians have capitalized on the issue of health for personal benefit. Politicians may gain a political benefit from emphasizing health issues in their platforms, or could benefit financially through the contributions of pharmaceutical companies. Either way, politicians prey on the public's fixation on health care by continually making it an issue. As a result, our society feels more ill.

CASE STUDY

The Politics of Stem Cell Research

In November 1998, scientists successfully isolated and cultured human embryonic stem cells. For the previous twenty years, this achievement had eluded researchers, so the scientific community was abuzz. This announcement proved to be the beginning of an intense and unrelenting debate between those in favour of embryonic stem cell research and those who oppose it. No other health issue has generated such a level of political activism in the United States and elsewhere.

Some scholars consider the activism surrounding stem cell research as the most significant case of public engagement in recent history. This grassroots movement led to a radical transformative experience. Staunch advocates of stem cell research include scientists and patients who believe that embryonic stem cell research is the key to developing new treatments and cures for some of humanity's most pernicious afflictions—for example, brain diseases such as Alzheimer's and Parkinson's, and more general health disorders such as heart disease and diabetes.

The most vocal dissent over stem cell research comes from those who have a shared desire to heal but feel that this research crosses ethical boundaries. The political jostling as to how to pursue this type of research has sparked a health social movement that has shaped and influenced policy more than any other similar movement in the past three decades. The unpredictable alliances and partnerships around the common cause of curing disease have broken through the gridlock of partisan politics, uniting people from various political parties and backgrounds. The leaders of this movement understand the power of community voices and use that to gain leverage.

Source: Solo & Pressburg (2007).

Chapter Summary

At the beginning of this chapter, students were asked to consider how we balance the duty of the state to protect the health of citizens against the right of individuals to define and pursue their own health as they see fit. How much power should the state have over us and how can we influence the state to ensure that it always serves our interests? Keeping these questions in mind, the goal of this chapter was to introduce students to the different theories of social justice and how these movements aim to maximize health equality and health care rights. This chapter demonstrated the roles of health advocacy and health activism, and explored the ideologies and ideas that underpin them. In addition, this chapter examined several health social movements that have emerged to improve situations for individuals and for specific populations.

To summarize, the first section discussed the term *social justice* and its many different connotations. The section highlighted that, in its most basic sense, social justice is a philosophical construct that determines the mutual obligations between an individual and society. Students were introduced to four specific theories of social justice—libertarian, utilitarian, Marxist, and Rawlsian—and how each of these theories varies in their analysis of health care. The analysis of these theories focused particularly on the question of health as a basic human right.

The chapter then moved on to discuss the politics of social justice, contrasting health activism with health advocacy and examining how these methods challenge social injustice. We then talked about social movements—what they are and how they differ from other types of interest and pressure groups. Finally, the discussion concluded with an investigation of health social movements and their ability to challenge the way we think about individual and collective identity. Students learned about three types of health social movements: health access movements, constituency-based health movements, and embodied health movements.

There are two central messages that students should take away after reading this chapter. First, students should consider how much control the state should have over our health and what role individuals have in negotiating this matter. The hope is that students now have a deeper understanding of what citizens are capable of doing and how like-minded individuals can come together to influence change. Second, we should consider what it means to create a health care system that reflects the values of social justice. Increasingly, there are attempts to frame health in the context of social justice, as demonstrated in the case of asthma. Overall, a critical look at health activism, health advocacy, and health movements allows us to better understand the connections among politics, social justice, and health.

STUDY QUESTIONS

1. Why do we need so many different definitions of social justice? How do they differ?
2. How plausible is the assumption that those affected by an issue will mobilize to react to, change, or improve it?
3. What role should the state play in vaccinations?
4. What should Canada's policy on refugee health care be? Does advocacy make a difference in influencing the state on this issue?
5. What are the primary similarities and differences among the various types of HSMs?

SUGGESTED READINGS

Crossley, N. (2006). *Contesting psychiatry: Social movements in mental health*. London: Routledge.
Dumit, J. (2006). Illnesses you have to fight to get: facts as forces in uncertain, emergent illnesses. *Social Science & Medicine, 62*(3), 577–90.
Laverack, G. (2013). *Health activism: Foundations and strategies*. London: Sage Publications Ltd.
Nahuis, R. & Boon, W. P. (2011). The impact of patient advocacy: The case of innovative breast cancer drug reimbursement. *Sociology of Health & Illness, 33*(1), 1–15.

SUGGESTED WEB RESOURCES

Garrett, J. (2005, August 24). Rawls' Mature Theory of Social Justice: http://people.wku.edu/jan. garrett/ethics/matrawls.htm
Onyegbula, I (2013). Refugee Healthcare Cuts in Canada (Spoken word poem): www.youtube. com/watch?v=zHthlErCOLU
Patient Commando: http://patientcommando.com

GLOSSARY

Classic utilitarianism   A political theory stating that all relationships are voluntary and, as such, the distribution of goods and services should do the most good for the greatest number of people.
Constituency-based health movements   Focus on health discrepancies between members of different demographics or constituencies, e.g., those of a certain race, gender, or sexuality (see Brown et al., 2004).
Embodied health movements   Bring together people who experience particular illnesses or diseases to advocate to increase awareness, raise funds, or alter policies.

Health access movements Health social movements that focus on ensuring adequate access to medical care for everyone in society (see Brown et al., 2004).

Healthism The idea that, through making proper lifestyle choices, one can be proactive in maintaining one's health or becoming healthier. An emphasis on an individual's responsibility for their health.

Libertarianism A political ideology that emphasizes individual rights and argues for minimal state intervention into the lives of individuals.

Marxism A political theory centred on the idea that socio-economic divisions within a society drive its evolution. Generally speaking, Marxists believe that all members of society should have access to the basic needs of life (e.g., food, water, medical care, housing, employment).

Rawlsian theory of social justice The political philosophy of John Rawls (1971). Centres on the concept of a "social contract" in which individuals define their own concept of a just society. Ideally this society would distribute wealth and power equally among all of its citizens.

Social movements Groups of individuals mobilized around a common cause.

REFERENCES

Allsop, J., Jones, K., & Baggott, R. (2004). Health consumer groups in the UK: A new social movement? *Sociology of Health and Illness, 26*(6), 737–56.

Born, K., Yiu, V., & Sullivan, T. (2014). Provinces divided over mandatory vaccination for school children. HealthyDebate.ca, 22 May 2014. Web.

Brown, P. (2011). *Contested illnesses: Citizens, science, and health social movements.* Oakland, CA: University of California Press.

———— & Zavestoski, S. (2004). Social movements in health: An introduction. *Sociology of Health & Illness, 26,* 679–94.

————, Zavestoski, S., McCormick, S., Mayer, B., Morello-Frosch, R., & Gasior Altman, R. (2004). Embodied health movements: New approaches to social movements in health. *Sociology of Health & Illness, 26*(1), 50–80.

Castells, M. (1996). *The rise of the network society, the information age: Economy, society and culture.* Malden, MA: Blackwell Publishers.

Caudarella, A., & A. Evans, Ending health care for refugees has put children in grave danger," *Ottawa Citizen,* 15 May 2014. http://www.theglobeandmail.com/globe-debate/ending-health-care-for-refugees-has-put-children-in-grave-danger/article18679568/

Epstein, S. (1996). *Impure Science.* Berkeley, CA: University of California Press.

Furedi, F. (2005). Our unhealthy obsession with sickness. Spiked. 23 March 2005. http://www.spiked-online.com/newsite/article/1174#.VXkBmPlVhBc

Geist-Martin, P., Berlin Ray, E. C., & Sharf, B. F. (2003). *Communicating health: Personal, cultural, and political complexities.* Belmont, CA: Thomson/Wadsworth.

Masson, D. (2012). Changing state forms, competing state projects: Funding women's organizations in Quebec. *Studies in Political Economy, 80,* 79–103.

Morgen, S. (2002). *Into Our Own Hands: the Women's Health Movement in the United States, 1969–1990.* New Brunswick: Rutgers University Press.

Orsini, M. (2008). Health social movements: The next wave in contentious politics? In M. Smith (Ed.), *Group politics and social movements in Canada* (pp. 475–98). Peterborough, ON: Broadview Press.

Peffer, R. G. (1990). *Marxism, morality, and social justice.* Princeton, NJ: Princeton University Press.

Phillips, S. D. (2004). Interest groups, social movements and the voluntary sector: En route to reducing the democratic deficit. In J. Bickerton & A. G. Gagnon (Eds), *Canadian politics* (4th ed., pp. 323–47). Peterborough, ON: Broadview Press.

Rawls, J. (1971) *A Theory of justice.* Cambridge, MA: Harvard University Press.

————. (2001) *Justice as fairness.* Cambridge, MA: Harvard University Press.

Rescher, N. (1966). *Distributive justice: A constructive critique of the utilitarian theory of distribution* New York: Bobbs-Merrill.

Rimal, R. N., Ratzan, S., Arntson, P., & Freimuth, V. S. (1997). Reconceptualizing the "patient": Healthcare promotion as increasing citizens' decision-making competencies. *Health Communication, 9,* 61–74.

Smith, M. (2014). *Group politics and social movements in Canada* (2nd ed.). Toronto: University of Toronto Press Higher Education, 2014.

Solimano, A. (Ed.). (1998). Alternative theories of distributive justice and social inequality: Liberal, socialist, and libertarian perspectives. *Social inequality: Values, growth and the state.* MI: University of Michigan Press.

Solo, P. & Pressberg, G. (2007). *The promise and politics of stem cell research.* Westport, CA: Praeger Publishers.

Tarrow, S. (2005). *The new transnational activism.* New York, NY: Cambridge University Press.

Warmington, R. & Lin, D. (2014). Healthcare is political: Case example of physician advocacy in response to the cuts to refugees' and claimants' healthcare coverage under the Interim Federal Health Program. *University of Ottawa Journal of Medicine, 4*(1), 45–8.

World Health Organization. (1948). World Health Organization constitution. *Basic documents,* 1.

Zoller, H. (2005). Health activism: Communication theory and action for social change. *Health Communication, 15,* 341–64.

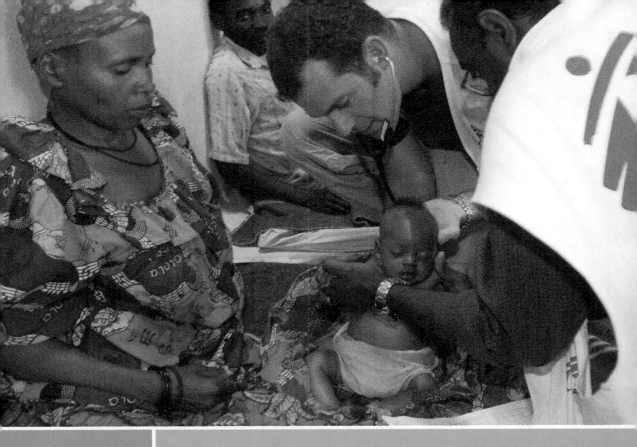

7

Globalization and Health

Leigh-Anne Gillespie and James Gillett

LEARNING OBJECTIVES

In this chapter, students will learn

- how globalization relates to individual health
- the specific drivers of globalization such as global market forces, technological developments, international trade, migration, and health
- how the effects of globalization shape responses to current and emergent health concerns and crises
- the concept of "One Health" and its use in understanding the ethical dimensions of local and international responses to health concerns and crises

Introduction

What is **globalization**? Globalization is a relatively recent term but the processes it describes stretch back as far as when people first began to migrate, trade, socialize, and communicate with one another around the globe. The current use of the term is often credited to Theodore Levitt, a professor in the Business School at Harvard. In 1983, he identified that many corporations were beginning to move beyond the conventional regional, national, and even multinational boundaries that regulate and structure economic activity. He suggested that a "globalization of markets" was emerging, transforming economies and social lives across the globe (Levitt, 1983). With advances in technology, especially in the spheres of communication, transportation, and economic production, corporations began to act as if there were a single global market for the buying and selling of goods and services. Corporations like Coca-Cola and McDonalds recognized the possibility of selling the exact same product, produced in the exact same way, to virtually everyone around the world, regardless of citizenship or geographic location (Ger & Belk, 1996).

The current use of the term *globalization* is more expansive and nuanced. The term has been used so extensively and in so many different ways that it is difficult to form a precise definition. From a critical social science perspective, it is helpful to look at the concept of globalization as a series of related complex and dynamic processes. In very broad terms, the process of globalization refers to the unrestrained flows of capital, commodities, ideas, technologies, people, and even pollution across international borders (Di Chiro, 2004). This rise of global flows contributes to "globality"—the process by which the entire planet is experienced and conceptualized as a single social space (Pal, 2010). This idea is more practically illustrated in the idea of "glocalization," a term popularized by sociologist Roland Robertson: the global expressed in the local, and the local as a particularization of the global (Beyer, 2007).

This process is akin to the rise of global flows that challenge and strain existing social relations and institutional structures. Along this line, Appadurai (1996) identifies five dimensions to the process of globalization which influence different social spheres:

- *Ethnoscapes* (the geographical flow of groups such as tourists, immigrants, and refugees)
- *Technoscapes* (the flow of goods and ideas through modes of communication and other technologies of transportation)
- *Mediascapes* (the flow of an increasing number of images around the globe through the media)
- *Ideoscapes* (ideas, terms, and images constructed locally and spread globally)
- *Financescapes* (the unpredictable and fluid flow of commodities and economic exchange)

The five different spheres are not mutually exclusive but rather intersect. Across each it is possible to identify the global flows that make the fabric of social life more fluid and interconnected. In short, everything affects everything.

Globalization and Health

According to Joseph Stiglitz, the Nobel laureate in economics, the process of globalization is "neither good nor bad" (2003, p. 20). Rather, it is the consequences of these global flows that are beneficial or detrimental. For instance, on the positive side, as our society becomes more global, we become more aware of the issues and problems in different parts of the world. We understand how issues that affect us may also affect the entire planet, as in the case of climate change. At the same time, the opening of global marketplaces also creates economic inequalities. Small groups of people control most of the wealth and power; Freeland (2012) calls these individuals "plutocrats," the new global super-rich. In each of these instances, both good and bad, the consequences of globalization influence the health of individuals and populations.

To analyze this issue further, the chapter now explores three key dimensions of globalization. Using case studies, we will delve into specific ways that an increasing global society intersects with the health of individuals, populations, and non-human species. The first dimension that will be explored considers the political and economic flows of globalization. How do these benefit the wealthy while placing the health of the most vulnerable at risk? We illustrate the health consequences of this global political economy through the case of a lead poisoning epidemic in Northern Nigeria. The second dimension is the emergence of an international and global ethic of responsibility in responding to epidemics and other health crises. Organizations dedicated to humanitarian efforts, such as Doctors Without Borders, have proliferated with globalization. Most of these groups address, either directly or indirectly, the health of individuals in developing countries, especially during crises. The third dimension concerns global cultural politics in which the meaning of health and illness shifts in response to global flows of knowledge and information. The chapter traces the emergence of One Health, a movement that advocates for an understanding of health based on the interdependency between human and non-human species in a broad ecological and global context. Across the three dimensions, students will be asked to consider the ethical and moral questions arising from an increasingly globalized world. These types of questions are not just of interest to philosophers; students are also invited to engage in the ethical and moral considerations of globalization and health raised in this chapter.

Global Political Economy

In early 2012, human rights organizations began reporting on a lead poisoning epidemic occurring in Northern Nigeria. Thousands of children and adults were affected as a result of contaminated working conditions in gold mines (Human Rights Watch, 2012). At first glance, the epidemic can be attributed to the high levels of lead in the soil extracted during mining operations. The mining corporations, in their eagerness to extract the gold, did not sufficiently educate their workers or protect them from the harmful effects of the lead. While the facts here are correct, this understanding is only part of the overall story. It neglects to consider the ethical and moral dimensions of unfair labour practices, including the use of children as workers. Moreover, there are social, political, and economic factors tied to the process of globalization that situate this crisis in a broader context. To understand this concept, it is necessary to briefly discuss what we mean by a global political economy and how it relates to health.

The field of **political economy** derives from a long tradition of trying to understand the relationship between democratic governments and the economy. Dating back to the eighteenth century, early political economists were concerned with the interdependent relationship between politics and economics. Continuing in this tradition, taking a political economic perspective means assessing how the state and the market are intertwined at any specific historical moment (Hall, 1997). Currently, we live in a market-focused society where the role of government is in tension with, and potentially being replaced by, the marketplace. Further, economic relations are happening on a global scale. They are shaped by the global flows that we described earlier: corporations can do business almost anywhere with anyone while being independent of most, if not all, regulations set by government or international organizations. This unbridled global economic activity often has detrimental effects on health.

This unregulated global marketplace came under scrutiny during the 2008 financial crisis. Skeptics questioned the distributive efficiency of markets—that is, whether the marketplace alone could provide the means necessary for people to live healthy and dignified lives. The crisis prompted widespread concern that markets had become detached from moral values (Sandel, 2012). In a lecture presented at the Canadian Museum for Human Rights, environmental activist and author Vandana Shiva (2014) suggests that we have "shrunk our humanity" by giving legal personhood to corporations. A corporation is not a person. It is a construction we have created for doing business. But its rights have been elevated beyond the rights of real human beings. Corporations have privatized nearly every life-giving force, commodity, and process on the planet. In Shiva's view, consumerism demeans what it means to be human. According to Sandel (2012), "the logic of buying and selling no longer applies to material goods alone but increasingly governs the whole of life. It is time to ask whether we want to live this way" (p. 6).

To understand the influence of private financial corporations and public international economic institutions such as the World Trade Organization (WTO), the World Bank (WB), and the International Monetary Fund (IMF), it is necessary to understand **neoliberalism**. This expression of a global political economy drives policies in governments, corporations, and international governing bodies. As described by Harvey (2005, p. 2),

> [n]eoliberalism is a theory of political economic practices that proposes that human wellbeing can best be advanced by liberating individual entrepreneurial freedoms and skills with an institutional framework characterized by strong private property rights, free markets and free trade. The role of the state is to create and preserve ... those military, defense, police, and legal structures and functions required to secure private property rights and to guarantee, by force if need be, the proper functioning of markets. Furthermore, if markets do not exist (in areas such as land, water, education, healthcare, social security or environmental pollution) then they must be created, by state action if necessary.

According to Gaynor and Vogt (1997), in a democratic society in which government and the marketplace are intertwined, people in positions of influence will often tend toward self-interest. Looking critically at the effects of neoliberalism on a global scale raises questions like the following: Who are the actors involved and what interests do they pursue? What is the role of the government and corporations in giving advantage to some while neglecting others? What are the implications of globalization in identifying how a problem is defined, and what solutions can solve the problem?

Using the following case study, we will apply a political economy approach to analyze the important social, political, and economic forces that affected the Nigerian lead-poisoning epidemic. What caused this event? As Pringle and Cole (2012) explain, while lead-rich ore was a natural occurrence, the neoliberal context was not. The Nigerian lead-poisoning epidemic occurred within a context of poverty, inequality, high gold prices, and lack of essential health care provision. High gold prices, as a result of the recent global financial crisis, created an opportunity for poor local villagers and subsistence farmers to supplement meagre incomes. This will be explored further in the case study below.

Under the present rules of the world economy, accumulation of profits often comes at the cost of violating human rights. Many human beings struggle to meet their basic needs. In 2010, 18 percent of the world's population lived in extreme poverty, and 64 percent of these people lived in just five countries: India, China, Nigeria, Bangladesh, and the Democratic Republic of Congo (World Bank, 2014).

CASE STUDY

The 2010 Nigerian Lead-Poisoning Epidemic

In Yargalma, a small village in northern Nigeria, a mysterious illness befell large numbers of village children in February 2010. Although local health workers did their best to try to save the children, the antimalarial drugs they used proved totally ineffective. Many children died and many more arrived at the clinic, complaining of a range of symptoms including lethargy, fever, vomiting, weight loss, partial paralysis, and seizures. Within a few weeks, volunteers from the international health group Médecins Sans Frontières (Doctors Without Borders) arrived, but they too could not treat the disease. After blood samples were sent to a German lab for analysis, the results showed that many children had shockingly high levels of lead in their blood—up to thirty times beyond what is normally considered a "fatal" level. In the meantime, many more children in the region died.

Eventually, it became clear that the first deaths had occurred just as Yargalma villagers had stepped up gold-extraction activities in the village. As a result of the global financial crisis, the price of gold had shot up and poor subsistence farmers hoped to use this opportunity to improve their meagre incomes by extracting flakes of gold from the soil. As they dug up the earth, they were inadvertently creating the conditions for a lead poisoning epidemic.

The story of Yargalma and the surrounding region cannot be disentangled from wider global events. The same global financial crisis that had encouraged local farmers to engage in this dangerous form of informal mining had also caused many governments to prioritize economic recovery over public health programs (Beaglehole & Bonita, 1998). That these governments chose this path was no mere fluke: international financial institutions like the World Bank and IMF had long pushed the notion that economic development along the lines of the free market was a necessary precondition for participating in the global economy. As a result, "wasteful spending" on public health services and government regulation (of activities like mining) was cut. The dearth of domestic services meant that international agencies, like Médecins Sans Frontières, had to fill the gap.

Source: Pringle and Cole (2012).

A driving idea behind globalization is **free market capitalism**. This concept stresses that countries will thrive when they participate in the world economy and allow global economic pressures to penetrate their domestic economies (Pal, 2010). But the goals of increased efficiency, enhanced quality, and improved allocation are not always realized; participation in the global free market often adversely affects poorer countries by worsening conditions of poverty and inequality (Haque, 2002). As Blin and Marín (2012) explain, "the only law [a capitalist market] obeys is profit and, under the guise of freedom and the purpose of serving the consumer, it generates intense predatory activity that favours the wealthy and powerful and crushes the weak and the poor" (p. 9).

Many countries are forced to participate in the world economy on mostly unfavourable terms (George, 1999). For example, while rich countries can protect their markets (with tariffs, duties, quotas, subsidies, or export credits), trade barriers make it difficult for poor countries to export their products and compete in world markets (Pogge, 2013). Pharmaceuticals are another example. Intellectual property rights, which lead to high prices for medicine, prohibit poor people from buying advanced medicine. Consequently, many people die. While medicine can be made more cheaply through companies that produce "generic drugs," it is now more difficult to do so under new rules of the WTO (Pogge, 2013).

As in the case of lead poisoning in Nigeria, the imperative for global corporations to profit comes at the expense of the lives of those most vulnerable. Developing countries are often unable, either politically or economically, to exert control over working conditions or ensure environmental responsibility. The health of citizens is jeopardized accordingly. International humanitarian organizations try to raise awareness and lend support to initiatives which address the income inequalities and human rights violations that result from global political economic flows. This chapter now turns to **global humanitarianism**, a movement that has expanded in response to situations like that in Nigeria. These humanitarian groups emphasize that health is a basic human right for all people, regardless of location, and that violations of this right require response.

Global Ethic of Responsibility

In 2014, the World Health Organization (WHO) published its report on global humanitarian responses, detailing the need for relief in the most vulnerable countries (WHO, 2014). In this assessment, it was estimated that over 81 million people were in need of humanitarian assistance and aid. According to the report (p. 7), the key factors behind the need for assistance are

> related to displacement, chronic food insecurity, and malnutrition. The main factors driving these priority needs are multi-hazard environments characterized by insecurity, disasters associated with natural hazards, climatic variation and environmental degradation, extreme chronic poverty, and political instability.

In the case of the Democratic Republic of the Congo, for example, there are 6.4 million people in the country in need of assistance. Aid for these individuals would require over $830 million (US dollars). In 2014, over 200 humanitarian organizations were involved in the WHO strategy, planning to use over $400 million to "improve access to water and hygiene, promote education, combat the food crisis, and increase means of subsistence."

As one of the first humanitarian organizations, the International Committee of the Red Cross (ICRC), has been providing aid for over 150 years. Initially formed to help victims of war, the organization is one of the most recognizable symbols of humanitarian relief. Other well-known humanitarian organizations that attend to health and medical care include Doctors Without Borders/Médecins Sans Frontières (MSF), World Vision, and the United Nations International Children's Emergency Fund (UNICEF). As indicated in the report by the WHO, these organizations are only fractions of the total number of humanitarian organizations currently working around the world. The processes of globalization—the rise of global flows—have set the conditions for the proliferation of humanitarianism. People are more aware of and feel greater responsibility to respond to the strife between people, cultures, and societies around the globe. The communication of information through mass and social media globally connects people and fosters a desire to assist those in need, especially if they are portrayed as victims of injustice or violence. Interestingly, studies of responses to global crises demonstrate that the media sometimes intentionally highlight and prioritize certain injustices or disasters; this action influences the level and nature of aid and humanitarian relief provided (Jakobsen, 2000). As a result of globalization, people increasingly understand health as a human right—one that can be protected through the strategies of international organizations.

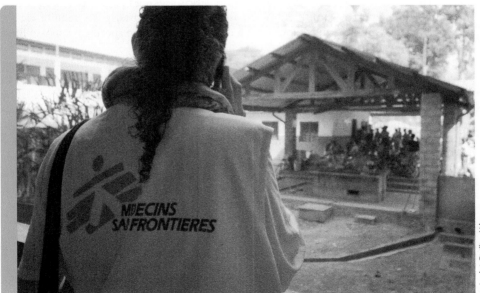

© André Quillien/Alamy

Médecins Sans Frontières/Doctors Without Borders is a humanitarian non-governmental organization, one of many organizations that respond to public health crises internationally. In 2013, the Canadian chapter of the organization engaged 210 doctors in international projects. To what extent should governments take responsibility for health crises globally? What form should health-related humanitarian aid take?

The rise of this global ethic of responsibility raises questions about what we owe to distant strangers. Should we give priority to helping vulnerable populations in developing countries or first tend to local challenges? As Buchanan and DeChamp (2011) note, until recently, health as a collective concern mostly referred to national health. While governments are the primary agents of national health, many health problems occur globally: infectious diseases, pollution of the oceans, global warming, and bioterrorism, to name a few (Buchanan & DeChamp, 2011). Chronic diseases, once felt disproportionately in industrialized countries, are now a major source of death and disability in resource-poor countries (Gostin & O'Neill, 2008). Physical distance can shape the way we respond to neglect; for example, we may care less about a starving child in Asia than about those in our own neighbourhood (Glover, 2011). "Moral distance" also influences our response to social injustice. Because of our tribalism, we may perceive people who are physically close as psychologically distant when we differ from these individuals on levels such as ethnicity, religion, or culture. As a result we care more about people we are "close to" even when they are on the other side of the world (Glover, 2011). Many important factors, such as poverty, increase our empathy for those living far away whom we have never met., For example, extreme poverty is certainly a "moral scandal": this violation of human rights is avoidable (Glover, 2011). Since rich countries benefit from the plight of the poor, this creates a humanitarian imperative as well as a claim of justice (Glover, 2011). Eradicating extreme poverty is one of the Millennium Development Goals (MDGs), a series of global changes that the UN is seeking to enact (United Nations Development Programme, 2014). However, as Pogge (2014) notes, goals require clearly appointed agents; thus, we must move from a detached wish-list to specific responsibilities of named, competent actors.

It is evident that this global ethic is complex and highlights the challenges of helping people on the global and local scales. Furthermore, social movement organizations—like in the case of HIV/AIDS activism—problematize this dualism between the local and global by demonstrating how they are interconnected (Gillett, 2011). There is some agreement on the primary conception of global justice, however, and the core of that is human rights (Pogge, 2013). While health is not yet considered a human right, and it may not have intrinsic value (that is, we do not value health in itself), it is nonetheless of moral importance. Without health we cannot enjoy any other human rights (Buchanan & DeChamp, 2011). In some cases, governments fall short of fulfilling basic health entitlements, which should protect individuals from serious, preventable health conditions. When this happens, people of wealthier states have an obligation to unite to supply aid to help every state meet its obligations regarding the health of its citizens (Buchanan & DeChamp, 2011).

What moral obligation does humanitarian medicine have when working with crumbling health care systems, negligent governments, or unstable political systems? As noted previously, international humanitarian response has been shaped by multiple forces, notably by globalization. Despite the proclaimed efficiency of global economic markets, they do not address basic human needs such as safe food, shelter, water, or livelihoods (Pringle & Cole, 2012). Consequently, public health emergencies in poorer countries are offloaded to international humanitarian organizations. This raises some serious ethical issues. For example, humanitarian medicine can undermine a government's responsibility to provide essential services and erode the remains of the existing health care system (Pringle & Cole, 2012). As Hunt (2011, p. 606) notes, "The moral dimension of humanitarian work is rendered more complex by the international and trans-cultural nature of this work." A paradox of the humanitarian enterprise is that, despite efforts to relieve suffering, humanitarian workers often face cruelties intrinsic to the humanitarian predicament. Clashes of rights and unmet expectations are part of the humanitarians' tragedy (de Waal, 2010). A study conducted by Schwartz et al. (2010) explored the ethical challenges encountered by health care professionals participating in humanitarian aid work. These challenges emerged from four main themes:

1. Scarcity of resources and the need to allocate them
2. Historical, political, social and commercial structures
3. Aid agency policies and agendas
4. Perceived norms around health professionals' roles and interactions

In this section, students learned how global inequality—and the social, economic, and political forces that create and maintain it—necessitates international responsibility for global health phenomena. What kind of world would we live in if others' suffering found absolutely no echo in us (Rességuier, 2014)? The moral obligation to act, propelled through compassion for far-away suffering, has become "one of the strongest political emotions in contemporary life" (Fassin & Pandolfi, 2010, p. 16). Students also learned that, while critical to saving lives and alleviating suffering, the provision of health care by international humanitarian organizations is fraught with ethical issues. As Ten Have (2014) observes, global suffering still persists despite humanitarian assistance. What is often forgotten is life before and after victimhood.

Global Cultural Politics

The processes of globalization and the rise of global flows intensify social relations between groups of people and between humans and other species. Since the early formation of human societies, we have been dependent on other species—animals in particular—for our survival. What has remained consistent since our early history is that humans have raised animals for food, taken them on as companions for emotional support and protection, and put them to work in a wide range of capacities. However, the nature of this dependent relationship has changed over time.

The first part of this section examines how our current relationship with other species has direct implications for our health. The second section considers the cultural framework we use to understand our relationship with other species. This framework directly influences our ability to respond to and prevent negative health outcomes as a result of our interspecies dependency. With globalization, we have new ways to conceptualize our relationship as a component of a complex interspecies ecological system. This new knowledge holds promise for shifting—and hopefully improving—the systems we have in place to address health and health care problems.

Consider the food industry, for example. The mode of production for raising animals as food has shifted from hunting and gathering to factory farms operated by multi-billion dollar corporate industries (Emel & Wolch, 1998). The gap between the production of food and its consumption has never been greater. Children are taught in schools that milk comes from cows and bacon from pigs; otherwise they may never make the connection in their everyday life. Governments and industries have had to create resource-intensive agencies devoted to systems of traceability, ensuring, with varying degrees of success, that "functional livestock" are raised, slaughtered, and made available to the public safely (Rude et al., 2006). The current global structure of food production makes it more and more difficult to trace the chicken that is sold in a fast food restaurant back to an actual chicken. Recent health scares and epidemics like SARS and H1N1 are attributed to poor controls and international regulations over food production. The global food system has fostered the ideal conditions in which a virus can jump from one species to another (Mykhalovskiy & Weir, 2006). Food production industries are criticized for using hormones and pesticides that contribute to the incidence and prevalence of food intolerances and illnesses like cancer. Furthermore, the demand for meat, through the global fast food industry in particular, has fueled production of beef, chicken, and pork at levels once thought impossible. Forecasts suggest that our current levels of food production are unsustainable, and that they are significantly contributing to climate change, threatening the integrity of our physical environment (Tilman et al., 2001).

Our relationship with other species is not entirely negative in terms of health, however. Companion animals perform a role in the lives of people that is distinct from previous generations. Once, dogs and horses were a necessity for transportation or protection. Now they are considered family members, used in recreation and leisure, and even as personal adornments or status symbols (Gilbert & Gillett, 2012). While companion animals have always worked in capacities like the military and police forces in particular, their functional role in society, especially for health care, has expanded (Cole & Gawlinski, 2000). Dogs, horses, and even cats, rabbits, and monkeys are increasingly being used in animal-assisted therapy and animal-assisted health care interventions (Halm, 2008). At universities, for instance, dogs are trained to assist students in managing the pressures of campus life. In a more medical context, psychiatric service dogs are highly trained canines that are used as a treatment for mental illnesses such as post-traumatic stress disorder (Nimer & Lundahl, 2007). Unlike typical service dogs that have assisted people with disabilities for decades, canines with specific mental illness training hold promise as an adjunct treatment. These animals could possibly provide an alternative to conventional biomedical treatments (Kruger & Serpell, 2006). On the darker side, however, we often violate principles of animal welfare. For instance, companion animals continue to be used in medical research as test subjects in clinical control trials of medications (Joffe & Miller, 2008). However, there is a growing critical analysis of the ethics of using companion animals in this capacity.

Clearly, we are interdependent on species other than ourselves in very complex ways. As a result of globalization, our existing paradigms for understanding and responding to issues related to health are ill-equipped to consider the interspecies nature of our existence. The biomedical paradigms that are dominant in health care and public health—the institutions that are responsible for treating illness and preventing large-scale health epidemics—take the human body as the primary focus and pay little attention to social, cultural, political, or ecological considerations (Borrell-Carrió, Suchman & Epstein, 2004). In response to this narrow focus on the human body, and against a backdrop of increased attention to globalization, paradigms have emerged to challenge biomedicine. The chapter now turns to **One Health**: a recent movement that proposes a paradigm shift which situates health and health care within a global, interspecies, and ecological context.

In the late 1880s Rudolf Virchow coined the term "zoonosis" in response to his observations that it was possible for disease to spread from animals to humans. Virchow's conclusion stemmed from his research on slaughterhouses and the need for more careful public mon-itoring of practices in the emerging meat industry (Zinsstag et al., 2011). Along with Canadian physician William Osler, the efforts of Virchow led to the concept of **One Medicine**. One Medicine sought to bring together veterinary medicine and human medicine under one set of practices, an early acknowledgement of the interdependency between the health of spe-cies (Tjaart, 1998). However, the dominant biomedical model of the early twentieth century prevented a concept like One Medicine from influencing the policies and practices of govern-ments and industry with regards to human health (Conrad et al., 2009). The rise of veterinary medicine as a distinct and independent profession further divided human and non-human health care practices. Hence, for decades the idea of integrating (or at least linking) human health and animal health remained on the margins of medicine and public health.

In the late 1960s a veterinarian named Calvin Schwabe began a campaign to reintroduce the concept of One Medicine to highlight the important connection between the health and illness of animals and that of humans (Cardiff, Ward, & Barthold, 2007). The efforts of Schwabe, among others, led to the formation of One Health as a revised, updated version of One Medicine. One Health better reflected the increasing tension around global epidemics that affect humans and other species. The movement toward a One Health paradigm has grown considerably across many disciplines and aspires to integrate approaches to health and health care globally.

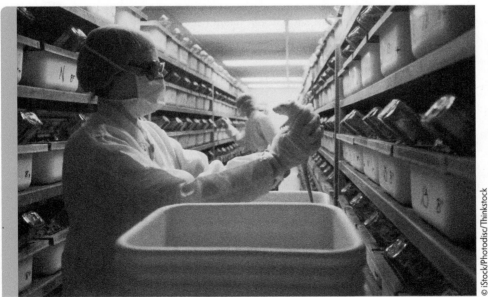

© iStock/Photodisc/Thinkstock

Human beings are increasingly interdependent on non-human species for our health, in very complex ways. This fact raises important political-economic, social, biomedical, philosophical, and ethical questions about the way in which humans' lives are entangled with those of other living beings. The health implications for interspecies relationships stretch around the globe.

CASE STUDY

One World, One Health

Recognizing the interconnectedness of species and the importance of that connection for health and illness, a group of experts gathered in New York in the fall of 2004 to draw up a global, interdisciplinary strategy for combating threats to the health of living creatures, both human and animal. Composed of individuals from governments, international bodies, and conservation associations, the group developed a twelve-point manifesto outlining their vision for a holistic approach to managing and maintaining human and animal health. These twelve points have become known as the Manhattan Principles:

> Recent outbreaks of West Nile Virus, Ebola Hemorrhagic Fever, SARS, Monkeypox, Mad Cow Disease and Avian Influenza remind us that human and animal health are intimately connected. A broader understanding of health and disease demands a unity of approach achievable only through a consilience of human, domestic animal and wildlife health—One Health. Phenomena such as species loss, habitat degradation, pollution, invasive alien species, and global climate change are fundamentally altering life on our planet from terrestrial wilderness and ocean depths to the most densely populated cities. The rise of emerging and resurging infectious diseases threatens not only humans (and their food supplies and economies), but also the fauna and flora comprising the critically needed biodiversity that supports the living infrastructure of our world. The earnestness and effectiveness of humankind's environmental stewardship and our future health have never been more clearly linked. To win the disease battles of the 21st century while ensuring the biological integrity of the Earth for future generations requires interdisciplinary and cross-sectoral approaches to disease prevention, surveillance, monitoring, control and mitigation as well as to environmental conservation more broadly.

> We urge the world's leaders, civil society, the global health community and institutions of science to:
> 1. Recognize the essential link between human, domestic animal and wildlife health and the threat disease poses to people, their food supplies and economies, and the biodiversity essential to maintaining the healthy environments and functioning ecosystems we all require.
> 2. Recognize that decisions regarding land and water use have real implications for health. Alterations in the resilience of ecosystems and shifts in patterns of disease emergence and spread manifest themselves when we fail to recognize this relationship.
> 3. Include wildlife health science as an essential component of global disease prevention, surveillance, monitoring, control and mitigation.
> 4. Recognize that human health programs can greatly contribute to conservation efforts.
> 5. Devise adaptive, holistic and forward-looking approaches to the prevention, surveillance, monitoring, control and mitigation of emerging and resurging diseases that take the complex interconnections among species into full account.

6. Seek opportunities to fully integrate biodiversity conservation perspectives and human needs (including those related to domestic animal health) when developing solutions to infectious disease threats.

7. Reduce the demand for and better regulate the international live wildlife and bushmeat trade not only to protect wildlife populations but to lessen the risks of disease movement, cross-species transmission, and the development of novel pathogen–host relationships. The costs of this worldwide trade in terms of impacts on public health, agriculture and conservation are enormous, and the global community must address this trade as the real threat it is to global socio-economic security.

8. Restrict the mass culling of free-ranging wildlife species for disease control to situations where there is a multidisciplinary, international scientific consensus that a wildlife population poses an urgent, significant threat to human health, food security, or wildlife health more broadly.

9. Increase investment in the global human and animal health infrastructure commensurate with the serious nature of emerging and resurging disease threats to people, domestic animals and wildlife. Enhanced capacity for global human and animal health surveillance and for clear, timely information-sharing (that takes language barriers into account) can only help improve coordination of responses among governmental and nongovernmental agencies, public and animal health institutions, vaccine / pharmaceutical manufacturers, and other stakeholders.

10. Form collaborative relationships among governments, local people, and the private and public (i.e., non-profit) sectors to meet the challenges of global health and biodiversity conservation.

11. Provide adequate resources and support for global wildlife health surveillance networks that exchange disease information with the public health and agricultural animal health communities as part of early warning systems for the emergence and resurgence of disease threats.

12. Invest in educating and raising awareness among the world's people and in influencing the policy process to increase recognition that we must better understand the relationships between health and ecosystem integrity to succeed in improving prospects for a healthier planet.

It is clear that no one discipline or sector of society has enough knowledge and resources to prevent the emergence or resurgence of diseases in today's globalized world. No one nation can reverse the patterns of habitat loss and extinction that can and do undermine the health of people and animals. Only by breaking down the barriers among agencies, individuals, specialties, and sectors can we unleash the innovation and expertise needed to meet the many serious challenges to the health of people, domestic animals, and wildlife and to the integrity of ecosystems. Solving today's threats and tomorrow's problems cannot be accomplished with yesterday's approaches. We are in an era of "One World, One Health" and we must devise adaptive, forward-looking and multidisciplinary solutions to the challenges that undoubtedly lie ahead.

Source: Retrieved from www.oneworldonehealth.org

Building on the momentum of the One Health movement, a conference on the topic of integrated health and health care was held in 2004 in New York by the Wildlife Conservation Society. At this conference, experts from a wide range of disciplines formulated a set of twelve principles to help us understand the interconnectedness of humans, animals, and our complex and dynamic ecosystem. The twelve principles shown in the case study below provide a comprehensive overview of the key tenets of One Health. There is a recognition that in a globalized world there needs to be a coordinated rethinking of the way we currently address health and health care problems. This new concept encourages an approach that looks at ecosystems and their relationships across national and international borders. One Health suggests that we critically examine current practices around the use and management of wildlife and domestic animals.

Attempts within One Health to reshape of how we think about the wellbeing of the planet has translated into a wide range of programs and initiatives that put the ideas of the Manhattan Principles, among other related ideas, into practice. In 2010, the Canadian organization Veterinarians Without Borders published a series of case studies that follow One Health principles (Veterinarians Without Borders, 2010). In the introduction (p. 3) they write,

> [t]he global initiative to address the one health of the one world that we share as multiple species is being carried forward through advances in theory and practice around the world. This compendium is intended to bring together stories of some of the initiatives that have been informed by one health thinking, and which have begun the journey toward a more integrative understanding of health and wellbeing.

The compendium includes One Health case studies, including the outbreak of Escherichia coli (E. coli) in Ontario, Vampire Bat Rabies in South America, Ebola in Africa, and SARS in Asia. Each case study identifies the disease, the ecosystem dynamics that are involved, responses to the problem using One Health, and suggestions for how governments, industries, academics, and community members can develop policies directed at improving health for all.

The One Health movement emerged in response to the health issues of our increasingly globalized society. With globalization, we have become more interconnected. It has become more possible, and in some cases more necessary, for people to cross borders. Furthermore, the demand for food production has increased and, in response, has been organized politically and economically in a way that jeopardizes the sustainability and integrity of our ecosystems. Our ability to come together in response to large-scale health crises on a global and local scale allows us to develop new ways of thinking about common issues. The rise of the One Health movement is an example of how the processes of globalization enable new paradigms to reframe our understanding of health within in a global, interspecies, and ecological framework.

Chapter Summary

The forces of globalization are powerful. In this chapter, students have read about the broader political and economic structures that influence global health. Our thinking

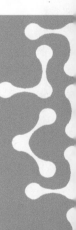

about these issues is better when we understand the magnitude and contours of the structures that play central roles in producing a problem. As discussed, national and global institutions set the rules, and the current global institutional architecture generally works against the poor. We can begin to appreciate how an alternative design of institutional arrangements could approach this problem more productively. Students have also learned how globalization extends beyond economics to include cultural and social changes. Global health can be viewed as a product of globalization. The interconnectedness of all life forms demands collaborative, global solutions to address the changing nature of the problems we face. There is an ethical imperative to work together to foster a healthier, global society.

STUDY QUESTIONS

1. How might you explain globalization to someone who had never heard the term?
2. What is neoliberalism and how does it impact people's health at the local level?
3. How can the emergence of the One Health movement be explained with reference to wider globalizing processes?
4. Why do some people find the proliferation of international humanitarian organizations problematic?
5. With reference to globalization, how can we explain the tremendous health inequalities between countries?

SUGGESTED READINGS

Caporaso, J.A. & Levine, D.P. (1992). *Theories of political economy*. Cambridge: Cambridge University Press.

Heymann, J., Earle, A., & McNeill, K. (2013). The impact of labor policies on the health of young children in the context of economic globalization. *Annual Review of Public Health, 34*, 355–72.

Singer, P. (2004). *One world: The ethics of globalization* (2nd ed.). New Haven, CT: Yale University Press.

SUGGESTED WEB RESOURCES

Dr. Peter Daszak's TEDMED Talk: What diseases come from animals? www.tedmed.com/talks/show?id=7047

Case Studies for Global Health: www.casestudiesforglobalhealth.org

Humanitarian Health Care Ethics: http://humanitarianhealthethics.net

GLOSSARY

Free market capitalism A open economy where vendors can buy and sell without any external interference such as government restrictions, international trade laws, or other taxes.

Global humanitarianism Addressing human rights violations and inequality on a global scale. Global humanitarian groups aim to ensure that the basic human rights of all individuals are met.

Globalization The process by which countries, people, and corporations are brought into closer contact with one another. Through globalization, we can more easily travel and exchange ideas, money, and resources.

Neoliberalism A theory of political economy derived from liberalism. Emphasizes capitalism, individual wealth, and private property. For neoliberals, markets are inherently good, self regulating, and necessary. Government interventions, such as taxes or redistributive processes for wealth, are not encouraged.

One Health An updated version of One Medicine. Stresses the importance of maintaining the health of all species and our overall ecosystem in an increasingly globalized society.

One Medicine An attempt to unite human and veterinary medicine as a result of the acknowledgement that humans and animals are interrelated.

Political economy The relationship between an interdependent government system and economy. Political economists inquire into the relationship between the state and the market at a given moment in time.

REFERENCES

Appadurai, A. (1990). Disjuncture and difference in the global cultural economy. *Theory, Culture & Society, 7,* 295–310.

Beaglehole, R. & Bonita, R. (1998). Public health and neoliberalism: Response to a commentary. *European Journal of Public Health, 8,* 331–33.

Beyer, P. (2007). Globalization and glocalization. In J. A. Beckford & N. J. Demerath (Eds), *The SAGE handbook of the sociology of religion* (pp. 98–118). London: Sage Publications.

Blin, A. & Marín, G. (2012, April). The commons and world governance: Toward a global social contract. Retrieved from http://rio20.net/wp-content/uploads/2012/10/Commons-and-World-Governance.pdf

Borrell-Carrió, F., Suchman, A. L., & Epstein, R. M. (2004). The biopsychosocial model 25 years later: Principles, practice, and scientific inquiry. *The Annals of Family Medicine, 2*(6), 576–82.

Brassington, I. (2012). What's wrong with the brain drain? *Developing World Bioethics, 12,* 113–120.

Buchanan, A. & DeCamp, M. (2011). Responsibility for global health. In S. Benatar & G. Brock (Eds), *Global health and global health ethics.* Cambridge: Cambridge University Press.

Burkle, F. M. (2010). Future humanitarian crises: Challenges for practice, policy, and public health. *Prehospital and Disaster Medicine, 25,* 191–99.

Cardiff, R. D., Ward, J. M., & Barthold, S. W. (2007). "One medicine—one pathology": Are veterinary and human pathology prepared? *Laboratory investigation, 88*(1), 18–26.

Cole, K.M. & Gawlinski, A. (2000). Animal-assisted therapy: The human–animal bond. AACN *Advanced Critical Care, 11*(1), 139–49.

Conrad, P., Mazet, J., Clifford, D., Scott, C., & Wilkes, M. (2009). Evolution of a transdisciplinary "One Medicine–One Health" approach to global health education at the University of California. *Preventive Veterinary Medicine, 92*(4) 268–74.

de Waal, A. (2010). The humanitarians' tragedy: Escapable and inescapable cruelties. *Disasters, 34,* S130–S137.

Di Chiro, G. (2004). "Living is for everyone": Border crossings for community, environment and health. In G. Mitman, M. Murphy, & C. Sellers (Eds), *Osiris,*

Volume 19: Landscapes of exposure: Knowledge and illness in modern environments (pp. 112–29). Chicago: University of Chicago Press Journals.

Emel, J. & Wolch, J. (Eds). (1998). Witnessing the animal moment. *Animal geographies: Place, politics and identity in the nature–culture borderlands*, (1–24). London: Verso.

Fassin, D. & Pandolfi, M. (2010). Introduction: Military and humanitarian government in the age of intervention. In D. Fassin & M. Pandolfi (Eds), *Contemporary states of emergency: The politics of military and humanitarian interventions* (pp. 9–25). Brooklyn: Zone Books.

Freeland, C. (2012). *Plutocrats: The new golden age.* Toronto: Random House LLC.

Gaynor, G. & Vogt, W. B. (1997). What does economics have to say about health policy anyway?: A comment and correction on Evans and Rice. *Journal of Health Politics, Policy and Law, 22,* 475–96.

George, S. (1999, March). A short history of neoliberalism: Twenty years of elite economics and emerging opportunities for structural change. Retrieved from http://www.globalexchange.org/resources/econ101/neoliberalismhist

Ger, G. & Belk, R. W. (1996). I'd like to buy the world a Coke: Consumptionscapes of the "less affluent world." *Journal of Consumer Policy, 19*(3), 271–304.

Gilbert, M. & Gillett, J. (2012). Equine athletes and interspecies sport. *International Review for the Sociology of Sport, 47*(5), 632–43.

Gillett, J. (2011). *A grassroots history of the* AIDS *epidemic in North America.* Spokane: Marquette Press.

Glover, J. (2011). Poverty, distance and two dimensions of ethics. In S. Benatar & G. Brock (Eds), *Global health and global health ethics.* Cambridge: Cambridge University Press.

Gostin, L. O. & A. L. T. O'Neill. (2008). Global health law: A definition and grand challenges. *Public Health Ethics, 1,* 53–63.

Groenhout, R. (2012). The "brain drain" problem: Migrating health professionals and global health care. *International Journal of Feminist Approaches to Bioethics, 5,* 1–24.

Hall, P. (1997). The role of interests, institutions, and ideas in the comparative political economy of the industrialized nations. In M. I. Lichbach & A.S. Zuckerman (Eds), *Comparative politics: Rationality, culture and structure* (pp. 174–207). Cambridge: Cambridge University Press.

Halm, M. A. (2008). The healing power of the human–animal connection. *American Journal of Critical Care, 17*(4), 373–76.

Haque, M. S. (2002). Globalization, new political economy, and governance: A Third World viewpoint. *Administrative Theory & Praxis, 24,* 103–24.

Harvey, D. (2005). *A brief history of neoliberalism.* New York: Oxford University Press.

Hidalgo, J. S. (2013). The active recruitment of health workers: A defence. *Journal of Medical Ethics, 39,* 603–09.

Humanitarian Health Ethics. (2014). *Case study: Coping with outbreaks of disease with limited resources.* Retrieved from http://www.humanitarianhealthethics.net

Human Rights Watch. (2012, February 7). *Nigeria: Child lead poisoning crisis.* Retrieved from http://www.hrw.org/news/2012/02/07/nigeria-child-lead-poisoning-crisis

Hunt, M. (2011). Establishing moral bearings: Ethics and expatriate healthcare professionals in humanitarian work. *Disasters, 35,* 606–22.

International Committee of the Red Cross. (2014). *History of the* ICRC. Retrieved from http://www.icrc.org/eng/who-we-are/history/index.jsp

Jakobsen, P. V. (2000). Focus on the CNN effect misses the point: The real media impact on conflict management is invisible and indirect. *Journal of Peace Research, 37*(2), 131–43.

Joffe, S. & Miller, F. G. (2008). Mapping the moral terrain of clinical research. *Hastings Center Report,* 38(2), 30–42.

Kruger, K. A. & Serpell, J. A. (2006). Animal-assisted interventions in mental health: Definitions and theoretical foundations. *Handbook on Animal-Assisted Therapy: Theoretical Foundations and Guidelines for Practice, 2,* 21–38.

Levitt, T. (1983). The globalisation of markets. In R. Z. Aliber and R. W. Click (Eds) *Readings in International Business: A Decision Approach* (pp. 249–266). Cambridge, Massachusetts/London: The MIT Press.

Mykhalovskiy, E. & Weir, L. (2006). The global public health intelligence network and early warning outbreak detection: A Canadian contribution to global public health. *Canadian Journal of Public Health,* 42–4.

Nimer, J. & Lundahl, B. (2007). Animal-assisted therapy: A meta-analysis. *Anthrozoos: A Multidisciplinary*

Journal of the Interactions of People & Animals, 20(3), 225–38.

OECD – Organisation for Economic Co-operation and Development (n.d.). Retrieved from http://www.oecd.org/social/poverty/migration-andthebraindrainphenomenon.htm

Pal, L.A. (2010). *Beyond policy analysis: Public issue management in turbulent times (4th ed.).* Toronto, ON: Nelson Education Ltd.

Pogge, T. (2013, December 23). *Human rights and human duties: What do we owe to compatriots and distant strangers?* Retrieved from www.youtube.com/watch?v=2ZbQsk-IzhQ

———. (2014, April 10). Hunger games. Lecture conducted from McMaster University, Hamilton, ON.

Pringle, J. D. & Cole, D. C. (2012). The Nigerian lead-poisoning epidemic: The role of neoliberal globalization and challenges for humanitarian ethics. In C. Abu-Sada (Ed.), *Dilemmas, challenges, and ethics of humanitarian action: Reflections on Médecins Sans Frontières' perception project* (pp. 48–69). Montreal: McGill-Queen's University Press.

Rességuier, A. (2014, February 20). Feeling what the other feels—for a sympathetic ethics. [Web log comment]. Retrieved from http://www.alnap.org/blog/95

Rude, J., Iqbal, J., & Brewin, D. (2006). This little piggy went to market with a passport: The impacts of US country of origin labeling on the Canadian pork sector. *Canadian Journal of Agricultural Economics/Revue canadienne d'agroeconomie, 54*(3), 401–20.

Samuels, W. T. (1977). The political economy of Adam Smith. *Ethics, 87,* 189–207.

Sandel, M. J. (2012). *What money can't buy: The moral limits of markets.* New York: Farrar, Straus, and Giroux.

Schillorn van Veen, Tjaart W. (1998). One Medicine: The dynamic relationship between animal and human medicine in history and at present. *Agriculture and Human Values, 15,* 115–20.

Schwartz, L., Sinding, C., Hunt, M., Elit, L., Redwood-Campbell, L., Adelson, N., … DeLaat, S. (2010). Ethics in humanitarian aid work: Learning from the narratives of humanitarian healthcare workers. *American Journal of Bioethics, 1,* 45–54.

Shiva, V. (2014, April). Fragile freedoms. *Ideas.* Lecture conducted from the Canadian Museum for Human Rights, Winnipeg, MB. Retrieved from http://www.cbc.ca/player/Radio/Ideas/ID/2449853936

Stiglitz, J.E. (2003). *Globalization and its discontents.* New York: W.W. Norton.

Ten Have, H. (2014). Macro-triage in disaster planning. In D. P. O'Mathúna, B. Gordijn., & M. Clarke (Eds), *Disaster bioethics: Normative issues when nothing is normal* (pp. 13–32). London: Springer.

Tilman, D., Fargione, J., Wolff, B., D'Antonio, C., Dobson, A., Howarth, R., … Swackhamer, D. (2001). Forecasting agriculturally driven global environmental change. *Science, 292*(5515), 281–84.

United Nations Development Programme. (2014). *Millenium development goals.* Retrieved from http://www.undp.org/content/undp/en/home/mdgoverview

Veterinarians Without Borders (2010). One Health for one world: A compendium of case studies. Retrieved from http://aitoolkit.org/site/DefaultSite/filesystem/documents/OHOW_Compendium_Case_Studies.pdf

World Bank Group. (2014). Prosperity for all/Ending extreme poverty: A note for the World Bank Group spring meetings 2014. Washington, DC: World Bank.

World Health Organization. (2014). *Overview of global humanitarian response.* Retrieved from https://docs.unocha.org/sites/dms/CAP/Overview_of_Global_Humanitarian_Response_2014.pdf

Zinsstag, J., Schelling, E., Waltner-Toews, D., & Tanner, M. (2011). From "One Medicine" to "One Health" and systemic approaches to health and well-being. *Preventive Veterinary Medicine, 101,* 148–56.

Part III

Health Care Paradigms, Systems, and Policies

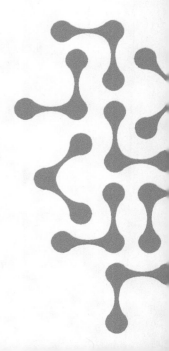

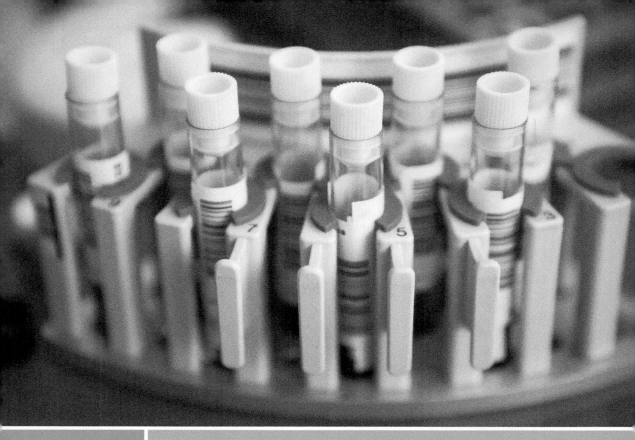

8

Modern Biomedical Culture

Elena Neiterman

LEARNING OBJECTIVES

In this chapter, students will learn

- the biomedical model of health
- major socio-cultural processes that facilitated the establishment of biomedicine's dominance in Western culture
- the process of medicalization and its conceptual framework
- the concept of iatrogenesis
- how critics question the role of biomedicine in contemporary life

Introduction

What do most people in Canada do when they feel sick? Where do they go when they have a medical emergency? Do they meditate? Do they go to a sacred temple or a church to pray? Do they ask a local wizard to use his magic to cure their illness? Most likely, they do not do any of that. Instead, they go to see a doctor or, in the case of emergency, run to the nearest hospital to get medical help. But why do they prefer a doctor to a local wizard? Is it because they trust doctors more than wizards when it comes to their health? If so, why? After all, most people have never even met a wizard, so why would they assume that a wizard has less to offer when it comes to curing their illness?

The goal of this chapter is not to convince students to use wizards as primary care providers, but to analyze the assumptions that we hold with regards to medicine, doctors, and the "right way" to deal with illness. This chapter suggests that much of our understanding of health draws overwhelmingly on beliefs about the role of biomedicine in contemporary world. The term *beliefs* is chosen deliberately; after all, most people have never sought proof that biomedicine is the best way to go about curing all illnesses. For example, most people rarely test different kinds of health care providers, such as naturopaths or homeopaths, before seeking help from medical doctors. Instead, we are born into a society that positions biomedicine at the top of the healing/medical hierarchy. Our culture downplays alternative health care practices and belief systems about health and illness. Popular understandings of health, illness, and healing are shaped by the biomedical culture. The terms that we use to describe our body or illness, the strategies that we utilize to become healthy, and our choices of medical help are all borrowed from the knowledge system of biomedicine.

This chapter expands upon the description of modern biomedical culture as found in Chapter Four. It examines how biomedical science has become the primary basis of Western understandings of health and illness. It analyzes the social and cultural transformations that allowed such a transition to occur and touches on how biomedical culture can intrude into people's everyday lives. It considers the medicalization of daily life and popular reliance on biomedicine to cure both physical and social ills. Finally, the chapter discusses how biomedicine changed the cultural landscape of our society. Introducing the concept of iatrogenesis, it examines the impact of biomedical culture on our bodies, our social lives, and our cultural beliefs and practices.

The Rise of Biomedicine

Medicine as a form of healing practice is not modern at all. Since ancient times, people have been practising healing. People have used herbs and various potions to treat ill individuals and even performed minor and major surgeries for thousands of years (Bloom, 2002; Thane, 2005). For instance, Hippocratic medicine, as practised in the ancient world, heavily emphasized diet and exercise as a part of treatment regimen for individuals whose health needed improvement (Bloom, 2002). In ancient Egypt, knowledge of anatomy and neuroscience was remarkable; local physicians were capable of performing successful brain surgeries (Elhadi et al., 2012). It would probably not be too far-reaching to suggest that there have been healers since the beginning of human society.

Drawing parallels between ancient and contemporary medicine is surely interesting. Some of our contemporary knowledge about medicine is based on the works of Galen,

Hippocrates, and other great thinkers of the past (Bloom, 2002; Thane, 2005). But there are also some stark differences between the old and new medical cultures. First, we generally believe that modern medicine knows more about the body, the origins of diseases, and the course of treatment than ancient medicine. Second, we would like to hope that our diagnostic procedures, the lab tests and technology that we use to diagnose diseases, allow us to identify illness more accurately and precisely. Because of our advanced understanding of the body, we are now capable of performing very complex surgeries like organ transplants. Finally, we can now also identify and treat a greater number of diseases.

But the major distinction between the biomedical model and "old" medical culture is not simply that we know more about the body. After all, knowledge in any field has evolved over the past thousands years. We now send rocket ships into space and are trying to make sense of quantum mechanics something our ancestors did not do thousands of years ago. The major difference between **biomedicine** and the "old" type of medicine lies in the way biomedicine understands the world and generates medical knowledge (Bloom, 2002). The ideas shown in Figure 8.1 characterize the biomedical model that separates biomedicine from other forms and types of healing practice. In the following paragraphs, we summarize each of these ideas and explain how they shape popular understandings of health, illness, and the body.

Mind–body dualism is a philosophical theory about the relationship between the mind and the body. Originating from the works of René Descartes, a seventeenth-century French philosopher, mind–body dualism postulates that mind and body are two separate entities.

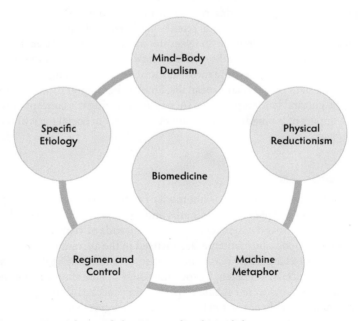

FIGURE 8.1   **Five Ideas of the Biomedical Model**

Source: Freund, McGuire, & Podhurst (2003).

The body represents the physical matter of an individual, whereas the mind is the non-physical entity that provides us with the ability to think, feel, and comprehend the world.

The assumption that body and mind were two discrete entities encouraged medical doctors to focus exclusively on the physical body when trying to identify and treat diseases. The psychosocial factors of illness were consequently removed from the process of diagnosis and treatment, essentially ignoring the social determinants of health (Mehta, 2011).

The separation of mind and body is probably one of the pivotal differences between the "old" and "new" medical sciences. This separation also helps to distinguish between biomedicine and complementary and alternative medicine (see Chapter Eleven). In order for "old" medicine to understand the progression of illness, practitioners focused on the individual's soul, their willingness to recover, and the psychosocial factors that contribute to illness. Hippocrates (470–360 BCE) and Galen (130–200 CE) both subscribed to these theories. In addition, older medical approaches often emphasized the healing power of faith and religion (Bloom, 2002). Biomedical culture, however, focused its sole attention on the body—its anatomy, its biophysical processes, and its ailments.

Another basic tenet of biomedicine is **physical reductionism**, an approach to studying a phenomenon by breaking it into smaller parts. For instance, breaking down aspects of the world into molecules or atoms can help biologists study human life through these smaller, more basic elements (Beresford, 2010). In contemporary medicine, physical reductionism is a general approach to understanding the origins and causes of diseases (Beresford, 2010).

CASE STUDY

The Placebo Effect

For true believers in the separation of mind and body, how can we explain the placebo effect? When patients receive placebos, they feel better solely because they *believe* that they are receiving medical treatment. There are many documented cases of the placebo effect (Finniss, Kaptchukb, Miller, & Benedetti, 2012). Randomized controlled trials, which are considered the most methodologically rigorous approach to validate the effectiveness of a treatment, often use double-blind designs to combat the placebo problem. In the double-blind study, neither the experimenter nor the research subjects know whether they are receiving the actual treatment or a placebo. The goal is to minimize personal bias (on behalf of both the researcher and the subject). This ensures that it is the actual treatment, rather than people's assumption about treatment, that creates a difference between those who are being treated and those who are not.

The placebo effect is evident not only in clinical trials for various drugs but also in surgical procedures. One study looked at the differences between patients who received an actual knee surgery and those who received a "sham" knee surgery (i.e., a placebo surgery). Researchers found no real differences between the two groups (Moseley et al., 2002). Physicians used these results to analyze the efficacy of the treatment.

Students may want to ask themselves how the placebo effect challenges the analytical separation of mind and body. What makes the placebo effect possible? Why do we need to worry about the objective efficacy of treatment if the mere perception of its efficacy can actually help?

The quest to identify and study pathology has moved away from the body to the medical lab, where scientists search for the signs of the disease in question under a microscope. Reductionism is not necessarily a bad thing, however, and we tend to practise it in our everyday life. When faced with a large problem, many people prefer to solve it piece by piece. For example, one can address complicated math equations by solving them in smaller steps. But some critics suggest that, by focusing on the little parts, we may sometimes miss the larger picture (Beresford, 2010), especially when it comes to our health. For instance, studying pathology under a microscope may disregard the importance of the larger socio-political context that produces disease in society. It can also demean individuals and negate their lived experience with an illness.

The third idea that informs biomedical thinking is that each disease has a **specific etiology**. Etiology literally means the origins of the cause (coming from the Greek *aitia*—cause). According to biomedical thinking, every disease has its own causes and origins. Medicine, in turn, must discern these causes in order to provide proper treatment for that particular ailment. The attempts to classify various diseases into different groups or subgroups—a subfield of medicine called nosology (Szasz, 2007)—are probably as old as the practice of medicine. Addressing the etiology of a disease draws attention to the disease itself. This focus on the disease defines our journey through the health care system and determines what interventions will be used to address the issue. Consequently, the role of the doctor is to treat the disease, not the individual. For instance, if a person has been diagnosed with high blood pressure, the doctor will prescribe a treatment for hypertension. As there are standard pharmaceutical drugs for high blood pressure, one hypertensive person will typically receive the exact same treatment as any other person suffering from high blood pressure. However, if the individual person, not the disease, was the focus of attention, treatment might be personalized to an individual's unique circumstances. Interventions could address where someone lives, what they eat, what kinds of stress they encounter on a daily basis, and many other factors that could all influence their blood pressure.

The **machine metaphor** is yet another idea that is fundamental to biomedical thinking. According to this idea, popularized in children's anatomy books, the body can be viewed as a machine. All parts are essential for the operation of the whole, yet each part performs its own unique function. As such, all parts should be taken care of properly. One can see the parallels between this idea and the organization of our health care system. When one hears strange noises while driving a car, it generally makes sense to take it to the mechanic. When the body makes strange noises while one is driving, most people would take their body to the doctor to identify what is wrong. Just as a car requires regular service and oil changes, so the body, too, requires a yearly physical to make sure that it functions well. Depending on the specific problem that a car has, one would choose a mechanic or garage that specializes in that particular area. Similarly, problems in one's body might bring a person to the office of a medical specialist in respirology, cardiology, ophthalmology, or other "ologies" that are uniquely suited to deal with the part of the body that needs medical attention.

While this approach to treating health problems seems highly efficient, it utilizes a very mechanistic perception of the body. Yet, our relationship with our body is intimately related to our body as a whole, not necessarily our lungs, kidneys, or other organs individually. Breaking the body into separate parts dissociates our organs, body systems, and any associated treatments from one another. In Chapter Eleven (on complementary and alternative medicine), students will notice that many other systems of healing do not share this reductionist view of the body. Instead, complementary and alternative medicine generally emphasizes the wholeness of the body and the relationships among various organs and systems.

Finally, the last basic idea of biomedicine to consider is that of **regimen and control**. According to this view, diseases can be managed via close control of one's body and through the use of specific regimens. As individuals, for instance, we are constantly reminded that proper nutrition, regular exercise, abstinence from drugs, and moderate alcohol consumption will make our bodies less susceptible to illness. We are told to take care of our bodies, and that if we fail to take proper care, we can be held directly responsible for the consequences. Consider, for example, what people would say

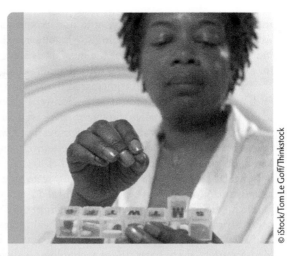

© iStock/Tom Le Goff/Thinkstock

The idea of regimen and control is a fundamental trope in modern biomedical culture. The effects of this idea are visible in notions like nutritional maintenance, and in physical artifacts, such as pill cases that divide dosages by day. What story does a weekly pill case tell? For whom is such a device intended? What can it tell you about biomedicine?

about an individual who is a smoker and who receives a diagnosis of lung cancer, or someone who did not use protection during sexual intercourse and contracts a sexually transmitted disease. If, despite our best efforts, we fail to protect our bodies and we do get sick, then doctors are faced with the task of controlling or combatting the disease. They prescribe the course of treatment and monitor the progress of this treatment. Ultimately, most people believe that we can avoid or manage illness with the appropriate regimen and control.

These five basic ideas of biomedicine not only form a wider knowledge framework that is used by medical doctors, they are embedded within our culture (see Chapter Four). These ideas shape our understanding of health and illness, what we should do in case we do not feel well, and what we regard as the "right way" to deal with health problems. For these reasons, if a person suddenly does not feel well, they will most likely go to see a doctor rather than a local wizard. For the same reasons, most people would be more inclined to use condoms, not prayers, to protect themselves from a sexually transmitted disease. What is important to understand is that the choices (of doctor versus shaman or condom versus prayer) are driven by the cultural assumptions that we hold about health, illness, and the body. These assumptions, in our society, are derived from the biomedical framework.

How did biomedicine become central in forming our understanding of health, illness, and the body? Researchers identify a number of historical transitions that solidified popular belief in biomedicine (Conrad & Leiter, 2004; Fox, 1994). First, the **secularization** of society, which decreased reliance on religious doctrine, allowed people to search for non-religious causes of illness (Conrad, 2007). For instance, if one's disease was considered a punishment from God for sinning, then trying to understand its causes, resisting it, or even treating it were virtually futile. Without God's help, one could not hope to cure or combat it. Hence, prayer and confession would be the most likely ways to make oneself feel better, rather than, for example, a treatment plan or early diagnosis.

The second process that contributed to the contemporary dominance of biomedical science was the rise of the medical profession—the allopathic medical doctor. **Allopathic** refers to the fact that these healers use treatments based on remedies that produce effects opposite from the diseases they are treating. For example, an allopathic physician uses drugs that decrease blood pressure to combat hypertension (high blood pressure). Allopathic doctors had a long history of competing with other healers, such as homeopaths, naturopaths, and local healers, for clientele. Eventually, they were able to organize and to position themselves as a distinct group of professionals. Medical doctors were subsequently able to redefine allopathic medicine as science, firmly linking it to the scientific progress of biomedicine, while using various techniques to exclude other health care providers.

Today, many people consider biomedicine to be at the edge of scientific progress. Media outlets share news about technological developments in medicine, research into the potential cures for various diseases, and novel, sophisticated treatments. Many people are deeply convinced that biomedicine is the answer to many human problems. We donate money and support to finding the cure for diseases such as Alzheimer's, Parkinson's, or cancer. The next section of this chapter examines how biomedicine entered our culture and daily lives.

Medicalization of Society

As discussed in earlier chapters, the influence of biomedical culture extends far beyond the specific medical treatment a person might receive when feeling unwell. Most of us would be truly surprised if we tried to record the extent to which our daily lives are influenced by biomedicine. Ideas about what to eat, how to sleep, whether to brush our teeth, how much we should exercise, and even what we wear are all influenced by medical advice about "proper care" for the body. For example, on a nearly daily basis, the media carries information about the latest research regarding the medical benefits or disadvantages of drinking coffee or red wine, eating cheese, running, walking, or smiling.

Virtually all aspects of our lives have been somehow influenced by biomedicine. The intrusion of biomedicine into everyday life is known as medicalization. According to Conrad (2000), medicalization is "a process by which nonmedical problems become defined and treated as medical problems, usually in terms of illnesses or disorders" (p. 324).

Three Levels of Medicalization

Medicalization can be said to occur on three levels: *conceptually* (which involves the adoption of medical vocabulary), *institutionally* (as organizations begin to approach a problem as medical), and through *interactions* (where providers and/or patients frame a problem as medical) (Conrad & Schneider, 1980). To understand how medicalization can occur at these levels, we can use the example of almost any medical condition. For instance, one of the most common diagnoses for children in North America today is attention deficit hyperactivity disorder (ADHD). While it probably would not be too far-reaching to suggest that children have always had behavioural problems, only recently has the cause of such behaviours been conceptualized in medical terms (Conrad, 2007). When the medical profession labelled children's hyperactive behaviour with the diagnosis of ADHD, the problem of hyperactivity in children became a medical issue. The subsequent introduction of special support programs for children diagnosed with ADHD, the accommodations provided by educational institutions, and the availability of treatment options all exemplify medicalization of hyperactivity at the institutional level. Finally, when the child is referred to a health care professional to be assessed for the presence of ADHD, and the doctor and/or parent agree that the child has ADHD, the medicalization of this child's behaviour is occurring at the level of interactions.

Researchers have identified many conditions that have been medicalized over the past decades (Conrad, 2000; Conrad & Leiter, 2004; Fox, 1994; Zola, 1994). For instance, normal physiological conditions such as aging, pregnancy, or childbirth (Davis-Floyd, 1994; Estes & Binney, 1989; Katz Rothman, 1993) are now under the purview of the medical profession. Medicalization not only creates new treatments for these conditions, it also changes the way people think about and understand them.

Take, for example, the way we now see and understand pregnancy and childbirth. For as long as humans have existed, women have given birth to children. Pregnancy and childbirth have always been somewhat dangerous: a lack of proper nutrition and clean water, hard physical work performed by women, the absence of hygiene, and widespread infections make

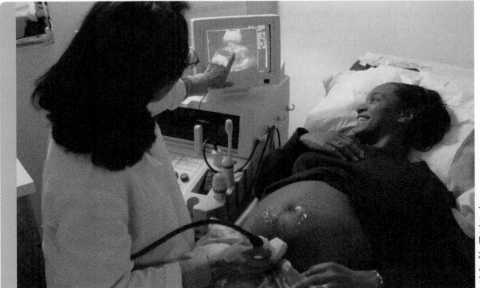

Fetal ultrasounds are one example of the ways in which modern biomedical culture has altered how pregnancy and childbirth are experienced. The intervention of medical imaging technology has become a normal part in the course of being pregnant in many Western societies.

Keith Brofsky/Thinkstock

pregnant and birthing women particularly vulnerable to illness. Pregnancy and childbirth can take quite a toll on women's bodies. Some scholars suggest that women's mortality rates prior to the twentieth century were higher than those of men because of the dangers associated with childbearing (Gorman & Read, 2007). Nevertheless, pregnancy and childbirth were not understood as illnesses or medical conditions. Midwives, local women who lived in the community, would provide assistance during childbirth. But the rise of biomedical discourse, the struggle for political and professional dominance, and the willingness of some women to medicalize pregnancy and childbirth rapidly transformed these events into medicalized conditions requiring constant medical supervision (Davis-Floyd, 1990; Katz Rothman, 1989; Riessman, 1983). In the process, lay healers like midwives diminished in status.

Thus, the medicalization of childbirth has dramatically altered the experience of birthing for women. It changed the very "physics" of birth—on the advice of midwives, women used to take a sitting or squatting position during labour. When physicians replaced midwives in childbirth, however, the birth position changed—women were now expected to lie down and be covered so that their modesty would be preserved. This position was also more convenient for the physician, who could maintain professional boundaries by staying at the "bedside" of the patient (Featherstone, 2001). The medicalization of childbirth also changed the dynamic of birth. The physician has become an active agent who supervises the birth, monitors progress, and identifies the course of "treatment." The birthing woman is now a passive recipient of that treatment (Davis-Floyd, 1990). Finally, the medicalization of childbirth has changed the nature of birth itself, which is no longer managed for women and by women in a community setting. Instead, the birth process has been hospitalized. Women's knowledge of their own bodies has been replaced by scientific evidence, medical wisdom, and various technological devices that allow physicians to look inside women's bodies and follow the development of the fetus (Katz Rothman, 1993). Today, we can hardly think about pregnancy and childbirth without envisioning a hospital and a health care professional. Expectant mothers are bombarded with endless medical advice on proper diet and exercise during pregnancy. Even though some women are choosing midwifery care as a more "natural" option to give birth, we no longer envision pregnancy and childbirth as non-medicalized conditions.

Another telling example of medicalization is the translation of many deviant behaviours into medical conditions. Behaviours that were once considered to be sins or deviations from a social norm have now become health problems. Alcoholism, kleptomania, and other conditions that were previously subject to social reprimand are now considered to be mental health problems that require medical attention and biomedical treatment (Conrad & Schneider, 1980; Szasz, 2007). The list of mental health problems has grown dramatically over the past sixty years. When the first *Diagnostic and Statistical Manual of Mental Disorders* (DSM) was published in 1952, it included a list of 106 psychiatric disorders. In 2013, the American Psychiatric Association published the most recent version of the DSM, the DSM-V, which includes a total of 297 disorders (Rosenberg, 2013). How did it happen that in just sixty years we have identified over 190 new medical conditions in the field of mental health?

It would be naive to suggest that this change is solely due to the fact that our knowledge of mental illness has advanced significantly. At some level this might be true. But such a simple approach ignores the impact of social and cultural shifts that have helped medicalize deviant behaviours. Thomas Szasz was one of the most vociferous and articulate critics of the medicalization of mental disorders. Despite being a qualified psychiatrist himself, much of his writing sought to demonstrate that mental health disorders cannot truly be considered illnesses. According to Szasz (2007), the presence of illness can always be detected in the body. When a medical examiner performs an autopsy, the diseased organ (e.g., heart, liver, or lungs) can be clearly identified. In the case of mental illness, such pathology cannot readily be identified. Hence, Szasz (2007) claimed, mental illness does not qualify as a real illness and should not necessarily be treated by doctors. He asserted that the concept of mental illness is simply society's attempt to designate certain behaviours as "good" or "bad"—a designation useful for controlling people who deviate from what we consider to be normal (Szasz, 2007). For critics like Szasz, the expansion of the DSM is the result of vigorous attempts by psychiatrists to gain more control over people's lives.

It is, of course, true that many individuals in our society suffer from mental health problems. It is also highly likely that people had experienced mental health problems before the establishment of biomedicine. When scholars criticize medicalization, they do not question whether mental problems exist. Rather, they examine how these problems are defined and how they are addressed. Examining the ways that these social problems are conceptualized also opens up the possibility of utilizing different solutions. For instance, if we are to assume that mental health problems, such as depression, are medical issues, then the solution lies in medications, counselling services, and mental health care facilities. However, if we see depression as a consequence of social inequality or other social issues, the solution would be found in a different (non-medical) realm.

According to the Canadian Mental Health Association (2014), approximately 20 per cent of Canadians will experience a mental illness during their lives. Is it possible that so many of us will experience mental suffering because we live in a society that creates illness? The stress that we experience while working, studying, dealing with income instability, sitting in traffic on the way to and from work, and trying to squeeze in too many daily tasks can negatively impact our wellbeing. It is hard to feel healthy and content when one is constantly worrying about the future, how to support oneself or a family, or coping with other instabilities in life.

Using these ideas, if we assume that mental problems are not personalized medical issues but wider social problems that affect many individuals within the population, one goal would be to address the social causes of mental illness such as people's living and working conditions. Creating more green spaces for relaxation, making our contemporary life less hectic, and creating more stability in the lives of individuals could help alleviate some of these social stresses. Yet as long as mental health problems are defined in medical terms, the solution to these problems will lie predominantly in the medical realm—one that focuses on individuals rather than on society more broadly.

There are certainly many areas where one could argue that biomedicine has improved our lives tremendously. For instance, many people suffering from mental health problems would have been jailed or marginalized in the past. Now they have the opportunity to receive treatment and get help. Nevertheless, many scholars in the social sciences take a more critical stance towards medicalization, partly because they see medicine as a form of **social control** (Conrad, 2007; Szasz, 2007; Zola, 1994). Substituting for the role of religion in our society, medicine has become a moral enterprise. The role of physician is not only to diagnose and treat illness, but also to label people as patients or malingerers; this process serves to legitimize or delegitimize their experience. In some situations, the medical model may blame

CASE STUDY

DES

A drug called DES (Diethylstilbestrol) was routinely prescribed to pregnant women in the United States and other countries to prevent miscarriages. It is estimated that between 1941 and 1971, close to 3 million women were prescribed this drug.

The negative consequences of exposure to DES were identified in the early 1970s, when the young women and daughters of mothers treated with DES were noted to have much higher rates of vaginal tumours. DES was identified as a carcinogen that affected both women taking the drug and their children. It also was linked to birth defects in infants whose mothers were exposed to the drug (Hammes & Laitman, 2003). These negative health effects are still affecting an unknown number of mothers and their children. Currently research is looking into long-lasting effects of DES that may be borne by grandchildren.

Since the discovery of the negative effects of DES, affected individuals have launched a number of lawsuits and political movements. DES Action is a global voluntary social movement of mothers and children who were affected by exposure to DES. Operating since 1982, the mission of the organization is to "identify, educate, empower and advocate for DES-exposed individuals" (DES Action Canada, 2014). The DES story serves as an example of why many people urge a more cautious attitude toward biomedical treatments.

people for not following medical advice and (thus) getting sick. In our society, individuals meet with health care professionals the moment they are born. They are closely monitored by health care providers throughout their infant years and into adolescence. Doctors constantly provide advice about how to act, and people are not even officially dead until a medical doctor makes a pronouncement. Hence, throughout our whole lives medical professionals shape our understanding of health, illness, our bodies, and the world more broadly.

Why does biomedicine's power make some people uneasy? One reason is that the production of knowledge—medical knowledge included—is not an exact science. Medical knowledge is constantly evolving, and sometimes previous ideas about the type of illness and the condition of treatment are proven to be false. Recall the example of homosexuality (mentioned in Chapter Three)—for many years medicine conceptualized it as a mental illness, prompting many individuals to undergo humiliating and harmful treatments to try to "correct" them. Although we now recognize homosexuality as a part of normal human experience, this was not always the case. But because physicians are held in high esteem in our society, we tend to believe doctors and follow their instructions on how to lead our lives.

Medical Knowledge Is Constantly Evolving

Some dramatic lessons from history remind us to avoid blindly accepting medical ideologies. Medical doctors were active participants in eugenics, a popular movement in the beginning of the twentieth century that aimed to genetically purify the human species by preventing the reproduction of "bad stock" (Lombardo, 1996). In Nazi Germany, doctors conducted experiments on prisoners in concentration camps. In North America, doctors sterilized women who were deemed "unfit" to reproduce, often without women's knowledge or consent. Between 1929 and 1972, close to 3000 women were sterilized in Alberta, many of whom were poor women, teenage mothers, or Aboriginal women (Grekul, Krahn, & Odynak, 2004). Other chapters in this book give many more examples of how blind adherence to biomedical ideas can have very dangerous consequences.

Students should note that the subjects of unsafe medical experiments and practices are often marginalized individuals. Recently, researcher Ian Mosby (2013) discovered that Aboriginal children across Canada were intentionally malnourished during the 1940s and 1950s. Such experiments aimed to study the effect of malnutrition and vitamin deficiency on children's development (Mosby, 2013). Instead of providing already starving children with a proper diet, the Canadian government decided to use these children as test subjects. They were divided into control and experiment groups with some being given "experimental" doses of essential dietary components as milk, iron, iodine, or vitamin B while others acted as the "control"—receiving no additional food despite their clear malnourishment (Mosby, 2013).

Clearly, vulnerable populations were a target audience for medical doctors in the early twentieth century. Eventually, though, the power of biomedicine affected not only marginalized groups but also society as a whole. As the twentieth century unfolded, doctors became the central authority for matters of health (Coburn, Torrance, & Kaufert, 1983; Freidson, 1970). They had unparalleled power over patients' bodies and treatment decisions. Medical doctors, arguably, drove the process of medicalization (Freidson, 1970). According to Freidson (1970), for instance, physicians in the United States were able to achieve control over the health care system by subordinating other health professions, gaining control via professional regulation, controlling clients, and establishing the notion of public trust in biomedicine.

Today, access to medical research is literally at our fingertips. A simple internet search can provide thousands of links regarding any health condition or medication. People can self-diagnose and go to their doctor with a long list of potential treatment options to discuss. Chapter Twelve highlights how many individuals now demand the opportunity to participate in decision-making processes regarding the course of their treatment. Although less-educated and older individuals continue to rely on their doctors in choosing the course of treatment (Brubaker, 2007; Lupton, 2003), doctors are no longer an unquestionable authority for many middle- and upper-class individuals. One might, of course, argue that liberation from doctors' totalitarian rule is the first step towards demedicalization of our culture, but our preoccupation with health and illness in everyday life suggests further medicalization of our lives.

Iatrogenesis

Iatrogenesis is a term coined by Ivan Illich. The word *iatrogenesis* derives from Greek and describes "physician-induced disease"; the concept illustrates the negative implications of widespread medicalization. Illich was a very outspoken critic of biomedicine, boldly stating that "the medical establishment has become a major threat to health" (Illich, 1976, p. 3). In his view, medicine forever changed our daily lives; our society itself is now iatrogenic. Illich (1976) identified three levels of iatrogenesis.

Clinical iatrogenesis refers to physician-induced illness that directly results from medical practice. Medical procedures can harm individuals or create a chain reaction that leaves them sicker than they previously were. For instance, if an individual contracts a drug-resistant bacterial infection, known as a "superbug," while in hospital, this additional medical problem is clearly a direct result of receiving medical treatment. Negative side effects from medications are another example of clinical iatrogenesis. By prescribing a pill to the patient, a doctor may be helping the individual deal with their problem but, if the patient experiences negative side effects from the drug, the physician may be indirectly harming the individual as well.

Social iatrogenesis, according to Illich (1976), is evident in society's growing dependency on the medical practice. Biomedicine actively encourages individuals to become consumers of medical care. Our society, he says, is a "morbid society" in which people are dependent on medical experts. Self-care is almost abandoned and is considered secondary to medical knowledge. Pharmaceutical companies promote the medicalization of conditions that were previously non-medicalized. According to Illich (1976), if we cannot make a free choice about whether to receive care at home or in a hospital, or if our choice to decline biomedicine is seen as deviant, we are living in an iatrogenic society. Our dependence on biomedicine is firmly entrenched in our society. We have an overarching health care system with its own institutions, hospitals, and clinics. We can anticipate seeing health care professionals at schools, camps, work, and other places where they perform their duties. The proportion of money that our government invests in the (biomedical) health care system is growing; this expansion might be described as an additional example of social iatrogenesis and an over-reliance on the medical establishment.

The final form of iatrogenesis that affects our society is *cultural iatrogenesis* (Illich, 1976). Our culture aims to escape pain, suffering, decline, and, ultimately, death. Biomedicine is the

CASE STUDY

Do We Live in an Iatrogenic Society?

Although many Canadian provinces allow minors to actively participate in medical decisions, minors' choices may be questioned if they decline treatment for an illness.

When a 15-year-old girl from Winnipeg known as A.C. refused a blood transfusion because the procedure was against her religious beliefs, child services removed her from her parents' guardianship and forced her to have the transfusion. The girl was a devoted Jehovah's Witness and her family launched legal action to question the right of the state to force medical treatments against an individual's will. Ultimately, the court sided with child welfare services and the state, suggesting that the patient was a minor who could not make her own decision. In 2009, the Supreme Court of Canada upheld this decision, arguing that the state was acting in the "best interests of the child."

While students may disagree with the teen's religious beliefs or her perspective on blood transfusion, it should still be possible to draw some parallels between this case and what Illich called social iatrogenesis. What are the "best interests of the child" in this case? Who defines what is best and on what criteria?

Source: National Post (2009).

method we use to erase these experiences from our lives. Today, facing pain and suffering is equated with masochism, a deviant behaviour. Illich argued that human culture always offers a script of behaviour that provides people with the right way to deal with illness and dying. The ability to empathize with these experiences is what makes us cultural beings and what connects our bodies to the bodies of people around us. Each of us, as a human being, is equipped with the genetic and social resources to face pain and death. And traditionally, the role of healing was to provide comfort and support to individuals going through the process of illness and/or dying.

In contemporary society, however, views on pain and dying have changed. Biomedical culture has replaced the human response to pain with a prescription for painkillers. It has undermined our ability to deal with impairment and a loss of function. Not only are we seeking to escape pain and suffering, we are also actively trying to escape death (Turner, 2007). According to Turner (2007), our psychological and emotional vulnerability to pain and death is what makes us human; it is what distinguishes us as a species and makes us unique. Our culture, Illich (1976) would suggest, is suffering from iatrogenesis—our traditional morals and norms are being replaced by biomedical concepts and practices.

Chapter Summary

The goal of this chapter was to demonstrate how the expansion of biomedical culture affects our lives. First, it examined how the biomedical model has distinguished itself from other forms of healing. It then discussed what social and cultural transitions facilitated this change and elevated the status of biomedicine in society. After discussing the history of the biomedical establishment, it analyzed the role biomedicine plays in contemporary culture. Students were asked to study the process of medicalization and how it affects our lives at three different levels. Finally, the chapter considered negative aspects of medicalization, iatrogenesis, and the social and cultural changes brought about by biomedicine.

There are three primary messages that students should consider upon reading this chapter. First, biomedicine is more than an approach to healing human bodies. Biomedical beliefs are firmly embedded in our culture; they shape our everyday lives and the way we understand the world around us. Second, the expansion of biomedicine and the process of medicalization cannot be reduced to a discussion of progress in a medical laboratory. Social and cultural notions about moral/immoral, normal/deviant and right/wrong form the knowledge base of biomedicine and drive biomedical research. Biomedicine is often perceived as an objective, science-driven enterprise, but it is wise to remember that it is also inherently social—the diseases we choose to study and the phenomena we label "a disease" are shaped by our cultural beliefs. Finally, we have to remember that the expansion of biomedicine is not always an exclusively positive phenomenon. Moreover, the intrusion of biomedical culture into our everyday life can eradicate our own culture. Scholars such as Turner (2007) and Illich (1976) argue that being vulnerable to pain, suffering, and death is a uniquely human experience. Biomedical culture aims to eliminate pain and suffering from the range of human experiences, and some scientists are even searching for the means to overcome death itself (Turner, 2007). If we can no longer die, will we still be human?

STUDY QUESTIONS

1. What is meant by the term *biomedicine*, and what are the keys beliefs of biomedical culture?
2. How can we best explain the dominant position enjoyed by biomedicine?
3. How has the basic experience of "being human" been shaped by the emergence of biomedicine?
4. Draw up a list of processes, conditions, and life experiences that have undergone medicalization. Draw up a separate list for demedicalization.
5. What does the term *iatrogenesis* refer to? Why are critics concerned about it?

SUGGESTED READINGS

Conrad, P. (1992). Medicalization and social control. *Annual Review of Sociology*, 209–32.
Lock, M. & Nguyen, V. K. (2010). *An anthropology of biomedicine*. Etobicoke: John Wiley & Sons.
Rose, N. (2007). *The politics of life itself: Biomedicine, power, and subjectivity in the twenty-first century*. Princeton: Princeton University Press.

SUGGESTED WEB RESOURCES

Conrad, P. (2013). The Medicalization of Society. Lecture given at Center for Health Policy at the University of New Mexico [Video file]: www.youtube.com/watch?v=9l8LJjy5B2g
Ben Goldacre's TEDMED Talk: What Doctors Don't Know about the Drugs They Prescribe: www.ted.com/talksben_goldacre_what_doctors_don_t_know_about_the_drugs_they_prescribe
Orlansky, I. Are We Over-Medicalized? TEDMED Talk [Video file]: www.ted.com/talks/ivan_oransky_are_we_over_medicalized

GLOSSARY

Allopathic A type of medicine that focuses on diagnosing an illness and treating it using remedies that counter its symptoms. For example, an allopathic doctor would prescribe a painkiller for a headache.

Biomedicine A system of healing that views illness as a biological manifestation affecting the individual. It relies upon ideas of mind–body dualism, physical reductionism, and specific etiology. It is considered the most legitimate form of healing by most Western governments and citizens.

Iatrogenesis Harm that results directly from medical treatment, such as the side effects of a prescription drug.

Machine metaphor A way of viewing the body, assuming that the body is but the sum of all of its "components" and "parts"—in a sense, the body is a machine made of individual mechanisms.

Mind–body dualism A theory postulated by René Descartes (seventeenth century) stating that the mind and the body are two separate, discrete entities.

Physical reductionism The act of analyzing a physical entity in light of its smallest parts. An example of this could be analyzing diseases on a microbiological level or studying the immunology of human blood types.

Regimen and control A basic tenet of biomedicine, stating that all illnesses and diseases can be prevented through a closely monitored, controlled, and regimented healthy lifestyle.

Secularization The process by which society has become increasingly detached from religious influence.

Specific etiology From -aita, the Greek word for "cause." Specific etiology suggests that illnesses have a unique, identifiable cause.

REFERENCES

Beresford, M. J. (2010). Medical reductionism: Lessons from the great philosophers. *QJM: An International Journal of Medicine, 103*(9), 721–24. doi: 10.1093/qjmed/hcq057

Bloom, S. (2002). *The word as scalpel: A history of medical sociology*. Oxford: Oxford University Press.

Brubaker, S. J. (2007). Denied, embracing, and resisting medicalization. *Gender & Society, 21*(4), 528–52. doi: 10.1177/0891243207304972

Canadian Mental Health Association. (2014). *Facts about mental illness* Retrieved from www.cmha.ca/media/fast-facts-about-mental-illness

Clarke, A. E., Shim, J. K., Mamo, L., Fosket, J. R., & Fishman, J. R. (2003). Biomedicalization: Technoscientific transformation of health, illness, and U.S. biomedicine. *American Sociological Review, 68*, 161–94.

Coburn, D., Torrance, G. M., & Kaufert, J. M. (1983). Medical dominance in Canada in historical perspective: The rise and fall of medicine? *International Journal of Health Services, 13*(3), 407–32.

Conrad, P. (2000). Medicalization, genetics and human problems. In C. E. Bird, P. Conrad, & A. M. Fremont (Eds.), *Handbook of medical sociology* (5th ed., pp. 322–33). Nashville, TN: Vanderbilt University Press

———. (2005). The shifting engines of medicalization. *Journal of Health and Social Behavior, 46*(1), 3–14.

———. (2007). *The medicalization of society: On the transformation of human conditions into treatable disorders*. Baltimore, MA: John Hopkins University Press.

——— & Leiter, V. (2004). Medicalization, markets and consumers. *Journal of Health and Social Behavior, (extra issue)*, 158–76.

——— & Schneider, J. W. (1980). *Deviance and medicalization: From badness to sickness*. Philadelphia, PA: Temple University Press.

Davis-Floyd, R. E. (1990). The role of obstetrical rituals in the resolution of cultural anomaly. *Social Science and Medicine, 31*(2), 175–89.

———. (1994). The technocratic body: American childbirth as cultural expression. *Social Science and Medicine, 38*(8), 1125–40.

DES Action Canada. (2014). *Our organization.* Retrieved from www.descanada.ca/anglais/anglais.html

DES Action USA. (2014). *About DES Action USA.* Retrieved from www.desaction.org/aboutus.htm

Elhadi, A. M., Kalb, S., Perez-Orribo, L., Little, A. S., Spetzler, R. F., & Preul, M. C. (2012). The journey of discovering skull base anatomy in Ancient Egypt and the special influence of Alexandria. *Neurological Focus, 33*(2), e2.

Estes, C. & Binney, E. (1989). The biomedicalization of aging: Dangers and dilemmas. *Gerontologist, 29*, 587–96.

Featherstone, L. (2001). The kindest cut? The Caesarean section as turning point, Australia 1880–1900. In M. Porter, P. Short, & A. O'Reilly (Eds), *Motherhood: Power and oppression* (pp. 25–40). Toronto, ON: Women's Press.

Finniss, D. G., Kaptchukb, T. J., Miller, F., & Benedetti, F. (2012). Biological, clinical, and ethical advances of placebo effects. *The Lancet, 375*(9715), 686–95.

Fox, R. C. (1994). The medicalization and demedicalization of American society. In P. Conrad & R. Kern (Eds), *The sociology of health and illness: Critical perspectives* (pp. 414–18). New York: St. Martin's Press.

Freidson, E. (1970). *Profession of medicine*. New York: Dodd, Mead and Company.

Freund, P. E S., McGuire, M. B., & Podhurst, L. S. (2003). *Health, illness and the social body: A critical sociology* (4th ed.). Upper Saddle River, NJ: Prentice Hall.

Gorman, B. K. & Read, J. G. (2007). Why men die younger than women. *Geriatrics and Aging, 10*(3), 182–91.

Grekul, J., Krahn, A., & Odynak, D. (2004). Sterilizing the "feeble-minded": Eugenics in Alberta, Canada, 1929–1972. *Journal of Historical Sociology, 17*(4), 358–84.

Hammes, B. & Laitman, C. J. (2003). Diethylstilbestrol (DES) update: Recommendations for the identification and management of DES-exposed individuals. *Journal of Midwifery and Women's Health, 48*(1), 19–29.

Illich, I. (1976). *Medical nemesis: The limits of medicine.* London: Penguin.

Katz Rothman, B. (1989). *Recreating motherhood: Ideology and technology in a patriarchal society.* New York/London: W.W. Norton & Company.

———— (1993). *The tentative pregnancy: How amniocentesis changes the experience of motherhood.* New York: Norton Press.

Katz, R. V., Kegeles, S. S., Kressin, N. R., Wang, M. Q., James, S. A., Russell, S. L., . . . McCallum, J. M. (2006). The Tuskegee Legacy Project: Willingness of minorities to participate in biomedical research. *Journal of Healthcare for Poor and Underserved, 17*(4), 698–715.

Lombardo, P. A. (1996). Medicine, eugenics, and the Supreme Court: From coercive sterilization to reproductive freedom. *Journal of Contemporary Health Law & Policy, 13*(1), 1–25.

Lupton, D. (2003). Power relations and the medical encounter. In D. Lupton (Ed.), *Medicine as culture: Illness, disease and the body in Western societies* (pp. 113–141). London: Sage.

McKinlay, J. B. & Arches, J. (1985). Towards the proletarianization of physicians. *International Journal of Health Services, 15*(2), 161–95.

Mehta, N. (2011). Mind–body dualism: A critique from a health perspective. *Mens Sana Monographs, 9*(1), 202–09.

Mosby, I. (2013). Administering colonial science: Nutrition research and human biomedical experimentation in Aboriginal communities and residential schools, 1942–1952. *Social History, 46*(91), 145–72.

Moseley, J. B., O'Malley, K., Petersen, N. J., Menke, T. J., Brody, B. A., Kuykendall, D. H., . . . Wray, N. P. (2002). A controlled trial of arthroscopic surgery for osteoarthritis of the knee. *New England Journal of Medicine, 347*(2), 81–88.

National Post. (2009). Teen cannot refuse blood transfusion, top court rules. *National Post* Retrieved from www.nationalpost.com/related/topics/Teen+cannot+refuse+blood+transfusion+court+rules/1735673/story.html

Navarro, V. (1988). Professional dominance or proletarization? Neither. *The Milbank Quarterly, 66* (Suppl. 2), 57–75.

Riessman, C.K. (1983). Women and medicalization: A new perspective. *Social Policy, 14,* 3–18.

Rosenberg, R.S. (2013). Abnormal is a new normal. Why will half of the U.S. population have a diagnosable mental disorder? Retrieved from www.slate.com/articles/health_and_science/medical_examiner/2013/04/diagnostic_and_statistical_manual_fifth_edition_why_will_half_the_u_s_population.2.html

Social Anxiety Institute. (2014). DSM-5 Definition of Social Anxiety Disorder. Retrieved June 13, 2015 from https://socialanxietyinstitute.org/dsm-definition-social-anxiety-disorder

Szasz, T. S. (2007). *The medicalization of everyday life: Selected essays* (1st ed.). Syracuse, N.Y: Syracuse University Press.

Thane, P. (2005). *A history of old age.* Los Angeles: Paul Getty Museum.

Turner, B. (2007). *Can we live forever? A sociological and moral inquiry.* London, London: Anthem Press.

Zola, I. K. (1994). Medicine as an institution of social control. In P. Conrad & R. Kern (Eds), *The sociology of health and illness: Critical perspectives.* (pp. 392–402). New York: St Martin's Press.

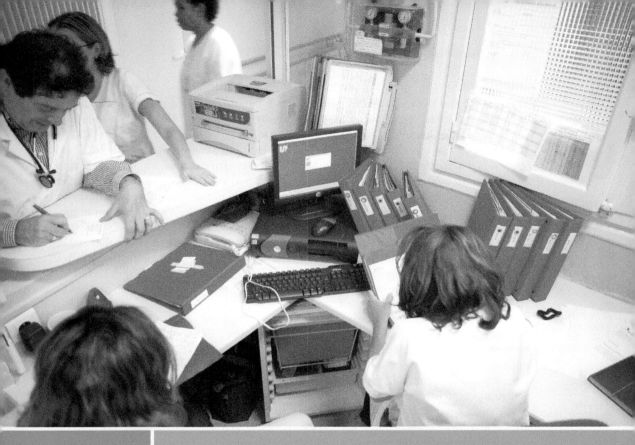

9

Health Care Systems, Public and Private

Michel Grignon

LEARNING OBJECTIVES

In this chapter, students will learn

- how health care systems are organized, managed, and funded
- the ways in which health care is financed
- the aspects of regulating health care
- that health care systems are a product of broader social contexts

Introduction

What we call "health care" is a relationship in which a group of individuals, known as "carers" or "providers," offers "personal services" to an individual "patient" (literally, the "one who suffers," from the Greek word *pathos*).

Of course, any service is personal to some extent, but services we call "personal" are specific in that the process matters more than the outcome. For example, when a person takes a taxi to go from A to B, they expect the driver to do just that, and they can monitor whether the driver is doing it as expected; there is nothing personal in such a relationship. The driver simply shuttles the individual between locations. But when a person asks a teacher to provide education to their children or asks a doctor for help when ill, it is not really possible to define a clear-cut outcome. Instead, we must rely on a due process. We trust that the teacher or carer will work in our best interests (Corduneanu-Huci et al., 2012). This element of trust is crucial to any care relationship. In technical terms, it is called a **principal–agent relationship**: we, as patients, are principals and we delegate decisions to an agent, such as a physician or nurse, who acts on our behalf.

There are several different classes of agents. An occupation is a regulated field of practice. In this sense, it is an institution, since it is regulated by a public body, such as the government. These regulations determine who can practise, what they can do, and, more importantly, what they are the only ones allowed to do. A profession is a self-controlled and monitored occupation. The profession itself controls training, licensing, disciplining, and sometimes even earnings. The word *profession* comes from the verb "to profess." Members have to take a public oath to work in the best interests of their principals. As a result, they are not usually paid a wage or salary. They earn fees, a very old feudal concept. The amount we pay doctors is not determined by supply and demand but, rather, by the social value and rank of the profession. As a result, patients are not allowed to shop around freely and pick anyone providing care. They have to interact with organized occupations and professions protected by the state. In this sense, the health care system is regulated (Bourgeault & Grignon, 2013).

As with any personal service, health care can be delivered in both a "formal" and "informal" context. When health care is delivered within pre-established relationships, such as through one's family or with a stranger, it is known as "informal" health care. "Formal" health care requires an explicit contract identifying the agent ("carer"), the principal ("patient"), and the duties of the agent toward the principal. With informal health care, the contract is implicit. For instance, parents care for their children when they are sick by virtue of being parents. However, what is formal and explicit varies across societies and time periods. For instance, 65 per cent of the elderly in Japan live with one of their children (Kinsella, 1999) versus 35 per cent in Portugal, and 3 per cent in Denmark (Iacovou, 2000).

What distinguishes health care from other personal services is that the patient is suffering from natural causes and that this state of suffering is seen as abnormal. What constitutes "health care" is highly contestable and largely a social construct. Different groups will have different views on what constitutes suffering, what is a natural cause, and what is pathological. For instance, in medieval Europe, many physical illnesses were viewed as moral problems. Being sick signalled that a person had an evil character and, as such, required punishment, not compassion. In contrast, many people now view abnormal behaviours as the result of a natural pathology such as a mental illness.

A health care system is a set of rules that presides over the functioning of the patient–carer relationship. These rules are, of course, social constructs and different societies will choose different rules (Grignon, 2012). These rules also determine how and where health care is delivered. Even though systems differ widely, we can distinguish three main characteristics of the health care relationship that are universal: licensure, health insurance, and contractors and funding.

Licensure

Since patient–carer health care relationships involve trust, there can be uncertainty regarding whether the health care professional acts with the best interests of the patient in mind. **Licensing** aims to eliminate such uncertainty by determining who can and cannot work as a health care professional. Professions and occupations control the process of licensure, providing credentials only to qualified practitioners. Drugs and medical goods go through a similar process known as authorization. Authorization is controlled by agencies such as the Canadian Agency for Drugs and Technologies in Health (CADTH), the Food and Drug Administration (FDA) in the US, and the European Medicines Agency (EMA) in the European Union.

Health Insurance

Because health care involves an abnormal state (sickness and suffering), it differs from other personal services in that not everyone will need it at one point in their life; it is different from education in that respect. This is a second element of uncertainty in health care and it justifies the existence of some kind of health insurance. Insurance programs are informal in many countries, and formal (through health insurance companies or public health insurance plans) in OECD countries.[1] As a result we rarely pay providers directly for what they do but rather pay into an insurance pool that will then pay providers for the services we receive. This is called a **third-payer relationship**: instead of paying a doctor directly, a third party, such as an insurance company, will fund the patient's health care services. This third party does not pay out of its own pocket. It simply redistributes to providers the money it has collected in the insurance pool. Therefore, patients indirectly pay for their own health care. The operation of collecting and pooling money from individuals is called financing health care. Whether private, such as **premiums**, or public, such as taxes—these contributions go to the insurance pool. There are rules that dictate the process of collecting and distributing these resources.

Contractors and Funding

Health care services are complex. They often involve several health care providers from different fields, such as occupational therapists, doctors, or nutritionists. The technologies and services used in medicine are advanced, and therefore costly. It is almost impossible for patients or their families to navigate all of this alone. A contractor is needed, someone who will organize a patient's care. This contractor can be the insurer or a separate organization such as a health management plan, a medical group, or a managed care organization. The contractor receives money from the insurance company and uses it to pay individual health care providers. The contractor is also expected to monitor quality on a statistical basis, keeping note of a doctor's performance.

To summarize: a health care system organizes the provision of health care to patients through three functions (financing, funding, and regulating), a variety of rules (licensure, authorization, insurance contributions), and a host of institutions (occupations, professions, insurers). The rest of this chapter describes these functions in greater detail.

Financing Health Care: How Health Care Insurance Works

We cannot predict when we will get sick. Medical treatments can be very expensive, so it makes sense to pool individual resources together so that those without health problems can help subsidize the sick. This is how insurance works: At the beginning of the year everyone contributes according to what their health care will cost on average. This is called an *actuarially fair premium*, and this pool of funds allows individuals to receive care without paying for it if they are sick. Insurance guarantees that, even when ill, a person can still afford other items (food, car, housing, leisure) rather than having to cut those expenses in order to pay for medical treatment. For obvious reasons, a lack of insurance—whether a person is excluded for financial or other reasons—can be quite harmful to an individual.

One specificity of health insurance is that it generally pays off through covering treatments regardless of their costs: few people would be satisfied with health insurance that merely provided a lump sum payment in case of illness, leaving the individual to absorb all costs above and beyond that sum. Because insurance covers the cost of treatment, whatever it might be, it is said to pay off through a reduction in the price of health care: the insured, when sick, find themselves in a world where the price of health care is much reduced compared to what they would have to pay if not insured.

Individuals are typically better off with full coverage (i.e., all their costs are covered) than with partial coverage. Insurers can even charge a fee to cover their administrative costs and individuals are still better off fully covered, even though it may mean paying more.

Full Coverage versus Co-payments

Insurance coverage can be problematic. When the cost of treatments is reduced, individuals may seek more services than they actually need. For example, they might opt for desired (but unnecessary) health care interventions such as additional blood tests or scans. Thus, the cost of treatments for all individuals will increase. This is known as the **moral hazard problem**. Thus, in theory, some people might actually be better off without purchasing insurance coverage. One option to counter moral hazard is to introduce **co-payments**: instead of covering the full cost of treatment, the insurer might pay only 90 per cent, leaving 10 per cent for the patient to pay. Because of the co-payment, people are less likely to purchase "unnecessary" care. Some private insurance plans (and even social insurance plans such as that found in France) leave co-payments to patients, meaning that up to 30 per cent of the cost of some treatments must be covered by individuals.

The question of an "optimal" co-payment rate in health insurance has been hotly debated for decades among economists (Nyman, 2000; Nyman, 2004). The primary and most well-established empirical observation is based is the following: on average, being insured means people utilize more health care services when sick—consulting more physicians, obtaining more prescriptions, and ordering more tests. Yet this does not necessarily mean that we have a moral hazard problem: a moral hazard problem would result from the insured using too much care, but the empirical difference between the insured and uninsured might also result from the non-insured using too little health care. A recent review of the literature on this topic (Grignon, 2014) indicates that not being insured causes poorer health, suggesting that not all is moral hazard and that introducing co-payments might create barriers to care that is needed. Also, we would have a moral hazard problem if (and only if) the decision to pursue more treatment when insured was made by patients themselves. Crucially, however, providers can influence people's decisions to pursue treatment; thus introducing co-payments will not necessary help. Rather, co-payments would likely only penalize the partially insured who are told by their doctor to spend more and get more. Overall, evidence suggests that the ideal solution is to introduce co-payments on the coverage of treatments that are highly predictable and controlled by the patient (such as prescription glasses, dental care, or cosmetic surgery), but not on treatments for highly unpredictable health problems requiring high technology, such as treatment for heart attacks.

Public versus Private

Once we agree that full coverage should be the norm for most treatments, we must next question whether coverage should be public or private. Public health insurance is also known as **universal coverage**. In a universal system, everyone (or at least everyone within a given group defined by age for instance, such as in the case of US Medicare) must enroll: opting

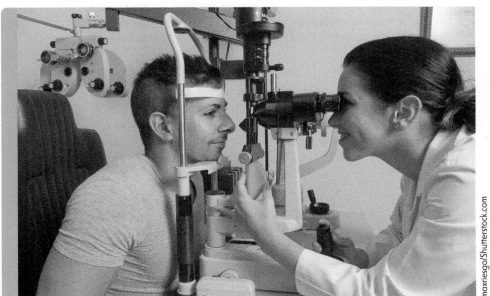

maxriesgo/Shutterstock.com

Many regular and predictable treatments that are controlled by the patient, such as having one's eyes tested in preparation for acquiring a new pair of glasses, are not covered by provincial health insurance schemes in Canada.

out of coverage is not permitted. Private health insurance, on the other hand, is **voluntary coverage**; one can decide whether to buy coverage or not.

Health care systems are not necessarily entirely public or entirely private. The US system is universal on paper (since the Affordable Care Act became a reality) but a substantial portion of the population is still uninsured. At the other end of the spectrum, some apparently voluntary schemes are so heavily subsidized (e.g., when employers sponsor and subsidize a plan for their employees) or so linked to a social contract that almost all eligible people enroll.

The next major distinction when it comes to insurance is between competition and monopoly: can insured individuals choose among plans or do they have to enroll with the only plan available to them? In practice, three situations exist: voluntary and competitive (the private model); compulsory and competitive (the American or the Swiss system); and compulsory and monopoly (the public model, as we have in Canada). No health system exemplifies voluntary and monopoly.

Historically, the financing of health care has followed three distinct models, as shown in Table 9.1.

Those in favour of a competitive system stress that it allows individuals to choose the coverage plan that best suits their individual needs. At the same time, however, critics highlight two fundamental problems with competition between health insurance providers:

1. **Switching plans.** Competition implies the option to switch plans. As such, insurers cannot sell long-term contracts that would allow individuals to pay the same fee over an extended period of time, say, for the next ten years. Short-term insurance plans can be helpful for acute illnesses such as heart attacks. However, chronic health issues require constant treatment over a number of years. Accordingly, long-term fixed premiums are

TABLE 9.1	Typology of Insurance Systems
Beveridge model	This model is named after Lord Beveridge, who wrote a report on the welfare state in Britain during World War II. It provides universal, compulsory benefits to all people but usually in a limited way. It is strictly rationed and controlled. This system is found in the UK and most Scandinavian countries as well.
Bismarck model	This model was named after Chancellor Bismarck of Prussia (Germany) at the end of the nineteenth century. This system builds on pre-existing social insurance funds. Such funds were usually created by occupational trades to cover the major financial risks of life (unemployment, illness, funerals) for its members. Each trade had its own pool and a set of rules for coverage.
American model	This model is more decentralized. Hospitals would set up their own insurance pools so that patients could afford the services these hospitals had to offer. Very often, hospitals sold their pools to local employers who would then encourage their workforce to enroll.

Note: A synthesis of these systems can be found in Kutzin (2001).

attractive for two reasons: we do not know whether we will be chronically ill years down the line, and we generally believe that fixed premiums are fairer. It is not right that some-one diagnosed with heart disease, diabetes, or dementia ends up paying more for treat-ments that are required for the rest of their life. Unfortunately, no competitive market for insurance offers that kind of long-term insurance. No competitive long-term care insurance guarantees that a person's premium will not increase if they suddenly require long-term care (Grignon & Bernier, 2012).

2. **Pooling.** Some individuals might not choose the plan they actually want but will opt for insurance preferred by people they want to be pooled with. This often means that, although many individuals want comprehensive health insurance, they may choose less comprehensive plans due to lower costs. Since the price of insurance depends on who buys it, a plan that attracts sicker individuals will generally cost more (since these indi-viduals are likely to utilize more health care services). If insurers can tell in advance what group will spend more on average, they will create different plans with different premiums for individuals to choose from. A standard result is that those who know they are healthier will want more stringent, cheaper plans (providing less coverage albeit at a much lower premium). They know that extremely sick individuals will not choose these plans and, therefore, the cost of such plans will not drastically increase. When individuals want to separate this much, the market collapses and insurance is no longer competitive. This is why the elderly (65+) are often covered by a public, compulsory, monopolistic (rather than competitive) insurer—in that age category, the stakes are important and insurance markets are likely to collapse (Evans, 1984; Hurley, 2010).

How Should Revenues Be Collected?

In a purely competitive market, insurers charge individuals an average fee based on their likelihood of illness. Typically, this means that individuals who have pre-existing health conditions must pay higher premiums. Other markets are regulated, with rules imposed on insurers so that they cannot use all the information they have about an individual; instead, they charge a community rating—within a given area or community, all members of the same sex and age group pay the same amount, regardless of their health status.

The insured will then try to self-select, as described above, using the stringency of the plan. When private insurers cover a group (e.g., all workers of a given employer) they use experi-ence rating: insurance fees are based on the total health care cost of the group divided by the number of workers in the firm. Mandatory insurers in a social insurance system where vari-ous groups of workers (usually by trade) belong to various schemes also use experience rating.

Lastly, public, compulsory, universal, monopolistic insurers can either charge a flat rate or offer a sliding scale based on a person's ability to pay (i.e., the rich pay more as contributions are a share of income). In the former case, the poor may not be able to afford the premium, and a public fund must help them; in the latter, the rich might want to opt out and stop paying more than they would in a purely private market. If enough high-income individuals share their sentiments, they can vote down the public insurance scheme, or get a right to opt out, forcing poorer individuals to pay more. For a good introduction on revenue collection in health care systems, see Evans (2002).

CASE STUDY

Germany and the Right to Opt Out

In some health care systems, individuals contribute toward health care on the basis of their ability to pay. Thus, rather than having all citizens pay an equal flat rate, the rich pay more than the poor. Although some wealthy citizens might not object to such a system (seeing it as fair, just, or even a responsibility that comes with wealth), others might feel that such a system penalizes them for "being successful" and generating more money. In these situations, wealthy individuals might push for the right to opt out of the public system, believing they can get cheaper or better care through the private market.

In Germany, for example, the wealthiest 10 per cent of citizens can opt out and buy private insurance instead of contributing to the public plan. Previously, individuals could opt out when young and opt back in as senior citizens. Now, however, the decision is irreversible and individuals must opt out once and for all.

How Health Insurance Works in the Real World and Why

Most rich countries have some form of universal, compulsory health insurance. In most low- and middle-income countries, which make up 82 per cent of the world population, there is minimal health insurance. Insurance is generally limited to the formal sector, which means that rural workers and the urban poor are not covered by a plan. This does not mean there is no insurance at all: very often, neighbours or relatives will come up with the large sum of money needed for a treatment when someone gets sick. Children, the elderly, and sometimes women may be excluded from these informal pools, however, as they may not be seen as "productive." Moreover, because these pools are small they cannot afford to cover truly expensive treatments such as those for cancer or cardiac diseases. In the absence of insurance, patients simply do not receive any modern treatments and opt for cheaper, "traditional" medicines.

Informal schemes are the birthplace of most modern insurance plans. In some informal insurance schemes in the past, a community would create a pool to pay the salary of a doctor to make sure he didn't leave. This is how medical insurance was started in rural communities in Saskatchewan in the 1930s. In 1947, the same province was also a pioneer in hospital insurance, instituting the first public (compulsory, universal) insurance pool in Canada to cover the costs of hospital stays. These costs were certainly modest compared to today, but they were still expensive compared to an individual's average income. The plan was established by a CCF government, the ancestor of the current NDP, under the leadership of Premier Tommy Douglas. Initially, Douglas's plan was resisted by doctors, hospitals, and businesses. However, the federal government offered a cost-sharing mechanism to provinces willing to set up hospital insurance. The federal treasury offered to fund half of the costs, and hospital insurance spread rapidly to all provinces. In 1962, Tommy Douglas launched another plan, this time to cover the cost of physician visits; again, this plan was resisted by doctors, who staged a massive strike. Again, the plan spread through federal cost sharing (1967). The last step in the formation of Canada's modern health insurance plan was the enactment of Medicare in 1984. Medicare prevented extra billing by doctors and hospitals: not only was health insurance public in Canada, it was also full coverage, with no out-of-pocket payment at the point of use.

Canada has never implemented any other public insurance plans: prescription drugs, long-term care and rehabilitation, and dental and eye services all remain unfunded. Thirty years after Medicare, Canada has a unique insurance system. Physician and hospital care are almost fully covered; there is some public coverage of prescription drugs for the elderly, the poor, and individuals who have to pay more than 5 or 10 per cent of their income for drugs; and there is almost no public coverage for dental care. Most other countries with public coverage finance less of each service (they allow extra-billing by doctors or leave co-payments to be paid by patients at the point of use), but cover more types of services, including dental care and prescription drugs. As a result, Canada ranks low in terms of public coverage (Evans, 2000; Marchildon, 2013).

Public health insurance in Canada is funded through the government's general revenues. All contributions (from taxpayers, corporations, consumers who pay duties, and sales taxes) go into a giant pot, some of which is used to pay for health care. It is therefore very difficult to know exactly who pays what for health care. However, because taxes are somewhat linked to income (income tax more than proportionally and sales taxes less than proportionally), it is fair to say that in Canada, the rich pay more for public health insurance than the poor (Corscadden, Allin, Wolfsin, & Grignon, 2014). In other countries, such as Switzerland and the Netherlands, everyone within age brackets and geographic boundaries pays the same amount. The poor pay the same unless they cannot afford it, in which case the government subsidizes the cost. In the Bismarck model, utilized in countries like Germany, each economic sector (agriculture, mining, steel manufacturers, and so on) sets up a separate pool called a "sickness fund." Each sector determines its own contribution rates and reimbursement policies. These funds tend to cover both treatment costs and income loss due to sickness. Because governments now allow individuals to enroll in whichever fund they want, the Bismarck model is evolving toward the general revenue model or the Swiss model, with sickness funds behaving like private insurers under community rating.

In Canada, dental care, prescription drugs, and vision care are not covered by public insurance. Instead, employers will often contribute a portion of each employee's paycheque and buy into a group insurance plan for private coverage. In Canada, approximately 15 per cent of total insurance expenditure is covered by private, employer-sponsored plans; 12 per cent is left for patients to pay, and 3 per cent is covered by donations (Marchildon, 2013).

Funding and Regulating Health Care

After determining how health insurance will be structured, it is important to consider the best way to pay health care providers. Should they be paid a wage for their time, should they be paid for each service they provide, or should they be given a flat-rate salary? Another important consideration is the regulation of health care services, as this can increase the price of treatments. While regulation can improve the quality of health care services, it may increase the price of health care in a competitive market.

All insurers, whether public, private, monopolistic, or competitive, must consider these issues. However, the insurance policy's approach will dictate how they deliver health care. Public insurance, for example, must respect the democratic process. As such, they will need to make decisions much more slowly than a private insurance company. Competition among insurance providers can influence how health care is delivered; competitive markets, many suggest, promote innovation and experimentation.

Insurers cannot afford to be cost-conscious if they are to succeed in a competitive market. The insured are potential patients who want access to the best providers and hospitals if they get sick. Accordingly, insurance programs must attract the best doctors, and this process can be quite costly. This increases the cost of insurance premiums.

At the other end of the spectrum is the public insurer who, in a position of monopoly, will have more clout to ration care. The public insurer is regulated by the elected government, so the public voters have a say in how health care is provided. Americans, for example, spend more than any other population on health care. Sixteen per cent of their national income goes to health care, compared to 11 per cent in Canada, (OECD, 2014). Accordingly, they get "more": shorter wait times and lavish access to high-technology diagnostics. Whether this system is actually efficient is still very much a disputed question.

How Much Regulation?

Licensure is the process that dictates who can act as a health care professional. The process aims to increase trust in the health care services relationship. Licences are often allotted on the basis of academic success, aiming to improve the quality of the workforce. For example, only good students are admitted to medical or nursing schools. To further improve worker accountability, licences can be revoked if a health care provider breaches, for example, their professional code of conduct. Non-licensed workers are less worried about being fired because, being paid their marginal value, they will find employment elsewhere at the same rate. Such a threat acts as a disciplining device, reminding the health care provider that they have an ethical obligation to their serve their patient, rather than themselves.

In theory, the process of regulation seems logical. But it is almost impossible to empirically assess whether licensure increases the quality of a health care provider's work. While there is little experimental data on this issue, the threat of being excluded from an esteemed group of professionals may improve quality and efficiency.

Licensure not only prevents non-certified individuals from practising, it also restricts mobility for those who are certified. A certified nurse working in Canada, for example, may not be licensed to work in the United States, or at least not before overcoming a protracted process to get their credentials recognized. Licensing also increases the cost of providing a service: locally licensed health care providers are protected from the competition of "foreign" workers. After all, patients can only negotiate with those who are legally allowed to work. In that sense, licensure works as a union.

Finally, licensure determines the scope of practice of a profession. If only doctors can provide a given array of services, it means nurses are prevented from providing them too, even though they might be as good at providing them in the majority of the cases. This restriction of scope also increases the cost of treatments in comparison with a purely competitive situation where doctors must compete with other types of health care professionals for patients and insurers. Overall, restrictions increase the cost of health care (and the incomes of providers) by between 10 and 20 per cent (Kleiner & Krueger, 2013).

Insurers, private or public, therefore look for more flexible tools of regulation to ensure quality without drastically increasing price. As mentioned in the introduction to this chapter, one aspect of the health care relationship that justifies licensure is the fact that outcomes are hard to observe (i.e., it is a personal relationship). For this reason, insurers are trying to find ways to monitor the results of patient–carer relationships. Health care systems have changed dramatically over the past thirty years as a result of the evidence-based movement. Prior to **evidence-based medicine (EBM)**, doctors, nurses, and hospitals were expected to do the right thing by virtue of being certified and accredited. There was no focus on the outcomes of the patient–carer relationship, only emphasis on the process of licensure. Health care providers were considered experts whose actions were usually beyond question, as detailed in Chapter Twelve. Insurers have used the evidence-based movement to their (and their customers') benefit in that they can now, at least in theory, monitor whether providers are indeed doing their best and working on behalf of their patients. Insurers use their large caseloads to monitor how various providers perform on average. They measure quality against recommendations in the EBM literature, acting as a "statistical buyer."

Paying Providers

Monitoring doctors, nurses, and hospitals is not simple, however. First, it requires a highly skilled workforce, able to understand medical decisions and access and analyze complex data. Second, it requires winning a power struggle with providers: it is often difficult to take action when providers do not deliver the required level of quality; action may include penalizing a provider or excluding them altogether, barring patients from seeing them. But providers can appeal to their patients' loyalty. Patients, too, can refuse to abide by such restrictions, remaining faithful to "their" doctor. Private insurers who tried to select doctors and hospitals in the US in the 1990s, during the so-called "managed care revolution," faced a backlash from patients. As a result, private insurers cannot really restrict access to a select few health care providers. They must be content with varying co-payments across providers in the hope that patients will choose a provider that the insurance company favours. In health care systems that are publicly funded, the government-sponsored scheme acts as the only third-payer (called a single-payer for that reason); in these systems, it is even more difficult for the payer to act upon the results of monitoring since, with no option but to work for the single-payer, excluding a provider means depriving them of their ability to work.

This is why insurers try to use payment schemes to encourage good practices without having to closely monitor providers. In essence, payment schemes work along the following lines: if providers are financially rewarded for working in the best interests of the patient and penalized for doing things poorly, they will do their best to get the rewards and avoid the penalties. Consequently, health care providers' behaviours should align with payers' and patients' interests. This system is meant to incentivize providers: an incentive is a device that makes people follow instructions of their own accord rather than because they are ordered to do so. Of course, such a system relies on the assumption that providers are mainly motivated by income or profit. This is a strong and potentially dangerous assumption: if good doctors are motivated by an ethical desire to do well and see financial motivation as greed, they might react negatively to the incentives and lose their motivation to do things well. In the long run, it might also attract profit-motivated or greedy individuals to the health professions, discouraging the self-motivated individuals that most people would prefer to have as health care providers (see Grignon, Paris, & Polton, 2004).

CASE STUDY

Financial Incentives in Blood Donation and Child Care

Intuitively, it makes sense to reward people for good deeds or to punish them when they misbehave. We are surrounded by many instances of financial consequences for our behaviours: late fees for overdue library books, "employee of the month" bonuses, and higher electricity rates during peak periods of use. All of these examples reflect the logic that money can be used to encourage people to behave in the "right" way.

Yet in some cases, providing financial incentives to individuals for doing the right thing does not always work and can even make matters worse. For instance, it has been suggested that paying donors for their blood may attract only donors who want the financial reward, deterring those who give out of a sense of ethical responsibility (Titmuss, 1971). While some empirical evidence (Slonim, Wang, & Garbarino, 2014) does not seem to support the claim, in theory paying donors for blood may actually decrease the quantity and quality of blood that is collected.

Another example is when childcare agencies fine parents who are late to pick up their children. These fines are meant to incentivize parents to be on time. However, this system can result in more parents being late, realizing that they can now merely pay for tardiness rather than incurring moral blame for doing something wrong (Gneezy & Rustichini, 2000). These examples demonstrate that financial incentives do not always work as planned.

An issue with incentives is that payers do not always know what they are supposed to incentivize. If they want to encourage productivity through increasing the number of patient visits or treatments, paying health care providers per service would be effective. Such a process is called a retrospective payment: doctors are paid for their services after they provide them. Yet retrospective payment might encourage providers to offer too many services, even ones that do not benefit the patient. Since doctors are paid only per visit or treatment, this model could also discourage prevention.

If payers want to encourage quality and prevention, they might choose to give providers a given amount per patient (per capita) in a scheme called **capitation**. Any time a patient enrolls with a doctor or organization, the latter receives a lump sum to provide care for a given period of time. Usually, this sum is provided annually and covers the year to come. If the doctor/organization works well and their patients are sick less often than the average person of the same demographic group, the provider keeps a profit from the capitation. Such an incentive is great for quality but comes with two problems. First, providers will tend to select patients who will likely be well in the coming year, rejecting people who might represent too much work. In this model doctors can effectively cherry-pick their patients, neglecting those who need the most care. Quite obviously such a situation is problematic, since a health care system is supposed to treat those in need first. Secondly, providers will make decisions that are good for health in the long run but might be painful for their patients in the short term. A capitated provider will be less responsive to suffering if it will not necessarily lead to of deteriorating health. For example, there might be little harm in not addressing abdominal pain in a child if it is likely to go away without any intervention, yet refraining from treatment might not be what parents (or the child) want; thus, capitation systems are often seen as callous.

The last payment option is salary, paying doctors and nurses to provide care to whoever needs it. Doctors will have no problems seeing a child with belly pain and providing good quality care, but, at the same time, critics argue that they might spend too much time with each patient, reducing their overall productivity.

As students can see, each payment scheme has benefits and drawbacks, and there is no consensus on what comprises an optimal system of health care. The only consensus is that payment schemes must blend a bit of fee-for-service, capitation, and salary. Each mode of payment can be used to accomplish a specific goal, whether increasing efficiency or quality of care. A relatively new model of these blended schemes is called Pay-for-Performance (or P4P), in which providers receive a bonus any time they reach a target performance, for instance a proportion of their caseload receiving immunization (Hurley & Li, 2014).

How Licensure and Payment Schemes Work in the Real World

The traditional model of health care sees medical doctors working in solo practices, charging fees for their services, and hiring nurses. This model is called professional dominance: doctors dominate other health professionals and are reimbursed retrospectively for all of their costs. Payers, either in competition or single-payers, do not have much choice but to pay whatever price doctors ask.

By contrast, hospitals are paid through two models. If a hospital is public, they receive a global budget. Private hospitals are paid retrospectively. There are two major types of private hospitals: not-for-profit and for-profit. The former, often run by charities, charge what they need to operate and re-invest surpluses into the hospital itself. The latter receive funding from investors and distribute dividends when they make a profit. A third, smaller, category is known as proprietary clinics. These smaller structures are owned by a group of doctors who specialize in highly specialized care. Any profits are usually distributed among the clinic's founders.

Since the 1990s, most health systems in the OECD have been experimenting with new payment schemes. One of the first systems to begin this experimentation was American Medicare which made the decision to stop paying hospitals for whatever they claimed and start paying them per diagnosis. Under these rules, patients are assigned a diagnostic label when they are admitted to the hospital. According to how they are categorized, the hospital will receive a payment that reflects the average cost of treating such a diagnosis. This system resembles capitation and has its disadvantages. Hospitals have an interest to select cases that require relatively little intervention. They will provide no-frills care, guaranteeing that the patient leaves the hospital alive. Sometimes they may seek to ensure that the patient is not re-admitted too soon if this is part of their payment scheme. Other health care systems that used to pay their hospitals a global budget are also moving toward diagnosis-related payment. These hospitals hope to increase productivity through a higher number of admissions and shorter stays.

Independent of payment schemes and their reforms, hospitals in OECD countries have followed a similar path toward specialization in high-technology, high-stakes cases. Hospitals used to admit and treat patients who could have been treated in the community, but they now treat complex cases that cannot be treated in primary care settings. There has also been a push toward discharging patients sooner, making sure that only acute care patients occupy hospital beds.

Starting in the 2000s, most OECD health systems have moved away from fee-for-service payment schemes and toward more prospective payment schemes for primary care doctors. For instance, whereas 80 per cent of physicians' incomes were composed of fees in Ontario in 2003, that proportion has fallen to approximately 50 per cent in 2013 and is still declining. The Ontario **single-payer model** has created strong financial incentives for doctors to join multidisciplinary teams with other health professionals, such as nurses and dietitians. These teams are paid a mixture of capitation and fee-for-service. Blending payment schemes is more costly as payers have to put more money on the table to convince doctors to move away from solo practices and fee-for-service. At the same time, younger doctors often welcome this new model since they tend to enjoy working in teams and sharing the burden of being on call after hours. The multidisciplinary team might signal the decline of professional dominance and the emergence of clinical governance.

The ability of health systems to move away from fee-for-service and toward prospective payments for multidisciplinary teams depends on the societal context in which the health system has developed. Societies relying on high-level negotiations between employers and workers, like Germany's heavily unionized economy, are moving more slowly toward innovative payment schemes. Countries like Canada, with decentralized labour relationships in general, are more welcoming to these changes.

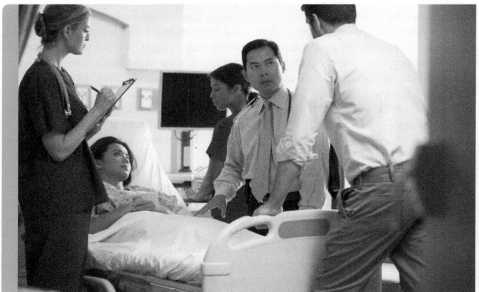

Strong incentives exist in some health systems—such as the system in Ontario—for physicians to work in teams.

Chapter Summary

A health system is a set of institutions and rules to regulate, finance, and pay for personal services called health care. There are very strong arguments in favour of public (compulsory, universal) insurance in health care due to market failures in competitive environments. There are no compelling arguments for generating revenues on a redistributive basis (the rich pay more) rather than a flat rate, except of course that the poor need to be helped. It is interesting to see that most countries (including the US) lean toward some form of universal, public insurance.

However, the form taken by that public insurance is very much the product of broader societal values and institutions. It seems to be resilient to change: for instance, the institution of employer-sponsored health insurance is now well entrenched as a societal value in the United States, even though it has its obvious shortcomings that the recent Affordable Care Act is trying to address. Most Americans who work and have a good plan would not agree to being pooled with less fortunate Americans into a national pool similar to the system in Canada. Similarly, even though we, in Canada, can see the benefits of a public plan for hospital and physician services, no government seems to be able (or willing) to expand that plan to other necessary medical services such as prescription drugs or dental care. Again, because 62 per cent of Canadians access these additional services through an employer-sponsored plan, it is hard to convince them to drop it in favour of a larger pool that would include the remaining 38 per cent less fortunate Canadians.

The same is true of regulating and funding, to a lesser extent; because the "ideal" or "proper" conclusions are less certain, we should not expect too much convergence of health systems. However, most systems are less strict in their definitions of scope of practice, licensure, and accreditation. Most systems are moving toward greater specialization of each type of provider as well as blended payment models. Systems are resilient in that area too, however: each jurisdiction maintains a local system of accreditation for its future providers through medical, dental, and nursing schools. They have specific mechanisms for the authorization of drugs and technologies. In that respect, the European Union constitutes a large-scale and bold experiment in which credentials are now recognized in all member countries (a German-educated doctor or nurse can practise freely in France or Portugal if they choose to do so, and authorized drugs are available for all 500 million Europeans, regardless of their home country).

Another aspect in which health systems are resilient is in their definition of what constitutes health care. Most systems follow a somewhat circular definition: health care is what is delivered by health care professionals. It is an obviously problematic definition but also a revealing one in that it confesses that health care is a social construct—society decides what qualifies as health care. Not everyone agrees, of course, and boundaries are highly disputed in all systems: kinesiology or traditional Chinese medicine are now regulated (if not covered) in Canada but are still marginal and almost clandestine in other jurisdictions. Kinesiology, for example, is not recognized as a health specialty in France: some physiotherapists might decide to practise it, but there is no official designation or credential. Midwifery, however, has been recognized for centuries in France but is still in its infancy in Canada; there are currently 20,000 practising midwives in France but fewer than 1,200 in Canada.

Lastly, health care systems are living organisms: health care is determined by innovation. New treatment possibilities appear almost every day. Many treatments that we now take for granted did not exist fifty years ago: for instance, angioplasty was first performed in 1977, and the first antidepressant medications were not marketed before the late 1950s. Moreover, innovation is adopted progressively and expands to more patients over the years: patients who were once deemed too frail to receive an intervention, most often because of their age, are now considered robust enough to receive it. The definition of what constitutes health care tomorrow is determined by decisions made in investments in research and development (R&D). Health care coverage also influences the progress of the field: a treatment that is not covered will be less likely to be widely adopted and, as a result, will not improve as much as a treatment that doctors use all the time. These decisions, in turn, reflect what societies want and what they can pay for; R&D in private firms is motivated by profit, helping those who can pay over those who are in the greatest need. For example, we are still waiting for a vaccine for malaria, an illness that mainly kills children in the developing world. We will likely only find a vaccine due to a generous private donor (perhaps the Bill & Melinda Gates Foundation). Pharmaceutical firms will not invest massively in a vaccine that no one will be able to buy. They would rather invest in cures for illnesses that affect the rich, elderly populations of the OECD, such as skin cancer.

STUDY QUESTIONS

1. Compare and contrast the arguments in favour of private and public forms of health insurance.
2. What factors led to the development of the modern Canadian health care system?
3. What are the primary differences between the Bismarck, Beveridge, and American models of health care?
4. Why does the licensure system exist? What are the arguments for and against it?
5. Why might someone support greater regulation for a health care system? Why might they oppose it?

SUGGESTED READINGS

Basu, S., Andrews, J., Kishore, S., Panjabi, R., & Stuckler, D. (2012). Comparative performance of private and public healthcare systems in low-and middle-income countries: A systematic review. *PLoS medicine, 9*(6), e1001244.

Marchildon, G. (Ed.). (2012). *Making medicare: New perspectives on the history of medicare in Canada.* Toronto: University of Toronto Press.

Star, P. (2011). *Remedy and reaction: The peculiar American struggle over healthcare reform.* New Haven: Yale University Press.

SUGGESTED WEB RESOURCES

Health Systems Reviews. European Observatory on Health Systems and Policies: www.euro.who.int/en/about-us/partners/observatory/publications/health-system-reviews-hits
The Waiting Room: Storytelling Project: www.whatruwaitingfor.com

YouTube Video: Impatient Optimists: Malaria (Bill & Melinda Gates Foundation): www.youtube.com/watch?v=sETIl3rn_Zo

YouTube Video: Universal health: From public coverage to private care (issues with health care funding in Africa, Asia, and Latin America): www.youtube.com/watch?v=YzNS5jd-LTY

GLOSSARY

Capitation A model of financing health care that pays providers a lump sum per patient to cover health care for a given period of time.

Co-payments The process in which patients pay for a portion of their services while insurers cover the remaining charges.

Evidence-based medicine (EBM) An approach to biomedicine that statistically evaluates how patients respond to treatments and what interventions are most effective. Evidence-based medicine is an empirical approach to medicine that is based on scientific research such as randomized controlled trials.

Licensing Using a system of formalized credentials to determine who can practise a given profession. For example, doctors must pass certification exams and complete medical school.

Moral hazard problem In health care, it arises when insured patients heavily utilize available health care resources. As a result, they drive up the cost of insurance for everyone involved.

Premium The fee charged for insurance coverage for a given period of time.

Principal–agent relationship A relationship in which the principal contracts an agent to work in the principal's best interests. Such a relationship involves an element of trust. Economists use this term to describe the relationship between a patient and health care practitioner.

Single-payer model How health insurance works in Canada. The government pays all health care providers directly for their services.

Third-payer relationship The process through which an insurance company, or another third party, pays the health care provider on behalf of a patient.

Universal coverage Health insurance that covers an entire demographic or population. Universal coverage is mandatory: citizens must enrol and cannot opt out.

Voluntary coverage Health insurance that individuals can opt to buy of their own volition. Such coverage is generally organized through private companies and is therefore competitive.

NOTE

1. The OECD, Organisation of Economic Co-operation and Development, is a group of 30 rich countries, representing 18 per cent of the world's population and 78 per cent of its GDP (the annual income).

REFERENCES

Bourgeault, I. & Grignon, M. (2013). A comparison of cross-professional boundaries in OECD countries. *European Journal of Comparative Economics*, *10*(2), 199–223.

Boyd, K. M. (2000). Disease, illness, sickness, health, healing and wholeness: Exploring some elusive concepts. *Journal of Medical Ethics: Medical Humanities, 26*, 9–17.

Corduneanu-Huci, C., Hamilton, A., & Ferrer, I. M. (2013). *Understanding policy change: How to apply political economy concept in practice.* Washington, DC: World Bank.

Corscadden, L., Allin, S., Wolfson, M., & Grignon, M. (2014). Publicly financed healthcare and income inequality in Canada. *Healthcare Quarterly*, *17*(2), 7–10.

Evans, R. G. (1984). *Strained mercy: The economics of Canadian healthcare*. Toronto, ON: Butterworths.

———. (2000). Canada. *Journal of Health Politics, Policy, and Law*, *25*(5), 889–97.

———. (2002). Financing healthcare: Taxation and the alternatives. In E. Mossialos, A. Dixon, J. Figueras & J. Kutzin (Eds), *Funding healthcare: Options for Europe* (pp. 48–75). Buckingham, PA: Open University Press.

Feachem, R., Neelam, G. A., Sekhri, K., & White, K. L. (2002). Getting more for their dollar: A comparison of the NHS with California's Kaiser Permanente. *British Meidcal Journal*, *324*(7330), 135–143.

Gneezy, U. & Rustichini, A. (2000). A fine is a price. *Journal of Legal Studies*, 29(1) , 1–17.

Grignon, M. (2012). A democratic responsiveness approach to real reform: An exploration of healthcare systems' resilience. *Journal of Health Politics, Policy and Law*, *37*(4), 665–76.

———. (2014). Access and health insurance. In: A. J. Culyer (Ed.), *Encyclopedia of health economics* (Vol.1, pp. 13–18). San Diego, CA: Elsevier.

——— & Bernier, N. (2012). *Financing options for long-term care in Canada*. Montreal: Institute for Research in Public Policy (IRPP).

———, Paris, V., & Polton, D. (2004). Influence of physician payment methods on the efficiency of the healthcare system. In F. Pierre-Gerlier, G. P. Marchildon, & T. McIntosh (Eds), *Changing healthcare in Canada: The Romanow papers* (Vol. 2). Toronto: University of Toronto Press.

Hurley, J. (2010). *Health economics*. Toronto, ON: McGraw Hill Ryerson.

——— & Li, J. (2014). Financial incentives and pay-for-performance. In G. P. Marchildon & L. di Matteo (Eds), *Bending the cost curve in health-care—Canada's provinces in international perspective* (pp. 35–64). Toronto: University of Toronto Press.

Iacovou, M. (2000). *Institute for Social and Economic Research, University of Essex: The living arrangements of elderly Europeans*. Retrieved from www.iser.essex.ac.uk/files/iser_working_papers/2000-09.pdf

Kinsella, K. (1999). Aging and the family: Present and future demographic issues. In Albers, C. (Ed.), *Sociology of the Family: Readings* (pp. 421–437). Buffalo, NY: Sage Publications.

Kleiner, M. M. & Krueger, A. B. (2013). Analyzing the extent and influence of occupational licensing on the labor market. *Journal of Labor Economics*, *31*(2), S173–202.

Kutzin, J. (2001). A descriptive framework for country-level analysis of healthcare financing arrangements. *Health Policy*, *56*(3), 171–204.

Light, D. & Dixon, M. (2004). Making the NHS more like Kaiser Permanente. *British Medical Journal*, *328*(7442), 763–5.

Marchildon, G. (2013). *Health in transition: Canada*. Copenhagen, Denmark: European Observatory of Healthcare Systems and Policies.

Nyman, J. (2000). *The theory of demand for health insurance*. Stanford University Press.

———. (2004). Is "moral hazard" inefficient? The policy implications of a new theory. *Health Affairs*, *23*(5), 194–99.

OECD—Organisation for Economic Co-operation and Development (2014). *Health database*. Retrieved from www.oecd.org/els/health-systems/health-data.htm

Slonim, R., Wang, C., & Garbarino, E. (2014). The market for blood. *Journal of Economic Perspectives*, *28*(2), 177–96.

Strandberg-Larsen, M., Schiøtz, M. L., Silver, J. D., Frølich, A., Andersen, J. A., Graetz, I., … Hsu, J. (2010). Is the Kaiser Permanente model superior in terms of clinical integration?: A comparative study of Kaiser Permanente, Northern California and the Danish healthcare system. *BMC: Health Services Research*, *10*(91), 1–13.

Titmuss, R.M. 1971. *The gift relationship*. London: Allen and Unwin.

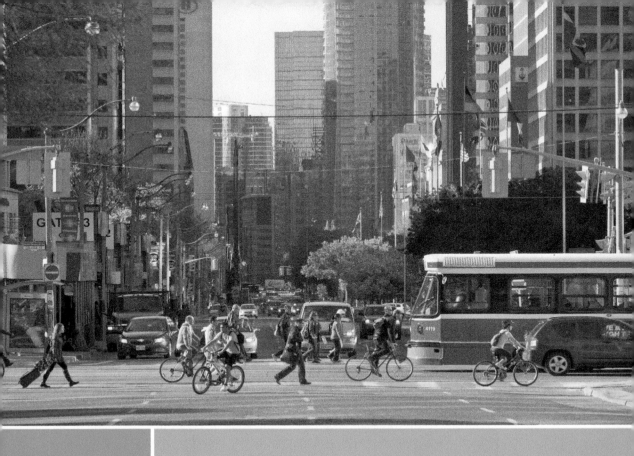

10

Social Determinants of Health

Anthony Lombardo

LEARNING OBJECTIVES

In this chapter, students will learn

- the broader social, economic, environmental, and political factors that shape health
- the importance of political and economic systems in health
- the influence of key determinants of health, including income, income inequality, social networks, and neighbourhoods
- to think critically about the causes of, and responses to, existing and emerging health issues

Introduction

Take a moment to ponder the following two questions: What makes people sick? On the other hand, what makes them healthy? According to typical messages in the media, people get sick because they do not do a good enough job of taking care of themselves. We eat "junk" food, spend too much time tweeting and posting on Facebook instead of exercising, and drink too much alcohol at parties. Conversely, we are told that we can keep healthy by following the Canada Food Guide, wearing a helmet when riding a bike, and using condoms. To some extent this is indeed true. However, this chapter will explore how health—or the lack thereof—is structured by forces well beyond what might be considered individual "choices." Indeed, the question of "choice" needs critical reflection itself. Although it is true that people make choices as individuals, the choices that we are able to make, and the options available to us, are functions of our social, economic, cultural, and political circumstances. In fact, "the primary factors that shape the health of Canadians are not medical treatments or lifestyle choices but rather the living conditions they experience" (Mikkonen & Raphael, 2010, p. 7).

These broader circumstances and contexts are known, collectively, as the social determinants of health. Figure 10.1 is a map of the many different influences on—or determinants of—health. In this chapter students will learn about the history of the social determinants of health concept. They will be introduced to some different approaches to understanding health. The chapter will then examine some key determinants of health and how they can be changed to influence health. Of course, this is a very broad area of study and this chapter can only introduce some key issues, debates, and examples. The goal is for students to think about health differently: why some people are healthy while others are not, the roots of these differences, and the nature of responses we should have to these health issues.

Canada's History with the Social Determinants of Health

Canada has been a leader in recognizing the importance of the social determinants of health and the related concept of **health promotion**. A first exploration of some of the social determinants of health occurred in the 1974 report *A New Perspective on the Health of Canadians* (Lalonde, 1981). From this report came the enduring **health field concept** (Lalonde, 1981), which aimed to direct attention to areas of importance for sustaining a healthy population. While Lalonde recognized that a focus on health care itself was important, he did not believe it should be the totality of the focus. Instead, he proposed the health field concept to shift the focus to a few other areas:

- **Human biology**—the biological and physiological aspects of health
- **Environment**—external factors like food safety and pollution, as well as the social environment
- **Lifestyle**—all other "decisions by individuals" that influence or impact their health, "over which they more or less have control" (Lalonde, 1981, p. 32)
- **Health care organization**—the nature of the health care system: the "quantity, quality, arrangement, nature, and relationships of people and resources in the provision of health care" (Lalonde, 1981, p. 32)

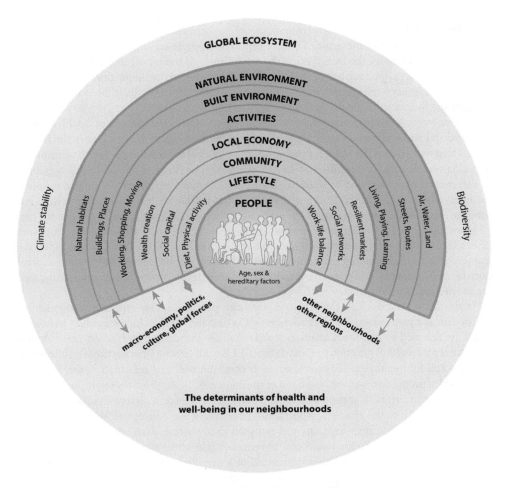

FIGURE 10.1   **The Determinants of Health and Wellbeing in Our Neighbourhoods**

Source: Barton & Grant (2006), Figure 1, p. 252.

The health field concept was important because it began to acknowledge factors beyond the individual that could impact health. However, note the description of lifestyle risks: "personal decisions and habits that are bad, from a health point of view, create self-imposed risks. When those risks result in illness of death, the victim's lifestyle can be said to have contributed to, or caused, his [sic] own illness or death" (Lalonde, 1981, p. 32). The keen observer might take some issues with this "lifestyle" category and notice how it seems completely divorced from the "environment" category. In other words, the health field concept does not seem to take into account how the environment, an aspect which individuals cannot control, might impact the "risky decisions" that individuals come to make.

Indeed, as it turned out, the government of the day (and successive ones) picked up on the "lifestyle" component of the health field concept. The lifestyle argument seemed to offer the most political "bang for the buck," while the others areas of the report did not offer as much traction for policy (Raphael, 2008). As such, the *Lalonde Report* unintentionally emphasized an individual's responsibility for their own health instead of promoting a broader consideration of the factors influencing individual health (Robertson, 1998).

Twelve years later, two more seminal documents in the development of health promotion and the social determinants of health were published. The *Ottawa Charter for Health Promotion* was released in 1986, following an international conference on health promotion. The *Charter* provided a definition of health promotion as "the process of enabling people to increase control over, and to improve, their health," where health was "seen as a resource for everyday life, not the objective of living" ("Ottawa Charter for Health Promotion: An International Conference on Health Promotion," 1986). Importantly, the *Charter* set out certain prerequisites for health that mirrored much of what are considered the determinants of health such as peace, shelter, food, income, and so on. In addition, the *Charter* called for numerous actions, including the construction of healthy public policy, the creation of supportive environments, stronger community action, the development of personal skills, and the reorientation of health services.

In the same year, the *Epp Report* (1986) was also published. This report called on health promotion as a response to health challenges of the day, aiming to reduce inequities in health. Later, in the mid-1990s, the Canadian Public Health Association published their *Action Statement for Health Promotion in Canada* (1996). Like the *Ottawa Charter*, these publications shared a call for healthy public policy, stronger communities, and reformed health care systems. Health promotion was the backbone of the response. Throughout these publications, we see a shared concern with acknowledging and addressing the social determinants of health.

However, despite the charters, reports, and statements, the concept of health promotion and its associated practices arguably did not gain prominence, particularly when they ran somewhat afoul of the 1990s neoliberal governance (Labonte, 1995 1997; Raphael, 2008). In the mid-1990s, then, came the introduction of a new perspective on health: **population health** (Evans & Stoddart, 1990). In brief, like health promotion, the population health framework emphasized the importance of the social determinants of health. It was interested in reducing expenditures on health care by redistributing funds to areas that would promote prosperity for all (Labonte, 1995).

Since its advent, though, this framework of population health has been subject to much criticism (Coburn & Poland, 1996; Coburn et al., 2003; Labonte, 1995, 1997; Labonte, Polanyi, Muhajarine, McIntosh, & Williams, 2005; Poland, Coburn, Robertson, & Eakin, 1998; Raphael & Bryant; Robertson, 1998). To summarize, the approach is said to prize epidemiology and empirical approaches to understanding health; it is both atheoretical and apolitical; it neglects the *unique* determinants, contexts, and circumstances under which people enact health behaviour; and it offers little opportunity for community involvement (Coburn et al., 2003; Labonte, 1995; Labonte et al., 2005; Labonte, 1997; Poland et al., 1998; Raphael & Bryant; Raphael, 2008; Robertson, 1998).

There was particular concern with the notion of redistributing funds from health care. On the one hand, health promotion is "explicitly political" (Robertson, 1998, p. 161; see also

Bambra, Fox, & Scott-Samuel, 2005; Raphael & Bryant, 2002). As such, it focuses on how the structural factors that create health inequalities should be corrected through a reallocation of resources. In other words, health promotion strives to reduce income inequality. However, population health, as above, favoured "producing wealth" as a means of improving the health of a population, without addressing the ways in which our political and economic systems create these inequalities (Coburn et al., 2003; Labonte, 1995, 1997; Labonte et al., 2005; Poland et al., 1998; Robertson, 1998). In this view, funds recovered from the health care sector should be redistributed to other areas to strengthen the *economy*, rather than to aid individual citizens. As some have pointed out, there is no guarantee that efforts to improve a nation's economy will actually result in population health improvements—but few governments would argue with an approach that emphasizes a reduction in health care spending (Labonte, 1995, 1997; Labonte et al., 2005; Poland et al., 1998; Robertson, 1998). Indeed, there is concern that population health was more palatable to neoliberal governance (a topic discussed shortly) and that it supplanted health promotion as the dominant means of understanding health, decreasing support for core health promotion tenets such as community empowerment and social justice (Coburn et al., 2003; Labonte, 1995; 1997; Poland et al., 1998; Raphael & Bryant, 2002; Raphael, 2008; Robertson, 1998).

Since the publication of the original "formulation" of population health, there has been considerable debate about what "population health" actually means and how it is done (e.g., Dunn & Hayes, 1999; Kindig & Stoddart, 2003; Kreuter & Lezin, 2001). The Public Health Agency of Canada (PHAC) defines population health as a "unifying approach for the entire spectrum of health system interventions—from prevention and promotion to health protection, diagnosis, treatment, and care—and integrates and balances action between them" (Public Health Agency of Canada, 2012). It also states that population health is an "approach that aims to improve the health of the entire population and to reduce health inequities among population groups. In order to reach these objectives, it looks at and acts upon the broad range of factors and conditions that have a strong influence on our health" (Public Health Agency of Canada, 2012). To this end, PHAC has defined 12 key determinants of health, as illustrated in Table 10.1. Echoing the publications highlighted above, PHAC states that population health requires upstream investment, multiple and multisectoral responses, citizen engagement, and accountability for health outcomes.

TABLE 10.1	Public Health Agency of Canada: Determinants of Health
• Income and social status	• Personal health practices and coping skills
• Social support networks	• Healthy child development
• Education and literacy	• Biology and genetic endowment
• Employment/working conditions	• Health Services
• Social environments	• Gender
• Physical environments	• Culture

Different Approaches to Understanding Health

People may tend to think of health and illness in biomedical and/or behavioural terms, perhaps because this perspective is often reflected in the media's portrayal of health issues (Hayes et al., 2007; Raphael, 2011). In a biomedical approach, illness is seen as a result of some form of biological or physiological problem—for example, a bacterial infection that can be treated with antibiotics. On the other hand, in a **behavioural approach**, health or illness are viewed as results of individual behaviours or actions. For instance, it is our "decision" whether or not to smoke, to eat healthy foods, to wear a seatbelt, or to go skydiving. At this point, students are encouraged to think about the assumptions made in these two models. Is there something missing in these approaches?

A major limitation of these models is that they do not account for the environments in which individuals get sick or make health behaviour choices. Such an approach assumes, of course, that individuals are in complete control of their choices—for instance, people do not eat healthily because they are poorly informed about nutrition or they simply prefer the convenience of fast food. Thus, we need a third model for thinking about health: the **socio-environmental model**. Unlike the other two models, this model considers the broader structural factors that shape individuals' health and health behaviours. For instance, instead of accepting an explanation that someone eats poorly because they want to, or because they do not "know any better," a socio-environmental approach would dig deeper. Perhaps a person eats poorly because they cannot afford to purchase healthy food. Maybe there is no place in their neighbourhood to buy healthier food, they cannot drive, and public transit is poor. From this perspective, we begin to see the factors that structure health beyond the individual.

How we think about the causes of health or illness is important because it influences our responses to health-related issues. If one assumes that health issues are caused by some type of biological or physiological issue, then the solution to illness is to "fix" that issue at a cellular level (or, by other means, like quarantine). If one assumes that health is a behavioural issue, then changing individuals' behaviour becomes the primary way to improve health; for instance, through anti-smoking posters. Yet neither of these approaches addresses the broader factors that come to influence health— that is, the social determinants of health.

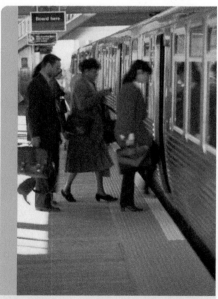

Steve Mason/Photodisk/Thinkstock

Thinking about the social determinants of health encourages us to consider health in terms of the factors that structure people's lives. One socio-environmental factor may be public transit. Access to adequate transit systems may have positive impacts not only on individuals' access to medical care, for example, but also on their ability to access healthy food providers, their stress levels, their transportation costs, and the level of air pollution in urban centres.

A strict focus on the individual-level behavioural and biomedical determinants of health has important consequences: it suggests that health issues are personal—not social—issues. Thus, adherents to this theory believe that solutions also reside at the individual level, rather than thinking about broader social changes which might improve health (Raphael, Curry-Stevens, & Bryant, 2008). A socio-environmental approach, on the other hand, encourages us to think about the "upstream" causes of health problems: instead of trying to heal people once they have already become sick (a "downstream" approach), we try to "heal" the circumstances that make people sick in the first place. Table 10.2 outlines how the three primary models of health understand health issues differently, and Table 10.3 notes how strategies to improve health differ depending on the framework used to understand the underlying issues.

TABLE 10.2 Leading Health Problems by Three Models of Health

Biomedical Model	Behavioural Model	Socio-Environmental Model
• cardiovascular diseases • cancer • HIV/AIDS • stroke • diabetes • obesity • hypertension etc.	• smoking • poor eating habits • physical inactivity • substance abuse • poor stress coping • lack of life skills etc.	• poverty • unemployment • powerlessness • isolation • environmental pollution • stressors • hazardous living and working conditions etc.

TABLE 10.3 Three Approaches to Reducing Heart Disease

Health Model	Causes of Problem	Principal Strategies to Address Problem
Biomedical	• hypertension • family history • hypercholesterolemia	• treatment • drugs • low salt/low cholesterol diet
Behavioural	• lifestyle • smoking • high-fat diet • low level of physical activity • high stress levels	• health education • health communication • self-help/mutual aid • advocacy for health public policies supporting lifestyle choices (e.g., workplace smoking bans)
Socio-Environmental	• living conditions • working conditions • social isolation	• policy change • advocacy • community mobilization • self-help/mutual aid

Key Determinants of Health

Income and Health

Of all of the determinants, income is likely the biggest contributor to health status (Mikkonen & Raphael, 2010; Wilkinson & Marmot, 2003). This section will consider some of the research evidence about the influence of income on health, as well as the effects of income inequality on health. It concludes with a reflection on the place of income and income inequality in the political "bigger picture."

Two common measures of health in a given population are life expectancies and self-reported health. Figure 10.2 shows life expectancy at birth in Canada as a function of neighbourhood income, using vital statistics data from Statistics Canada. Likewise, Figure 10.3 from the *National Population Health Survey, 1996–97* relates Canadians' self-reported health level by income level.

Looking at these figures, it is obvious that income has something to do with health. The trends show that life expectancy and self-rated health tend to change with differing income levels—that is, the higher the income, the better the life expectancy and/or self-reported level of health. Many research studies have considered this relationship in greater detail.

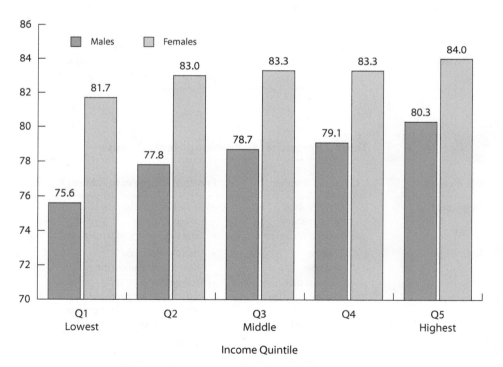

FIGURE 10.2   Life Expectancy at Birth, by Sex, Neighbourhood Income Quintiles, 2005–2007

Source: Greenberg and Normandin (2011), Chart 5, p. 6.

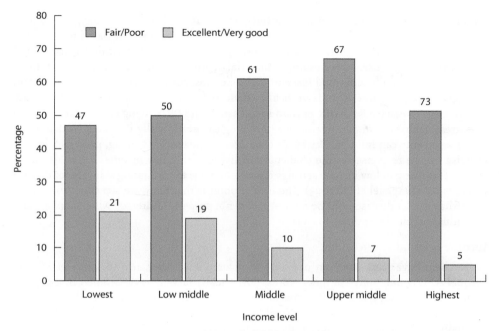

FIGURE 10.3 **Self-Rated Health, by Income Level, Canadians Aged 12+, 1996–1997**

Source: Federal, Provincial and Territorial Advisory Committee on Population Health (1999), Exhibit 1.1, p. 15.

For instance, Lantz et al. (1998), in an analysis of a representative sample of adults in the US, found that socio-economic disadvantage was linked with higher mortality rates. This relationship held even when controlling for the behavioural risk factors for mortality, such as smoking, diet, and physical activity. In a recent example using the Canadian Community Health Survey, Dinca-Panaitescu et al. (2011) found an inverse relationship between income and the prevalence of type 2 diabetes—that is, as income increases, the rate of diabetes decreases. Similarly, Diez Roux et al. (2001) found higher rates of coronary heart disease in socio-economically disadvantaged neighbourhoods in the US.

Income can also play a role in disease-specific outcomes. For example, Lowcock, Rosella, Foisy, McGreer, and Crowcroft (2012) investigated the severity of H1N1 flu in a sample of people from Ontario. They noted the importance of the social determinants of health; income-related variables were directly related to the rate of hospitalization for "severe" cases of H1N1. For instance, those who were hospitalized for H1N1 were more likely to have a high school education or less and were more likely to live in poorer neighbourhoods. Interestingly, key clinical risk factors for H1N1 (e.g., smoking, high BMI, use of antiretroviral medications) mediated these relationships, but only somewhat, suggesting that the socio-economic indicators played a greater role in influencing who did and did not develop severe H1N1 infections.

In another example, Raphael and Farrell (2002) set out to investigate explanations for rates of cardiovascular disease (CVD) in North America beyond the behavioural or biomedical model. Citing a World Health Organization study that suggested the best predictors of

CVD are social issues like civil unrest, poverty, and social and economic change, they took a materialist approach to trace three ways in which low income is associated with cardio-vascular disease. First, they cite research showing that **material deprivation** is associated with cardiovascular disease. For example, material deprivation can lead to more exposure to negative impacts on health (food insecurity, housing insecurity, insecure employment) and less exposure to positive impacts on health (education, recreation opportunities). Second, they present research associating **psycho-social stress** and CVD: living on a low income cre-ates stressors that can impact health on a physiological level. Finally, they suggest that living with low income can influence "risky" behaviours. For instance, smoking, poor diet, lack of exercise can be responses to the challenges of living with a low income. It has also been argued that living in low income settings is not conducive to facilitating self-care for disease management (Raphael et al., 2003). The overall point is that there are structural influences on cardiovascular disease—like poverty—that are not properly addressed when emphasizing individual-oriented responses to CVD.

Income Inequality and Health

Researchers have paid attention not only to income levels, but also to levels of income *inequality* in populations—in other words, how equally income is distributed in a popula-tion. Figure 10.4 is a graph of life expectancy by income inequality (measured by the Gini co-efficient, a measure of inequality). Notably, one can easily see that higher levels of income inequality are associated with lower life expectancies.

Seminal work in the mid-1990s investigated the relationship between income inequality and health in the United States. Kennedy, Kawachi, and Prothrow-Stith (1996), for instance, showed that income inequality rates in US states were related to increased chances of mor-tality, even when taking into consideration factors such as poverty and smoking. Similarly, Kaplan, Pamuk, Lynch, Cohen, and Balfour (1996) found that income inequality in US states was related to increased chances of mortality. Beyond this, inequality was associated with a number of other health-related issues, including homicide and violent crimes, smok-ing, physical inactivity, higher rates of unemployment, and imprisonment, among others. Continuing this line of inquiry, Lynch et al. (1998) analyzed data for 282 metropolitan areas of the US and also found similar results linking income inequality with mortality. All three studies share a similar conclusion: efforts to improve health should focus on reduc-ing income inequality. There are limitations to the methods used in these studies, and the strength of the link between income inequality and health has been questioned (e.g., Judge, Mulligan, & Benzeval, 1998). Nevertheless, it is worthwhile to consider this relationship, particularly in light of the role of the political economy, which is explored below.

The association between income inequality and health gave rise to questions about the mechanisms through which income inequality may influence health. Referring to the stud-ies cited above, Kawachi and Kennedy (1999) suggest that a "disinvestment in human capi-tal" arises from income inequality. Here, income inequality leads to a disparity in interests between the "rich" and the "poor," decreasing support for the social services that would best help the less well-off, such as education or health care. Indeed, as Kaplan et al. (1996) showed, there was lower social spending on education in US states with higher income inequality.

A second proposed pathway is the "erosion of social capital" (Kawachi & Kennedy, 1999). Social capital, which will be explored later in this chapter, has been shown to be protec-

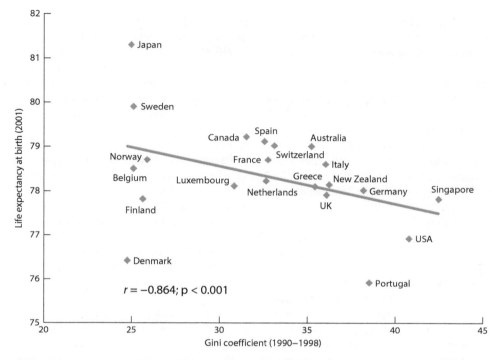

FIGURE 10.4   **Income Inequality and Life Expectancy at Birth Among Industrialized Countries**

Source: De Vogli, Mistry, Gnesotto, & Cornia, (2005), Figure 2, p. 160.

tive of health. To this end, Kawachi, Kennedy, Lochner, and Prothrow-Stith (1997) explored the idea that **social capital**—including levels of trust, civic participation, group membership, and so on—is a mediator in this relationship. They showed, for example, that income inequality was associated with reduced social cohesion and reduced social trust, which were subsequently associated with mortality. As a pathway linking income inequality and health, Kawachi and Kennedy (1999) suggest that income inequality erodes the protective effects of social capital on health. With low levels of social capital, community members are less likely to engage with the political system. This effect is particularly pronounced among the less well-off, meaning that public policies will not be implemented to support people with lower incomes. Finally Kawachi and Kennedy (1999) explore social comparison as another mechanism, in that frustrated expectations in achieving the cultural lifestyle ideal (e.g., the "American Dream") could have physiological health effects.

Contextualizing Income, Income Inequalities, and Health

Recognizing the importance of income and income inequality to health, there has been interest in the "bigger picture"—in other words, in the question of what creates these situations in the first place. Considering our systems of government is a good place to start. Most people probably have a basic understanding of how our government affects our health. In Canada, for example, there are federal departments like Health Canada and the Public Health Agency of Canada, and each province has some form of provincial health authority. Additionally, most municipalities have public health departments and run clinics for certain health issues.

Beyond this, systems of governance have a profound influence on individual and population health in more ways than one might imagine. Policy decisions from governmental bodies and broader economic structures in a given area all affect the health of a society. Indeed, health is innately political (Bambra et al., 2005; Robertson, 1998). The way a government understands health and public policy has great implications for how health concerns are addressed (Raphael & Bryant, 2006b; Bambra et al., 2005). Raphael and Bryant (2006a), in fact, refer to politics as the "missing dimension" in promoting health. In this section, students will explore some of the ways that politics can influence our health.

Certainly decisions about health policy have a direct impact on our health. For example, the structure of the health care system in the US means that Americans have more unmet health needs than Canadians. This is especially so for Americans who do not have private health insurance (Lasser, Himmelstein, & Woolhandler, 2006). While disparities in access exist in both countries, "low-income Canadians have better access to medical care than do low-income US residents" (Lasser et al., 2006, p. 1305).

However, it is important to recognize that it is not only health policy that can impact our health. Indeed, approaching the issue from a social determinants of health perspective highlights that policies of all types, even those that are not explicitly health-related, can affect our wellbeing. Take a moment to consider how policies about minimum wage, housing, or a publicly funded child care program influence could health. The nature of a state's political system determines the extent to which health figures into broader public policies (Raphael & Bryant, 2006a).

A political economy perspective on health focuses on the intersections among the state, the economy, and the general population (Raphael & Bryant, 2006a). A political economy approach is typically critical in nature; it seeks to expose the structures that create inequalities, often with an eye to changing them (Minkler, Wallace, & McDonald, 1994). As such, this perspective asks questions about how who has power in a given situation and who controls resources; it focuses on the production and distribution of wealth (Raphael & Bryant, 2006a; Minkler et al., 1994). Applied to issues of health, a political economy perspective examines how the distribution of wealth and resources determines the health of a given population (Raphael & Bryant, 2006a). This is known as a neo-materialist approach to understanding the social determinants of health (Raphael, 2006; Lynch, Smith, Kaplan, & House, 2000).

Some areas of focus for a political economy approach include the following: the social causes of preventable disease and injury; racial, class, and gender inequalities in health; the underdevelopment of health in developing nations; the privatization of health care; and political factors in the debates over health care reform. The balance of this section considers how a political economy approach provides a lens to look at some of the ways in which our systems of governance influence our health.

Political Regimes and Welfare States

One aspect of the relationship between a government and its economy has to do with a nation's welfare state—the extent to which the government provides social and health services to its citizens. Some examples of these policies and services include education, housing, employment, and public health resources (Eikemo & Bambra, 2008). Over time, a number of different conceptualizations of welfare state regimes have arisen, all of which are ways to categorize how various governments/political parties have supported welfare states (Eikemo & Bambra, 2008; see also Bambra, 2007). Different governments have different welfare state regimes; health outcomes of citizens will vary accordingly (Navarro et al., 2001; 2003; 2006).

Navarro et al. (2006) studied health outcomes under four different welfare state regimes over the period from 1950 to 2000. In particular they considered the nature of the welfare states across these different political traditions and the nature of their redistributive policies (policies that reduce income inequality by redistributing wealth between the "rich" and "poor").

1. **Social Democratic**—typically have the firmest commitment to redistributive policies with strong support for the welfare state and broader public policies aimed at supporting the citizenry (e.g., employment equity, child care, home care); they tend to have the lowest income inequality. Countries such as Sweden, Norway, Denmark, Finland, and Austria have strong social democratic traditions.
2. **Christian Democratic**—characterized by lower support for redistributive policies. These regimes do, however, provide some forms of social support, such as social security for older adults and universal health care coverage. These countries have a higher level of income inequality. Italy, the Netherlands, Belgium, and France are all examples of countries with Christian democratic traditions.
3. **Liberalism**—countries like Canada, the United States of America, the United Kingdom, and Ireland have been associated with liberalism, with low support for redistributive policies. Social services, when available, are generally weaker and are often means-tested. Levels of income inequality are higher within states with these traditions.
4. **Conservative/Fascist**—welfare states in these countries were not well supported. Expenditures on public and social services were extremely low; there was little support for redistributive policies. Perhaps not surprisingly, income inequality was greatest under this political tradition. Spain, Portugal, and Greece (before they became democracies) are examples of countries that belonged to the conservative/fascist category.

In their analyses, Navarro et al. (2001; 2003; 2006) found better health outcomes under political traditions that were committed to redistributive policies. For instance, they found that infant mortality rates were lowest among countries governed by parties that favoured redistributive policies and policies to promote social equality. Life expectancy was also positively associated with redistributive policies, although to a lesser degree than infant mortality. They further showed that longer periods of pro-redistributive policies were associated with policies supporting employment and social support as well as stronger funding for public health. Here too, debates remain about the relationship of political systems to health outcomes (see, e.g., Beckfield & Krieger, 2009; Muntaner et al., 2011; Brennenstuhl, Quesnel-Vallee, & McDonough, 2012), but it is a proposition worth considering.

Income Inequality, Social Capital, and Mortality Revisited

Coburn (2000; 2004) argued that we need to situate the relationship between income inequality, social cohesion, and mortality within the political forces that structure these issues. Of particular interest for Coburn is the neoliberalist (see Chapter Seven) tradition of many systems of government. Coburn (2000; 2004) argues that neoliberalism has a number of tenets that foster inequalities and weaken social cohesion. For instance, neoliberalism emphasizes the decommodification of social programs and "means-testing" for social programs. In other words, fewer social programs are offered and it becomes more difficult to access those that are available. Neoliberal traditions also tend to oppose policies that redistribute wealth. Additionally, they often emphasize the individual over the group, detracting from social cohesion and collective empowerment.

Thus, from this perspective, the income inequality and poor social cohesion that affects our health must be situated within the context of neoliberal political forces. Coburn argues that it is neoliberalism itself that first produces the higher levels of inequality and lower levels of social cohesion, ultimately worsening our health.

In sum, politics have quite a bit to do with health, but not always in ways that one might assume. As such, the political economy of health is a good perspective to keep in mind as students think through health issues and the responses to them. The chapter now turns to a consideration of some social determinants of health that are more "local" in nature.

Networks and Neighbourhoods as Social Determinants of Health

Our social networks and the places we live can have a profound effect on our health. This area of study is very large, but this section will introduce students to these ideas. It focuses on a few popular topics to provide an overview of these ideas. The following will consider the role of social networks, social capital, and our neighbourhoods and other physical environments.

Social Networks and Social Capital

Social networks are the social groups to which people belong such as families, friendship groups, work groups, and so on. Social capital is a concept with varying definitions, but as mentioned earlier, it typically considers issues related to the social fabric, like trust, civic participation, and group membership. Our health is affected by all of these factors.

Generally speaking, our networks help shape our health-related behaviours. For instance, a literature review by Sawka, McCormack, Nettel-Aguirre, Hawe, and Doyle-Baker (2013) showed that the social networks of young adults could influence levels of physical activity. In a similar way, Amirkhanian's (2014) literature review on men who have sex with men (MSM) found that men's social networks influenced their knowledge, attitudes, and behaviours, as well as social norms in the group.

Social support within networks, in particular, can have a protective effect on health in various ways. Among older adults, for instance, Gilmour (2012) analyzed the data from the Canadian Community Health Survey and found that seniors with lower levels of social support were lonelier and had poorer self-perceived health. Gilmour (2012) also showed that, even after accounting for differences in socio-demographics and health, social participation was shown to be protective for health.

Social support has also been shown to have protective effects on mental health. For instance, Fowler, Wareham-Fowler, and Barnes (2013), analyzing data from the Canadian Community Health Survey, showed that social interaction and a sense of belonging to community was linked with less severe and shorter episodes of depression. Kumar et al. (2012),

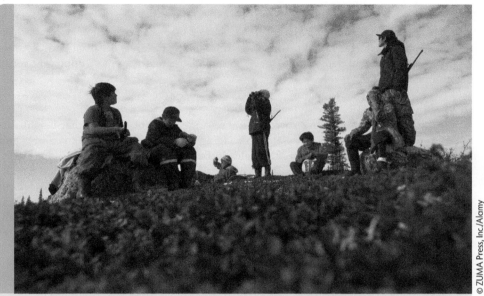

Levels of social support have been positively correlated with protective effects in mental health. This group of Innu boys from Mastastin Lake, Newfoundland and Labrador, is taking part in a hunting trip as part of an effort organized by leaders from Natuashish. In encouraging the formation of stronger cultural and social bonds, the communities hope to decrease negative health outcomes for their young members.

considering data from the Aboriginal People's Survey, found that a lack of social support was a risk factor for suicidal ideation among Métis women in Canada. Meanwhile, Fuller-Thomson, Battiston, Gadalla, and Brennenstuhl (2014), in their analysis of the National Population Health Survey, identified that social support might decrease the time to remission from depression.

Like social networks, social capital can be protective of health. For instance, in the US, Kawachi et al. (1999) investigated the relationship between self-reported health and measures of social capital (such as civic trust, norms of reciprocity, and group memberships). In states that had lower levels of social capital, fewer residents reported that their health was good or excellent. In a similar way, Lochner, Kawachi, Brennan, and Buka (2003) looked at data from over 300 neighbourhoods in Chicago and found that higher levels of social capital (using similar measures) were linked with lower death rates. This relationship held true even when controlling for the socio-economic status of the neighbourhood itself.

Research from Canada has shown similar findings. In Montreal neighbourhoods, for instance, Bassett and Moore (2013) found a protective effect of social capital against depression. Langille, Asbridge, Ksely, and Rasic (2012), looking at data from high school students in Nova Scotia, showed that social capital (measured as the perceived trustworthiness and helpfulness of others at school) was protective against both thinking about suicide and actually attempting suicide. In a study of older adults with chronic diseases in Hamilton, Ontario, Hand, Law, Hannah, Elliott, and McColl (2012) showed that a sense of neighbourhood cohesion was linked to social support, which was then linked to levels of social participation. As the next section will demonstrate, neighbourhoods represent a vitally important social determinant of health.

Neighbourhoods

Woven throughout the previous discussion was some sense of the role that neighbourhoods and our built environments play in shaping our health. Indeed, the facilities and services available to us may affect our health in both good and bad ways. Undoubtedly, access to health care services themselves will impact our use of them; for instance, a number of studies have considered the availability of, and access to, health care services within neighbourhoods. These studies have shown various findings about the impact of their utilization (e.g., Bell, Wilson, Bissonnette, & Shah, 2013; Bissonnette, Wilson, Bell, & Shah, 2012; Harrington, Wilson, Bell, Muhajarine, & Ruthart, 2012; Hiscock, Pearce, Blakely, & Witten, 2008; Law et al., 2005).

CASE STUDY

Age-Friendly Cities

The World Health Organization (WHO) launched the Age-Friendly Cities project in 2006 in 33 cities across the globe, including four cities in Canada. The purpose of the project was to identify specific features of an age-friendly city that support older adults' quality of life, and to produce a guide that would help cities become more age-friendly (World Health Organization, 2007). According to the WHO, an age-friendly city "encourages active aging by optimizing opportunities for health, participation, and security in order to enhance quality of life as people age" (World Health Organization, 2007, p. 1).

Age-friendly cities encompass a number of domains. For instance, there is an emphasis on making outdoor spaces, transportation, housing, and health services available and accessible for older adults. Thereby, individuals of all ages will benefit as well. However, age-friendly cities are not only about such architectural and urban planning issues. Understanding the importance of social capital, age-friendly cities also address issues of civic participation, respect, and social inclusion for older adults, reflecting again the importance of social support and capital for health.

In Canada, a first step towards promoting age-friendly cities occurred with the publication of the "Age-Friendly Rural and Remote Communities" guide (Federal/Provincial/Territorial Ministers Responsible for Seniors, 2007). The document was a report on ten small Canadian communities, each with a population of less than five thousand, and their efforts to become more age-friendly. Subsequently, many communities have adopted similar projects across the country. Age-friendly cities are a good example of a multisectoral, upstream response that involves transforming social, physical, and political environments to improve health.

The health effects of neighbourhoods are not, however, limited to just the availability of health care services. Richard et al. (2013), for example, looking at older adults living in Montreal neighbourhoods, found that proximity to local facilities such as public libraries, recreation facilities, and shopping centres was associated with increased social participation. Other studies have shown how neighbourhood design can facilitate or impede physical activity (Esliger, Sherar, & Muhajarine, 2012; Kaczynski & Glover, 2012; Pouliou & Elliott, 2010). In addition, Chaiton, Mecredy, Cohen, and Tilson (2013) showed that places to buy cigarettes in Ontario are more likely to be found in disadvantaged neighbourhoods and/or close to schools.

Recently, researchers have been interested in the relationship between neighbourhoods and eating behaviour, especially in relation to obesity. For example, Hollands et al. (2013) analyzed data from the Canadian Community Health Survey and the locations of fast-food outlets in Canada. The group found that the density of fast-food restaurants in a given area was linked with the average BMI of that area. In a similar way, He et al. (2012) showed that proximity to convenience stores was linked to poorer eating behaviours among grade 7 and 8 students.

There has also been particular interest in considering how the availability and proximity of fast food outlets can influence children's eating behaviour. Seliske et al. (2013) showed that students were more likely to eat lunch at food retailers close to the school when such retailers were available. In a similar way, a study of 8- to 10-year-olds in Quebec showed a relationship between the availability of unhealthy food around schools and poorer eating habits. On the other hand, the study found that children in areas with less access to unhealthy foods were less likely to eat out (Van Hulst et al., 2012). Meanwhile, research among young people in London, Ontario, showed that living close to places to play was associated with lower BMI scores and that having a fast-food outlet close to a school was associated with higher BMI scores (Gilliland et al., 2012).

As such, there is much interest now in how neighbourhoods, and environments more broadly, can be obesogenic in nature. That is, "the sum of influences that the surroundings, opportunities, or conditions of life have on promoting obesity in individuals or populations" (Swinburn, Egger, & Raza, 1999, p. 563). Egger and Swinburn (1997) propose an ecological approach to understanding obesity. They argue that energy intake and expenditure are influenced by biology and behavioural factors and therefore related to obesity at an individual level. However, the relationship between energy intake and expenditure is also affected by the environment. To this end, Egger and Swinburn (1997) suggest that we need to consider the micro and macro physical, economic, socio-cultural, and political environments and their influences on food and activity (Egger & Swinburn, 1997).

The broader point is that obesity prevention needs to look beyond solutions focused on the individual because, from a social determinants of health perspective, one can see that obesity can understood as to be a "normal response to an abnormal environment," rather than the reverse (Egger & Swinburn, 1997, p. 477). As discussed earlier, changing the way we understand a health issue can structure our response to it. Thus, Swinburn (2008) categorizes obesity as a market failure: while our markets create success for sellers and consumers, offering ample food choices, these markets also encourage the spread of obesity and do not provide for the long-term good of the social system. As such, Swinburn (2008) argues that governments must take a stronger lead in addressing the obesity epidemic through leadership, advocacy, funding, and policies that support multisectoral responses to the problem.

Governments must provide avenues to improve our neighbourhoods as they can better promote health.

Daily Experience as a Social Determinant

Thus far we have considered some of the key determinants that influence our health. This section brings together some of these concerns to consider two daily experiences: driving and eating.

Cars and Health

Woodcock and Aldred (2008) explore the ways in which the automobile affects our health. Some of the ways are obvious. When we drive, we are not getting the exercise we would get from walking or cycling. Moreover, driving also contributes to air pollution. Having more cars on the roads also increases the number of motor vehicle accidents, harming both drivers and pedestrians. While these consequences may seem obvious, the implications of "car culture" are more far-reaching; they link with aspects of our built environment and the ways in which we interact (or do not) with people. For instance, cars allow people to live farther away from each other, worsening social cohesion through urban sprawl. This creates challenges for both those who are car-less and the neighbourhood's public transit system, which will struggle to adequately reach all areas.

Woodcock and Aldred (2008) also highlight broader health implications of car culture. For instance, cars make a large contribution to the world economy, including the production and sale of cars, the quest for fuel, and infrastructure building and maintenance. "Supercentre" stores (like Walmart) are associated with heavy car use societies. They also note the vested interests of automobile companies in influencing global policies on issues like climate change and road safety, both of which impact health on a global scale. For example, dependency on oil can have dire implications for the health not only of nations that use oil but also of those that produce it. They also assert that car culture promotes aggression and control over the environment, which can increase stress and road rage. In short, car ownership—something one may think of as a particularly individual experience—can have far-reaching implications for the health of society as a whole.

Eating

People tend to think about eating behaviour as rather individualistic in nature. Individuals choose what to eat, where to eat it, and when to do it. Yet again, it is necessary to scrutinize the notion of choice in eating behaviour. For example, Raine (2005) argues that even personal eating behaviours are structured by factors beyond individual choice. There is no doubt that people make decisions about eating at the individual level. For instance, there are certain physiological aspects to eating: children tend to eat more; as we age, we tend to eat less. We may also have allergies to certain foods. People have certain preferences—some like chocolate, some do not—and we possess differing levels of nutritional knowledge. To that end, individuals also have differing understandings of what qualifies as "healthy" food and what does not. Finally, there may be psychological influences on what individuals eat—for instance, we might use food as a way of making ourselves feel better in times of worry, stress, or sadness.

However, Raine (2005) makes the important point that our eating behaviour is influenced by factors related to our social, physical, and economic environments. First, our interpersonal environments influence our eating behaviours: families, friends, and peers play a role in affecting what, when, and how much people eat. Physical environments also play a role in structuring how much and what type of food is available to eat, including the accessibility of fresh food. The economic environment influences food choices, from the ways in which foods are marketed to certain demographics (children, in particular), to food prices and whether income levels are sufficient for the purchase of healthy foods. Social environments also play an important role in influencing eating behaviours: for instance, we have shared understandings of using food for cultural and symbolic means, like holiday meals. Finally, policy also plays a defining role in eating behaviours. For instance, policies may set out guidelines for healthy eating and for protecting the quality and safety of the foods we eat. At the same time, though, policies about social assistance, advertising restrictions, and "junk food" taxation would also have a profound—and perhaps wider-reaching—influence on consumption patterns at a population level.

In sum, eating behaviours are "highly contextual" (Raine, 2005, p. S13). As such, efforts to influence eating behaviours need to go beyond attempts aimed solely at changing individual-level factors. The chapter now turns to a consideration of different models of intervention to help students not only think about the social determinants of health, but also learn how to address them.

Identifying and Addressing the Social Determinants of Health

Many of the efforts at promoting health focus on what people have commonly come to know as "lifestyle" risks and, as such, focus on encouraging the individual to adopt healthier behaviour (see, e.g., Glanz & Bishop, 2010). Many programs subscribe to the model of "knowledge-attitudes-behaviour-prevention." This model assumes that changing an individual's knowledge will subsequently change his or her attitudes, fostering "better" behaviour and therefore preventing ill health. However, as discussed previously, focusing solely on an individual's choices ignores broader social, environmental, and political influences that may structure individual choice. This model also does not leave any room for individual agency in "risky" behaviour (i.e., the ways in which individuals can rationalize so-called "risky" behaviour, or, in other words, how "risky" behaviour can be normalized for people in certain situations) (see, e.g., Rhodes, 1997).

This section introduces the ecological model of health promotion to consider the many determinants of any health issue. It then presents a case study on one initiative that has sought to change the broader determinants of health behaviours rather than focusing on the individual him- or herself.

Ecological models, as the name suggests, focus on the ecology—or environments—of health behaviours. Such models encourage us to consider not only the individual but also the contexts in which individuals make health decisions (see, for example, McLeroy, Bibeau, Steckler, & Glanz, 1988). The goal of these models, then, is to think about changes that can be made at an individual, community, or broader social level to support healthier behaviours.

Maibach, Abroms, and Marosits (2007) propose a "people and places" framework to stimulate thinking on different levels of intervention for health behaviour change. This model, as the name suggests, encourages us to think about both people and places in our health promotion planning, from smaller to larger levels of aggregation. At the "people" level, the framework outlines three attributes: individuals, social networks, and populations/communities. The individual level encompasses the knowledge, attitudes, skills, cognitions, and behaviours of individuals themselves. The social network level includes the characteristics of the network (size, connectedness, diversity of ties) as well as the nature of the network's level of social support and positive role models ("opinion leaders"). Finally, at the broadest level are populations and/or communities, encompassing concepts like social norms, cultural understandings, disparities, and sources of discrimination (income inequality and racism, in particular). This level of consideration also addresses other health-protective issues of social capital, social cohesion, and the collective efficacy of a community.

The "place" level in this framework is divided into "local" and "distal" levels; the former refers to our immediate environments like our homes, schools, workplaces, and cities, while the latter category refers to broader "places" like our provinces, countries and, indeed, our global community. The areas of focus in this framework are shared for both levels. The first consideration is the availability of products and services in a given place and how that may affect health; for instance, the availability of healthy food. The second consideration is the physical structures of an environment. For instance, does a city provide safe sidewalks for walking and parks for playing, or is there a lack of such opportunity for physical activity? The social structures of an environment are the third consideration, including the extent to which laws and policies support health. The final consideration here relates to the media and cultural messages of the place. For instance, what messages are promoted by the media (and advertising) about healthy food intake? Or what messages do celebrities give about how to live and act?

This model helps us consider both broader issues that may need addressing in order to promote health and also the methods by which we should address these levels (see also McLeroy et al., 1988).

CASE STUDY

100% Condom Program in Thailand

The 100% Condom Program in Thailand (Rojanapithayakorn & Hanenberg, 1996; Rojanapithayakorn, 2006) is a widely cited example of the importance and effectiveness of a multisectoral response to a public health issue. In the late 1980s and early 1990s, Thailand experienced a large increase in HIV prevalence, mainly as a result of heterosexual commercial sex work. In response, the Thai government initiated a program to increase condom use in commercial sex through empowering the commercial sex workers themselves. In fact, the goal was to "promote the use of condoms 100% of the time in 100% of risky sexual relations, and in 100% of the sex entertainment establishments" (Rojanapithayakorn, 2006, p. 42).

By altering broader structures that promoted unprotected sex, the program empowered sex workers in a number of ways. The program involved numerous sectors. First, owners of sex work establishments came to learn that unprotected sex in their establishments would result in sanctions. The health sector provided the sex workers themselves with sexually transmitted infection services, peer education, condoms, and lubricants. An enforcement aspect was also a key component. The health sector would report establishments where workers were not using condoms and the police would issue sanctions. Penalties included warnings, temporary closures, or cancellation of business permits; over time, commercial sex work clients understood that sex without a condom would no longer be possible.

Begun as a pilot project in one Thai province, the program was so successful that it was eventually adopted as a national program. Evaluation results demonstrate the important successes of the program: since its implementation, condom usage rates in sex work rose to over 90 per cent. Likewise, incidence rates of sexually transmitted diseases dropped by more than 95 per cent and the HIV prevalence rate also declined (Rojanapithayakorn, 2006).

Chapter Summary

Despite the rhetoric afforded to health promotion initiatives in Canada, it would seem that efforts at promoting health, for the most part, still reflect an emphasis on individual-level change. Gore and Kothari (2012) conducted a review of health-promoting initiatives in British Columbia and Ontario, Canada's most populous provinces, aimed at improving diet and physical activity between 1 January 2006 and 1 September 2011. The researchers identified the initiatives as belonging to three separate approaches: "lifestyle" (efforts at changing individual awareness, knowledge, behaviours), "environment" (efforts at changing the environment in which behaviours are enacted, e.g., schools, communities), and "structure" (acknowledging the social determinants of health and trying to address them directly). In Ontario, only 9 initiatives were structure based; 26 were environment based, and the rest (36) were lifestyle based. In BC, only 7 were structure based; 27 were environment based, and 38 were lifestyle based.

While the authors acknowledge that environment-based initiatives do account for context and circumstances, they do not actively attempt to alter the determinants of health that influence those contexts. The authors claim that "it is not realistic to try to improve healthy eating, reduce tobacco consumption, and increase active living through environment-based initiatives alone when the mechanisms that produce unhealthy environments are left untouched" (Gore & Kothari, 2013, p. e53). To this end, Raphael et al. (2008), argue that there are "profound barriers" that prevent a proper acknowledgement of the social determinants of health in the political agenda, including "dominant ideologies typical of the health sciences, public attitudes towards personal responsibility, and increasing market influences" (p. 232).

However, Raphael and Bryant have argued that the situation is not wholly lost. There are avenues to change political will (e.g., Raphael & Bryant, 2006a). A first option is advocacy, and they call upon those who work in promoting health to lobby governments for greater action on the social determinants of health. A second approach is community-based education and research that aim to raise awareness in communities about the importance of the social determinants of health, while also building capacity for communities to be involved in policy research and development. Raphael and colleagues (2008; 2012) issue a call to health care workers to educate, motivate, and advocate for political change to support and manage the social determinants of health (Raphael et al., 2008). Following on this last point, it is hoped that students will use the lessons from this chapter—and indeed, from this entire book—to think more critically about the causes of health issues and the ways in which we should respond to them.

STUDY QUESTIONS

1. How would you explain the concept of social determinants of health to someone who had never heard the term?
2. Think about your own personal situation—how do your social networks and neighbourhood contribute to your own health status?
3. What are the main differences between the biomedical, behavioural, and social models of health?
4. Why have efforts aimed at tackling the social determinants of health lagged behind those aimed at changing individual behaviour?
5. What is the welfare state? What role does it play in a person's health?

SUGGESTED READINGS

Ayo, N. (2012). Understanding health promotion in a neoliberal climate and the making of health conscious citizens. *Critical Public Health, 22*(1), 99–105.

Bell, A. C., Ge, K., & Popkin, B. M. (2002). The road to obesity or the path to prevention: Motorized transportation and obesity in China. *Obesity Research, 10*(4), 277–83.

Marmot, M. G., Shipley, M. J., & Rose, G. (1984). Inequalities in death—specific explanations of a general pattern? *The Lancet, 323*(8384), 1003–06.

SUGGESTED WEB RESOURCES

National Collaborating Centre for Determinants of Health: www.nccdh.ca
Bill Davenhall's TEDMED Talk: Your Health Depends on Where You Live: www.ted.com/talks/
    bill_davenhall_your_health_depends_on_where_you_live:
Code Red: http://thespec-codered.com
Unnatural Causes: Is Inequality Making Us Sick? (documentary and website):
    www.unnaturalcauses.org

GLOSSARY

Behavioural approach   Views illness as a result of personal behaviours that can be modified.

Health field concept A way to address health that addresses biology, the environment, lifestyle, and health care systems. The health field concept addresses factors beyond individual control (see Lalonde, 1981).

Health promotion Encouraging people to maintain and/or improve their personal health through public information campaigns (see Ottawa Charter for Health Promotion: An International Conference on Health Promotion, 1986).

Material deprivation A lack of basic "materials," such as housing, food, and employment, needed for a certain standard of life.

Population health Originally, an approach to health that stresses the importance of ensuring the health of the broader population and the social determinants of health. It aims to reduce income inequality to improve everyone's quality of life and, in turn, decrease the government's health care budget. The concept of population health changes with context.

Psycho-social stress Stress related to one's position in society. For example, living with a low socio-economic status may introduce the added stress of securing housing and feeding one's family.

Social capital Refers to the strength of a society's social fabric. This includes levels of trust, civic engagement, and a sense of belonging. These traits can have a positive influence on health.

Socio-environmental model Considers the impact of society and how its structures affect an individual's health. It also takes into account how social structures affect our behaviour and therefore our health.

REFERENCES

Amirkhanian, Y. A. (2014). Social networks, sexual networks and HIV risk in men who have sex with men. *Current HIV/AIDS Report, 11*(1), 81–92.

Bambra, C. (2007). Going beyond the three worlds of welfare capitalism: Regime theory and public health research. *Journal of Epidemiology and Community Health, 61*(12), 1098–1102.

———, Fox, D., & Scott-Samuel, A. (2005). Towards a politics of health. *Health Promotion International, 20*(2), 187–93.

Barton, H. & Grant, M. (2006). A health map for the local human habitat. *Journal of the Royal Society for the Promotion of Health, 126*(6), 252–53.

Bassett, E. & Moore, S. (2013). Social capital and depressive symptoms: The association of psychosocial and network dimensions of social capital with depressive symptoms in Montreal, Canada. *Social Science and Medicine, 86*, 96–102.

Beckfield, J. & Krieger, N. (2009). Epi + demos + cracy: Linking political systems and priorities to the magnitude of health inequities—evidence, gaps, and a research agenda. *Epidemiologic Reviews, 31*, 152–77.

Bell, S., Wilson, K., Bissonnette, L., & Shah, T. (2013). Access to primary healthcare: Does neighborhood matter? *Annals of the Association of American Geographers, 103*(1), 85–105.

Bissonnette, L., Wilson, K., Bell, S., & Shah, T. I. (2012). Neighbourhoods and potential access to healthcare: The role of spatial and aspatial factors. *Health & Place, 18*(4), 841–53.

Brennenstuhl, S., Quesnel-Vallee, A., & McDonough, P. (2012). Welfare regimes, population health and health inequalities: A research synthesis. *Journal of Epidemiology and Community Health, 66*(5), 397–409.

Canadian Public Health Association. (1996). *Action statement for health promotion in Canada.* Ottawa, ON.

Chaiton, M. O., Mecredy, G. C., Cohen, J. E., & Tilson, M. L. (2013). Tobacco retail outlets and vulnerable populations in Ontario, Canada. *International Journal of Environmental Research and Public Health, 10*(12), 7299–7309.

Coburn, D. (2000). Income inequality, social cohesion and the health status of populations: The role of neo-liberalism. *Social Science and Medicine, 51*(1), 135–46.

——. (2004). Beyond the income inequality hypothesis: Class, neo-liberalism, and health inequalities. *Social Science and Medicine, 58*(1), 41–56.

——, Denny, K., Mykhalovskiy, E., McDonough, P., Robertson, A., & Love, R. (2003). Population health in Canada: A brief critique. *American Journal of Public Health, 93*(3), 392–96.

—— & Poland, B. (1996). The CIAR vision of the determinants of health: A critique. Critical Social Science and Health Group. *Canadian Journal of Public Health, 87*(5), 308–10.

De Vogli, R., Mistry, R., Gnesotto, R., & Cornia, G. A. (2005). Has the relation between income inequality and life expectancy disappeared? Evidence from Italy and top industrialised countries. *Journal of Epidemiology and Community Health, 59*(2), 158–62.

Diez Roux, A. V., Merkin, S. S., Arnett, D., Chambless, L., Massing, M., Nieto, F. J., . . . Watson, R. L. (2001). Neighborhood of residence and incidence of coronary heart disease. *New England Journal of Medicine, 345*(2), 99–106.

Dinca-Panaitescu, S., Dinca-Panaitescu, M., Bryant, T., Daiski, I., Pilkington, B., & Raphael, D. (2011). Diabetes prevalence and income: Results of the Canadian Community Health Survey. *Health Policy, 99*(2), 116–23.

Dunn, J. R. & Hayes, M. V. (1999). Toward a lexicon of population health. *Canadian Journal of Public Health, 90*(Suppl 1), S7–S10.

Egger, G. & Swinburn, B. (1997). An "ecological" approach to the obesity pandemic. *British Medical Journal, 315*(7106), 477–80.

Eikemo, T. A. & Bambra, C. (2008). The welfare state: A glossary for public health. *Journal of Epidemiology and Community Health, 62*(1), 3–6.

Epp, J. (1986). *Achieving health for all: A framework for health promotion.* Ottawa N: Health and Welfare Canada.

Esliger, D. W., Sherar, L. B., & Muhajarine, N. (2012). Smart cities, healthy kids: The association between neighbourhood design and children's physical activity and time spent sedentary. *Canadian Journal of Public Health, 103*(9 Suppl 3), S22–S28.

Evans, R. G. & Stoddart, G. L. (1990). Producing health, consuming healthcare. *Social Science and Medicine, 31*(12), 1347–63.

Federal, Provincial and Territorial Advisory Committee on Population Health. (1999). *Toward a healthy future: Second report on the health of Canadians.* Ottawa N: Minister of Public Works and Government Services Canada.

Federal/Provincial/Territorial Ministers Responsible for Seniors. (2007). *Age-friendly rural and remote communities: A guide.* Ottawa N.

Fowler, K., Wareham-Fowler, S., & Barnes, C. (2013). Social context and depression severity and duration in Canadian men and women: Exploring the influence of social support and sense of community belongingness. *Journal of Applied Social Psychology, 43*, E85–E96.

Fuller-Thomson, E., Battiston, M., Gadalla, T. M., & Brennenstuhl, S. (2014). Bouncing back: remission from depression in a 12-year panel study of a representative Canadian community sample. *Social Psychiatry and Psychiatric Epidemiology, 49*(6), 903–10.

Gilliland, J. A., Rangel, C. Y., Healy, M. A., Tucker, P., Loebach, J. E., Hess, P. M., . . . Wilk, P. (2012). Linking childhood obesity to the built environment: A multi-level analysis of home and school neighbourhood factors associated with body mass index. *Canadian Journal of Public Health, 103*(9 Suppl 3), eS15–eS21.

Gilmour, H. (2012). Social participation and the health and well-being of Canadian seniors. *Health Reports, 23*(4), 3–12.

Glanz, K. & Bishop, D. B. (2010). The role of behavioral science theory in the development and implementation of public health interventions. *Annual Review of Public Health, 31*, 399–418.

Gore, D. & Kothari, A. (2012). Social determinants of health in Canada: Are healthy living initiatives there yet? A policy analysis. *International Journal for Equity in Health, 11*, 41.

—— (2013). Getting to the root of the problem: Health promotion strategies to address the social determinants of health. *Canadian Journal of Public Health, 104*(1), e52–e54.

Greenberg, L. & Normandin, C. (2011). *Health at a glance: Disparities in life expectancy at birth.* Ottawa N: Statistics Canada.

Hand, C., Law, M., Hanna, S., Elliott, S., & McColl, M. A. (2012). Neighbourhood influences on participation in activities among older adults with chronic health conditions. *Health & Place, 18*(4), 869–76.

Harrington, D. W., Wilson, K., Bell, S., Muhajarine, N., & Ruthart, J. (2012). Realizing neighbourhood potential? The role of the availability of health-care services on contact with a primary care physician. *Health & Place, 18*(4), 814–23.

Hayes, M., Ross, I. E., Gasher, M., Gutstein, D., Dunn, J. R., & Hackett, R. A. (2007). Telling stories: News media, health literacy and public policy in Canada. *Social Science and Medicine, 64*(9), 1842–52.

He, M., Tucker, P., Irwin, J. D., Gilliland, J., Larsen, K., & Hess, P. (2012). Obesogenic neighbourhoods: The impact of neighbourhood restaurants and convenience stores on adolescents' food consumption behaviours. *Public Health Nutrition, 15*(12), 2331–39.

Hiscock, R., Pearce, J., Blakely, T., & Witten, K. (2008). Is neighborhood access to healthcare provision associated with individual-level utilization and satisfaction? *Health Services Research, 43*(6), 2183–2200.

Hollands, S., Campbell, M. K., Gilliland, J., & Sarma, S. (2013). A spatial analysis of the association between restaurant density and body mass index in Canadian adults. *Preventive Medicine, 57*(4), 258–64.

Judge, K., Mulligan, J. A., & Benzeval, M. (1998). Income inequality and population health. *Social Science and Medicine, 46*(4–5), 567–79.

Kaczynski, A. T. & Glover, T. D. (2012). Talking the talk, walking the walk: Examining the effect of neighbourhood walkability and social connectedness on physical activity. *Journal of Public Health, 34*(3), 382–89.

Kalichman, S. C. (2010). Social and structural HIV prevention in alcohol-serving establishments. *Alcohol Research & Health, 33*(3), 184–94.

Kaplan, G. A., Pamuk, E. R., Lynch, J. W., Cohen, R. D., & Balfour, J. L. (1996). Inequality in income and mortality in the United States: Analysis of mortality and potential pathways. *BMJ, 312*(7037), 999–1003.

Kawachi, I. & Kennedy, B. P. (1999). Income inequality and health: Pathways and mechanisms. *Health Services Research, 34*(1 Pt 2), 215–27.

Kawachi, I., Kennedy, B. P., & Glass, R. (1999). Social capital and self-rated health: A contextual analysis. *American Journal of Public Health, 89*(8), 1187–93.

Kawachi, I., Kennedy, B. P., Lochner, K., & Prothrow-Stith, D. (1997). Social capital, income inequality, and mortality. *American Journal of Public Health, 87*(9), 1491–98.

Kelly, J. A., Murphy, D. A., Sikkema, K. J., McAuliffe, T. L., Roffman, R. A., Solomon, L. J., . . . Kalichman, S. C. (1997). Randomised, controlled, community-level HIV-prevention intervention for sexual-risk behaviour among homosexual men in US cities. Community HIV Prevention Research Collaborative. *Lancet, 350*(9090), 1500–1505.

Kelly, J. A., St Lawrence, J. S., Diaz, Y. E., Stevenson, L. Y., Hauth, A. C., Brasfield, T. L., . . . Andrew, M. E. (1991). HIV risk behavior reduction following intervention with key opinion leaders of population: an experimental analysis. *American Journal of Public Health, 81*(2), 168–71.

Kennedy, B. P., Kawachi, I., & Prothrow-Stith, D. (1996). Income distribution and mortality: Cross-sectional ecological study of the Robin Hood index in the United States. *British Medical Journal, 312*(7037), 1004–07.

Kindig, D. & Stoddart, G. (2003). What is population health? *American Journal of Public Health, 93*(3), 380–83.

Kreuter, M. & Lezin, N. (2001). *Improving everyone's quality of life: A primer on population health.* Seattle, WA: Group Health Community Foundation.

Kumar, M. B., Walls, M., Janz, T., Hutchinson, P., Turner, T., & Graham, C. (2012). Suicidal ideation among Métis adult men and women—associated risk and protective factors: Findings from a nationally representative survey. *International Journal of Circumpolar Health, 71*, 18829.

Labonte, R. (1995). Population health and health promotion: What do they have to say to each other? *Canadian Journal of Public Health, 86*(3), 165–68.

——— (1997). The population health/health promotion debate in Canada: The politics of explanation, economics and action. *Critical Public Health, 7*(1&2), 7–27.

———, Polanyi, M., Muhajarine, N., McIntosh, T., & Williams, A. (2005). Beyond the divides: Towards critical population health research. *Critical Public Health, 15*(1), 5–17.

Lalonde, M. (1981). *A new perspective on the health of Canadians: A working document.* Ottawa N: Minister of Supply and Services Canada.

Langille, D. B., Asbridge, M., Kisely, S., & Rasic, D. (2012). Suicidal behaviours in adolescents in Nova Scotia, Canada: protective associations with measures of social capital. *Social Psychiatry and Psychiatric Epidemiology, 47*(10), 1549–55.

Lantz, P. M., House, J. S., Lepkowski, J. M., Williams, D. R., Mero, R. P., & Chen, J. (1998). Socio-economic factors, health behaviors, and mortality: Results from a nationally representative prospective study of US adults. *Journal of the American Medical Association, 279*(21), 1703–08.

Lasser, K. E., Himmelstein, D. U., & Woolhandler, S. (2006). Access to care, health status, and health disparities in the United States and Canada: Results of a cross-national population-based survey. *American Journal of Public Health, 96*(7), 1300–1307.

Law, M., Wilson, K., Eyles, J., Elliott, S., Jerrett, M., Moffat, T., & Luginaah, I. (2005). Meeting health need, accessing healthcare: The role of neighbourhood. *Health & Place, 11*(4), 367–77.

Lochner, K. A., Kawachi, I., Brennan, R. T., & Buka, S. L. (2003). Social capital and neighborhood mortality rates in Chicago. *Social Science and Medicine, 56*(8), 1797–1805.

Lowcock, E. C., Rosella, L. C., Foisy, J., McGeer, A., & Crowcroft, N. (2012). The social determinants of health and pandemic H1N1 2009 influenza severity. *American Journal of Public Health, 102*(8), e51–e58.

Lynch, J. W., Kaplan, G. A., Pamuk, E. R., Cohen, R. D., Heck, K. E., Balfour, J. L., & Yen, I. H. (1998). Income inequality and mortality in metropolitan areas of the United States. *American Journal of Public Health, 88*(7), 1074–80.

Lynch, J. W., Smith, G. D., Kaplan, G. A., & House, J. S. (2000). Income inequality and mortality: Importance to health of individual income, psychosocial environment, or material conditions. *British Medical Journal, 320*(7243), 1200–1204.

Maibach, E. W., Abroms, L. C., & Marosits, M. (2007). Communication and marketing as tools to cultivate the public's health: a proposed "people and places" framework. *BMC Public Health, 7*, 88.

McLeroy, K. R., Bibeau, D., Steckler, A., & Glanz, K. (1988). An ecological perspective on health promotion programs. *Health Education Quarterly, 15*(4), 351–77.

Mikkonen, J. & Raphael, D. (2010). *Social determinants of health: The Canadian facts.* Toronto: York University School of Health Policy and Management.

Minkler, M., Wallace, S. P., & McDonald, M. (1994). The political economy of health: a useful theoretical tool for health education practice. *International Quarterly of Community Health Education, 15*(2), 111–26.

Muntaner, C., Borrell, C., Ng, E., Chung, H., Espelt, A., Rodriguez-Sanz, M., . . . O'Campo, P. (2011). Politics, welfare regimes, and population health: controversies and evidence. *Sociology of Health and Illness, 33*(6), 946–64.

Navarro, V., Borrell, C., Benach, J., Muntaner, C., Quiroga, A., Rodriguez-Sanz, M., . . . Pasarin, M. I. (2003). The importance of the political and the social in explaining mortality differentials among the countries of the OECD, 1950–1998. *International Journal of Health Services, 33*(3), 419–94.

Navarro, V., Muntaner, C., Borrell, C., Benach, J., Quiroga, A., Rodriguez-Sanz, M., . . . Pasarin, M. I. (2006). Politics and health outcomes. *Lancet, 368*(9540), 1033–37.

Navarro, V. & Shi, L. (2001). The political context of social inequalities and health. *International Journal of Health Services, 31*(1), 1–21.

Ontario Prevention Clearinghouse. (2006). *The case for prevention: Moving upstream to improve health for all Ontarians.* Toronto N: Ontario Prevention Clearinghouse.

Ottawa Charter for Health Promotion: An international conference on health promotion. (1986) Retrieved 27June, 2014, from www.phac-aspc.gc.ca/ph-sp/docs/charter-chartre/index-eng.php

Poland, B., Coburn, D., Robertson, A., & Eakin, J. (1998). Wealth, equity and healthcare: A critique of a "population health" perspective on the determinants of health. Critical Social Science Group. *Social Science and Medicine, 46*(7), 785–98.

Pouliou, T. & Elliott, S. J. (2010). Individual and socio-environmental determinants of overweight and obesity in Urban Canada. *Health & Place, 16*(2), 389–98.

Public Health Agency of Canada. (2012). What is the population health approach? Retrieved 27June, 2014, from www.phac-aspc.gc.ca/ph-sp/approach-approche/index-eng.php

Raine, K. D. (2005). Determinants of healthy eating in Canada: an overview and synthesis. *Canadian Journal of Public Health, 96 Suppl 3*, S8–14, S18–15.

Raphael, D. (2006). Social determinants of health: Present status, unanswered questions, and future directions. *International Journal of Health Services, 36*(4), 651–77.

————, (2008). Grasping at straws: A recent history of health promotion in Canada. *Critical Public Health, 18*(4), 483–95.

————, (2011). Mainstream media and the social determinants of health in Canada: Is it time to call it a day? *Health Promotion International, 26*(2), 220–29.

————, (2012). Educating the Canadian public about the social determinants of health: The time for local public health action is now! *Global Health Promotion, 19*(3), 54–9.

————, Anstice, S., Raine, K., McGannon, K. R., Rizvi, S. K., & Yu, V. (2003). The social determinants of the incidence and management of type 2 diabetes mellitus: Are we prepared to rethink our questions and redirect our research activities? *International Journal of Healthcare Quality Assurance, 16*(3), x–xx.

———— & Bryant, T. (2002). The limitations of population health as a model for a new public health. *Health Promotion International, 17*(2), 189–99.

———— & Bryant, T. (2006a). Maintaining population health in a period of welfare state decline: Political economy as the missing dimension in health promotion theory and practice. *Promotion & Education, 13*(4), 236–42.

———— & Bryant, T. (2006b). The state's role in promoting population health: Public health concerns in Canada, USA, UK, and Sweden. *Health Policy, 78*(1), 39–55.

————, Curry-Stevens, A., & Bryant, T. (2008). Barriers to addressing the social determinants of health: Insights from the Canadian experience. *Health Policy, 88*(2–3), 222–35.

———— & Farrell, E. S. (2002). Beyond medicine and lifestyle: Addressing the societal determinants of cardiovascular disease in North America. *Leadership in Health Services, 15*(4), i–v.

Rhodes, T. (1997). Risk theory in epidemic times: Sex, drugs and the social organisation of "risk behaviour." *Sociology of Health and Illness, 19*(2), 208–27.

Richard, L., Gauvin, L., Kestens, Y., Shatenstein, B., Payette, H., Daniel, M., . . . Mercille, G. (2013). Neighborhood resources and social participation among older adults: Results from the VoisiNuage study. *Journal of Aging and Health, 25*(2), 296–318.

Robertson, A. (1998). Shifting discourses on health in Canada: From health promotion to population health. *Health Promotion International, 13*(2), 155–66.

Rojanapithayakorn, W. (2006). The 100% condom use programme in Asia. *Reproductive Health Matters, 14*(28), 41–52.

———— & Hanenberg, R. (1996). The 100% condom program in Thailand. *AIDS, 10*(1), 1–7.

Sawka, K. J., McCormack, G. R., Nettel-Aguirre, A., Hawe, P., & Doyle-Baker, P. K. (2013). Friendship networks and physical activity and sedentary behavior among youth: A systematized review. *International Journal of Behavioral Nutrition and Physical Activity, 10*, 130.

Seliske, L., Pickett, W., Rosu, A., & Janssen, I. (2013). The number and type of food retailers surrounding schools and their association with lunchtime eating behaviours in students. *International Journal of Behavioral Nutrition and Physical Activity, 10*(19), 1–9.

Statistics Canada (1999). *National population health survey, 1996–1997.*

Swinburn, B., Egger, G., & Raza, F. (1999). Dissecting obesogenic environments: The development and application of a framework for identifying and prioritizing environmental interventions for obesity. *Preventive Medicine, 29*(6 Pt 1), 563–70.

Swinburn, B. A. (2008). Obesity prevention: The role of policies, laws and regulations. *Aust New Zealand Health Policy, 5*(12), 1–7.

Van Hulst, A., Barnett, T. A., Gauvin, L., Daniel, M., Kestens, Y., Bird, M., . . . Lambert, M. (2012). Associations between children's diets and features of their residential and school neighbourhood food environments. *Canadian Journal of Public Health, 103*(9 Suppl 3), eS48–eS54.

Wilkinson, R. & Marmot, M. (Eds.). (2003). *Social determinants of health: The solid facts* (2nd ed.). Copenhagen: World Health Organization.

Woodcock, J. & Aldred, R. (2008). Cars, corporations, and commodities: Consequences for the social determinants of health. *Emerging Themes in Epidemiology, 5*, 4.

World Health Organization. (2007). *Global age-friendly cities: A guide.* Geneva.

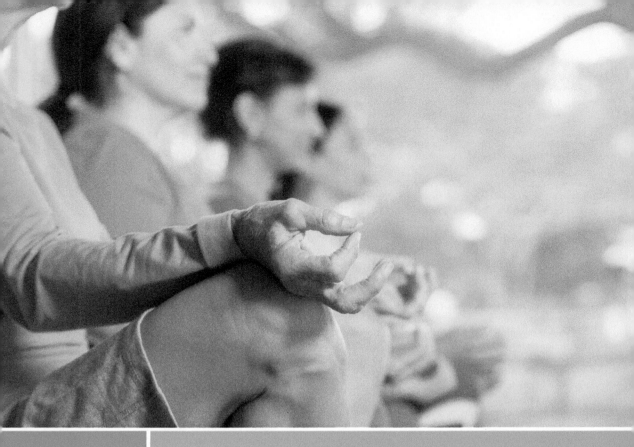

11

The Re-emergence of Other Healing Paradigms

Yvonne LeBlanc

LEARNING OBJECTIVES

In this chapter, students will learn

- the social construction of definitions and classifications of complementary and alternative medicines (CAM)
- the key philosophical concepts associated with CAM
- the historical evolution and (re)emergence of CAM within a biomedically dominant culture
- current utilization trends, patterns, and themes associated with the experience of CAM

Introduction

Similar to other Westernized societies, Canada hosts a variety of healing systems and techniques distinct from modern Western scientific medicine. Along with biomedicine, many Canadians use one or more "non-conventional" forms of healing, commonly referred to as "traditional," **"complementary,"** or **"alternative"** medicine (Kelner & Wellman, 2000). Basically, **complementary and alternative medicine (CAM)** is an term that refers to a diverse range of healing approaches, many with origins in ancient healing systems and indigenous cultures (Micozzi, 2006).

Although CAM has always been part of the fabric of health care, in the past few decades there have been massive changes in the public exposure to and availability of CAM. In pharmacies, health food businesses, and bookstores, one can find a range of herbal and homeopathic remedies and self-help books on health. Many health clinics provide a variety of therapies that include chiropractic services, massage, naturopathic medicine, reflexology, and Reiki. Television shows, the internet, and advertising have increased the visibility of CAM. Although predominantly a commercial enterprise, some forms of CAM are available to patients through the publicly funded health care system. For example, health professionals may offer therapeutic touch or acupuncture within their scopes of practice, and CAM practitioners often volunteer their services in palliative care and oncology units. Although alternative forms of healing have (re)emerged and are becoming increasingly popular, how CAM will continue to evolve remains unclear.

To gain a better understanding of this social phenomenon, this chapter introduces students to CAM-related terminology and concepts, as well as issues, patterns, and trends central to the practice and use of CAM. The chapter begins by considering the social construction of various definitions and classifications of CAM. Social constructionism is based on the idea that social meanings and knowledge are produced through interactions that occur within particular social and cultural contexts (Conrad & Barker, 2010). From this perspective, students will explore two concepts central to CAM: **holism** and **vitalism**. These principles raise important debates concerning the approach to client care and the legitimacy of CAM therapies and practitioners. Then, a review of the research on the resurgence of CAM will emphasize the important social and cultural conditions that have paved the way for greater public acceptance of various forms of CAM. An exploration of the issues of social legitimacy and the changing interface of biomedicine and CAM will follow. Last, the chapter reviews current patterns, trends, and themes demonstrating that CAM is widely used among health seekers and chronic illness sufferers. The experience of CAM can be simultaneously empowering and stigmatizing; it is also not without potential risk.

Defining Complementary and Alternative Medicine (CAM)

Meanings attached to alternative forms of healing are dynamic, open to interpretation, and shaped by individuals and groups from different social locations. As a result, CAM is often described in contrasting and conflicting ways. For example, between the 1960s and 1990s medical scholars often referred to CAM practices as "holistic," "folk," "traditional," or "alternative" (Low, 2004, p. 12). These medicines were defined as anything not taught in medical schools; as inconsistent with scientific thought; and as unacceptable within the parameters of conventional medical knowledge (Kelner & Wellman, 2000). Such "definitions of exclusion" assert the dominance of biomedicine by describing CAM as something external (Stone & Katz, 2005a).

In an attempt to depict the essence of a broad range of medicines that do not fit neatly within the conventional parameters of biomedicine, the Office of Alternative Medicine (1995), which later became the US National Center for Complementary and Alternative Medicine (NCCAM), provided a definition that more aptly captures the changing dynamics of **medical pluralism**. CAM is described as

> a broad domain of healing resources that encompasses all health systems, modalities, and practices and their accompanying theories and beliefs, other than those intrinsic to the politically dominant health system of a particular society or culture in a given historical period. CAM includes all such practices and ideas self-defined by their users as preventing or treating illness or promoting well-being. Boundaries within CAM and between the CAM domain and the domain of the dominant system are not always sharp or fixed. (Kelner & Wellman 2000, p. 4)

As Kelner & Wellman (2000) note, this definition attempts to level the playing field between CAM and conventional medicine.

By the early 1990s the underlying rationale was that "alternative medicine" was used more as an "adjunct to" rather than a "replacement for" conventional medical care (Micozzi, 2006, p. 9). Increasing consumer interest in non-conventional approaches to healing prompted some researchers to re-examine the nomenclature and introduce the term CAM (Kelner & Wellman 2000). While the term "alternative" implies that the approach is separate from and used in place of biomedicine, "complementary" infers working alongside and in partnership with conventional medicine (Stone & Katz, 2005a).

The difference in terminology reflects a change in the social acceptance of many forms of CAM within mainstream health care. In Canada, chiropractic medicine, once highly castigated, is one example. Chiropractors currently make up the third largest group of primary medical care practitioners after physicians and dentists (Clarke, 2012, p. 353). Further, the practice of midwifery recently became fully licensed and funded within Ontario's health care system (Bourgeault, 2000). Before the 1970s, the discipline was neither legally sanctioned nor officially recognized. Despite opposition from the medical profession and other more established health professionals, the "marginalized" practice has become widely accepted (Bourgeault, 2000). Additionally, naturopathy and homeopathy, once considered alternative practices, are now more commonly referred to as "complementary" (Sharma & Black, 2001).

More recently, the term **integrative medicine** has been used with respect to CAM. The central goal of integrative medicine is to work toward a form of health care that combines CAM and biomedicine. Boon, Verhoef, O'Hara, Finday, & Majid (2004) describe the integrative health care model in Canada as a seamless, pluralistic, and egalitarian system. Accordingly, the model champions an "interdisciplinary and non-hierarchal blending of both conventional medicine and alternative healthcare." This involves a collaborative team approach among practitioners and clients; the patient-centred, holistic treatment results in better and more cost-effective care (p. 55).

Integration tends to imply conforming to biomedical standards (Fries, 2011). This conformity involves a commitment to evidence-based medicine, requiring that only therapies tested by scientific methods, typically randomized controlled trials, are considered appropriate for integration. Only those that demonstrate scientific evidence of safety and effectiveness are deemed "evidence based." In general, healing systems and therapies that do not meet biomedical standards tend to be marginalized. Many mainstream biomedical practitioners insist that many forms of CAM are "pseudoscientific practices" lacking "real" scientific grounding and evidence; therefore, they have no place in conventional health care (Charlton, 2008; Ernst, 2008). But as Coulter (2012) notes, the criteria for integrating CAM and conventional medicine assumes that biomedicine is evidence based. In reality, many medical interventions would not hold up to the scrutiny of the evidence-based process and some of what is described as "evidence-based medicine" is, ironically, based on poor evidence (McAlister, van Diepen, Padwal, Johnson, & Majumdar, 2007; Greenhalgh, Howick, & Maskrey, 2014).

The degree to which CAM providers conform to evidence-based standards varies between and within groups. In an Ontario study, Kelner, Boon, Wellman, & Welsh (2002) evaluated whether chiropractic, homeopathy, and Reiki practitioners felt the need to demonstrate the cost-effectiveness, safety, and efficacy of their therapies and practices. They found that Reiki practitioners were the least interested in proving effectiveness. Most saw no need for providing proof of safety and all felt confident that Reiki therapy is cost effective. In contrast, chiropractic practitioners were most inclined to say that it is imperative to show effectiveness and believed that chiropractic care is cost effective. The homeopaths disagreed on the need for research on safety and effectiveness.

Although the integrative model is intended to bring together "the best of both CAM and biomedicine" (Baer, 2008, p. 52), there is less evidence to support that this is actually happening. As Kelner, Wellman, Boon, and Welsh (2004) point out, integration continues to mean different things to different stakeholder groups. For instance, even though CAM has been introduced into medical and nursing training programs, there is also evidence that the relationship in integrative care settings in Canada remains hierarchal rather than egalitarian (Hollenberg, 2006). This situation is not unique to Canada. Coulter (2004) argues that integrative medicine must be incorporated into predominantly hospital-based medical programs to be accepted in the US. Such a scenario implies an assimilation of CAM into the biomedical model, which Fadlon (2004) describes as the domestication of CAM into biomedicine. Researchers who have looked at integrative medicine in the UK (Cant & Sharma, 1999; Saks, 2001) and Australia (Baer, 2008) also contend that biomedicine is in the process of co-opting CAM practices. This empirical evidence suggests that conventional medicine is likely to dominate CAM in a system of integrative health care.

Classifying Complementary and Alternative Medicine (CAM)

The classification of CAM is also complex and controversial due to lack of knowledge and consensus about what CAM is or is not (Stone & Katz, 2005a). Researchers have developed various models aimed at describing the similar, underlying, or prevailing characteristics of groups of therapies. A widely used and accepted classification system, developed through the NCCAM, categorizes CAM therapies by type of therapeutic intervention. The categories include complete systems of theory and practice, mind/body medicine, biologically based therapies, manipulation and body-based therapies, and energy therapies.

TABLE 11.1	NCCAM Classification of CAM
Alternative Medical Systems	Complete systems of theory and practice including homeopathy, naturopathy, traditional Chinese medicine, and Ayurveda.
Mind–Body Interventions	Patient support groups, meditation, prayer, spiritual healing, therapies that use creative outlets such as art, music, or dance.
Biologically Based Therapies	Include the use of herbs, foods, vitamins, minerals, dietary supplements.
Manipulative and Body-Based Methods	Chiropractic or osteopathic manipulation, and massage.
Energy Therapies	The use and manipulation of energy fields.

Source: National Center for Complementary and Alternative Medicine (NC CAM), http://nccam.nih.gov/health/whatiscam

In Canada, Tataryn (2002) used a different approach to develop a typology based on the underlying philosophical similarities of various therapies. Forms of CAM are placed within one of four categories according to the each medicine's basic assumptions about health and disease. The four categories include:

- The body paradigm, which works through biologic mechanisms
- Mind–body therapies, which assume that stress, psychological coping styles, and social supports primarily determine health and disease
- Body–energy therapies, which assert that health and disease are functions of the flow and balance of life energies
- Body–spirit therapies, which presume that forces beyond the material universe (i.e. God or spirits) influence health and disease (p. 880).

These are but two of a number of classification systems. Such typologies can be beneficial when comparing CAM therapies and making decisions about their use (Tataryn, 2002). However, they become problematic for researchers when trying to make comparisons between various systems. This is largely due to differences in their conceptual frameworks (Boon et al., 2004). For example, homeopathy is considered an alternative medicine system in the NCCAM model but is an energy therapy according to Tataryn's (2002) typology. In another model it could be categorized as something else.

Key CAM Concepts

Holism and Holistic Approach

Definitions and classifications of CAM can be confusing. But some shared CAM concepts can provide the field with a common theoretical structure, lending coherence to an expansive range of healing practices. One such principle is holism. Holism is the idea that a person must be considered in his or her totality, as an extension of the environment, and that the whole of the individual is greater than the sum of his or her parts (Micozzi, 2006). To heal and achieve optimal health, it is necessary to attain balance or harmony between the individual and the broader environment. In a holistic approach, disease is perceived as the result of an imbalance of the physical, psychological, social, and spiritual dimensions of the person. Practitioners aim to treat the whole person and to facilitate the body's own healing response through an individualized plan of care. This is in contrast to reductionism, which is more commonly linked to biomedicine (see Chapter Eight). In a reductionist approach, the focus of treatment is on the diseased part of the body rather than on the individual as a whole (Lee-Treweek & Stone, 2005).

O'Connor (2000) further notes that an extension of the holistic approach is the attention to underlying causes; it is more important to identify and treat the underlying cause of illness than it is to treat the immediate symptoms. This model assumes that health can only be restored by treating this fundamental imbalance. Further, CAM systems hold moral assumptions such as beliefs in "the goodness of nature" and individual responsibility for "correct behaviour" in preserving health. In conjunction with harmony and balance, these views stress the interconnectedness of personal health, the whole person, the broader environment, and the universe (pp. 51–2).

Another extension of the holistic approach is the assumption that the therapeutic relationship between the practitioner and the client is inherently beneficial and acts as a catalyst for self-healing (Stone & Katz, 2005b). This is highly contested by many opponents of CAM. While CAM practitioners claim that the therapeutic relationship is an important tool for healing, critics argue that it is not more than a placebo—an inert substance like a sugar pill. When given instead of an active drug or treatment, physicians have found placebos make some people feel better (see the case study in Chapter Eight). The **placebo effect** refers to the phenomenon that some people will get better even when they have been administered a fake medication or treatment (Lee-Treweek & Stone, 2005). This implies that what a person perceives to be an effective treatment can be merely imaginary. Perceived effectiveness has more to do with one's belief in the remedy than the treatment itself. Opponents to CAM often use this argument to denigrate practitioners and individuals who believe in the effectiveness of the treatments. There has been little research into the synergistic effects of CAM to examine the combined impacts of treatment in conjunction with the therapeutic relationship (Barry, 2012).

Vitalism

Another concept central to the philosophy of many CAM practices is vitalism (Boon, 1998; Cant & Sharma, 1995). Vitalism refers to the idea that the human body is alive and well due to a special type of energy or force. Such a force "may be connected with a universal or cosmic source or reservoir" (O'Connor, 2000, p. 51). This term became popular in the elite universities of eighteenth- and nineteenth-century Europe (Micozzi 2006, p. 54). According to Canter (2008) the concept is etched in the belief that life cannot be fully explained by physical or mechanical laws. This same principle is assumed in the Greco-Roman notion of humours; the East Indian yogic idea of prana; "doshas" in Ayurvedic medicine; and the Chinese concept of chi or qi. Aristotle also believed in the "soul as a life force," and Descartes argued that a "spiritual entity" guides organisms. Vital energy enables self-regulation and gives the body/mind/spirit the capacity to heal itself (O'Connor, 2000).

Some of the healing practices that involve a belief in a "life force" are associated with formal religion. These methods can involve prayer, religious ceremonies, and rituals. Others are more directly linked to the idea of "spiritual healing" and hold more extensive or secular meanings than organized religious practices (White & Verhoef, 2006, p. 117). In this broader context, spiritual healing and mind–body CAM approaches are commonly linked. For example, energy therapies such as reiki are represented by some academic scholars as religious healing and by others as spiritual healing (McGuire, 1988; Glik, 1990; White & Verhoef, 2006).

More recently, CAM researchers have coined the terms *subtle energy* or *bio-field energy* to refer to this "life force energy" (Micozzi, 2006, p. 56). For proponents of the principle, personal perceptions of healing, such as sensations of heat, tingling, and vibrations, are proof that a

CASE STUDY

Reiki

Reiki is a healing practice that originated in Japan and was popularized in North America in the second half of the twentieth century. It operates on the basis that a person may feel unwell as a result of low or problematic life force energy. In order to help redress a person's life force imbalance, Reiki practitioners use their hands to manipulate that energy, encouraging a person's life force to flow smoothly. In this sense, Reiki is holistic, aiming to treat the body, mind, emotions, and spirit. Reiki practitioners aim to alleviate stress, improve mental wellbeing, and promote healing. Since the 1990s, Reiki has rapidly expanded; a proliferation of Reiki masters now offer their services around the world. Moreover, there are now many different subtypes of Reiki and individuals seeking out treatment may choose from a wide variety of Reiki practices.

Like many types of CAM, the efficacy of Reiki is subject to dispute. On the one hand, its practitioners cite testimonies of individuals who have been healed by Reiki as evidence of its effectiveness. The increased usage of Reiki in much of the world is also a testament to its success. Conversely, the scientific and medical establishment generally abhors the practice, seeing it as pseudo-scientific and even dangerous. These critics believe that the expansion of Reiki is primarily a result of the fact that people can be easily manipulated when it comes to their health; Reiki is problematic as it might convince people to eschew evidence-based treatments, thereby compromising their health. Finally, many people seem to fall into a third category—neither strong supporters nor vehement critics of the practice. They acknowledge that Reiki is different from traditional biomedicine but also view it as relatively harmless. These individuals believe that people should be able to pursue whatever health interventions they prefer. For this third group, Reiki's rapid growth can perhaps be explained by traditional biomedicine's shortcomings when it comes to healing the individual as a whole.

subtle energy exists. The institution of Western biomedicine, on the other hand, largely dismisses the concept of a "life force" (Micozzi, 2006). Socially, the notion of life force or subtle energy continues to spark a great deal of controversy over what constitutes a conventionally acceptable form of medicine. The extent of these debates both reflects and influences how much a healing system, therapy, or practitioner group is ridiculed for embracing the concept of a life force energy.

Resurgence of CAM

Prior to the 1900s, healing approaches in Western countries were pluralistic—that is, society accepted a wide variety of healing methods as being potentially beneficial (Saks, 2001). There were not always discrete boundaries between models. Through a series of legislative acts in the UK, the US, and Canada, the scope of practice of non-allopathic (see Chapter Eight) health care providers was restricted and statutory recognition of "irregular" medicine practices was blocked (Crellin, Anderson, & Connor, 1997; Saks, 2001; Winnick, 2005). Such "marginal" medical practices posed a threat to allopathic practice because practitioners functioned independently from conventional medicine and were able to treat patients within their specific modalities (Wardwell, 1994). Hence, the monopolization of allopathic medicine began by positioning centuries-old practices, such as midwifery and folk medicine, and newer modalities, like homeopathy and chiropractic medicine, outside the accepted norm (Crellin et al., 1997).

The contemporary evolution of CAM, then, began during the first half of the twentieth century, the "golden era of medical dominance" (Winnick, 2005). The idea of medical dominance, introduced by Freidsen (1970), refers to the power that the medical profession has over the health care system. He argued that the ability to gain and maintain a market monopoly sets allopathic medicine apart from other occupations. The medical profession was able to achieve this dominance in several ways. Medical practitioners established their expertise based on scientific knowledge, thereby attaining state support on the grounds of the benefit to society. In addition, the medical education process was standardized. Through these avenues, the profession gained legal support for control over their competitors (Winnick, 2005). This subsequently secured a degree of professional status that medicine has enjoyed for a number of decades (see Chapter Nine's discussion of licensure for more on this topic).

Some healing practitioner groups actively resisted. Fierce conflicts between various medical factions ensued and some groups made notable occupational advancements after years of legal wrangling. The main strategy that medical professionals used in their attempts to gain legitimacy and occupational status was to embark on legally sanctioned professionalization pursuits. **Professionalization** affords a group higher social status and control over the content and parameters of their work. In Canada, specific practices that have taken this route have been studied extensively. Some examples include chiropractic medicine (Coburn & Biggs, 1986), naturopathic medicine (Boon, 1998; Verhoef, Boon, & Mutasingwa, 2006), midwifery (Benoit, 1991; Bourgeault, 2000), and herbalism (Hirschkorn, 2005). More recently, attention has focused on other "emerging professions" such as massage therapy (Porcino, Boon, Page, & Verhoef, 2011).

Although each of these groups has its own unique history, the common thread between them lies in the compromise that groups make in order to become "legitimate mainstream

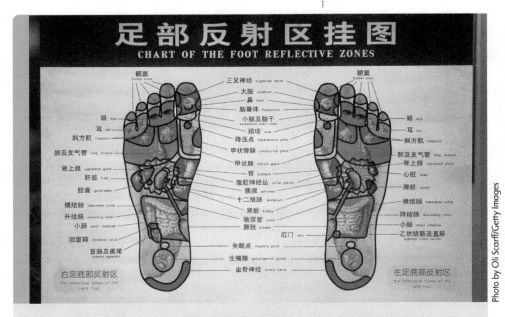

足部反射区挂图
CHART OF THE FOOT REFLECTIVE ZONES

Photo by Oli Scarff/Getty Images

While some complementary and alternative medical practices—such as naturopathy and chiropractic—have achieved increased status within mainstream health care in recent decades, other practices, such as reflexology, continue to operate outside the purview of biomedical standards.

practitioners." Fundamentally, more successful groups, such as chiropractic medicine, naturopathy, and midwifery, transformed their "lay" approaches to training and practice to fit within the scientific model and the conventional standards of professional biomedical practice (Coburn & Biggs, 1986; Bourgeault, 2000; Boon, 1998; Sharma, 1992; Porcino et al., 2011).

Still, the majority of CAM practitioner groups show little interest in pursuing state endorsed "health professionalization." However, this does not mean that they are passive about achieving social acceptance. As Coburn and Biggs (1986) have argued, professionalization is only one way to gain social legitimacy. CAM practitioner groups argue that they can "prove themselves" in other ways—through therapeutic relationships (Kelner, 2000) and by filling gaps within conventional health care (Hollenberg, Lytle, Walji, & Cooley, 2013; Vokey LeBlanc, 2010).

Conditions Influencing the Resurgence of CAM: 1960–1990

Through the first half of the twentieth century, the so-called "alternative" or "irregular" healing groups did not disappear entirely, although they were eclipsed by professional biomedicine (Wardwell, 1994). This situation began to change somewhat in the 1960s with the advent of the health and countercultural movements in the United States. More specifically, the "holistic health" and the "New Age" movements of that era were fundamental in challenging biomedical dominance. The holistic health movement evolved in response to a crisis in

Western health delivery. Problems with the biomedical system included rising health care costs, limited resources, ineffective treatment of chronic health care conditions, evidence of harmful effects of conventional treatment, dissatisfaction with medical encounters, and a growing consumer movement (Armstrong, 2002; Coburn, 2001; Gabe & Calnan, 2000; Illich, 1976; Lowenberg, 1989).

The holistic health movement in the US was part of what Lowenberg (1989) termed a "coalition of sixties movements" (p. 67). These included the feminist movement, which focused on women's reproductive rights, physician–patient relationships, public awareness of the harms associated with medicine, and the demystification of medical knowledge (Lowenberg, 1989; McGuire, 1988). Lowenberg (1989) notes that the human potential movement was also part of this trend. Pertinent in her description is the link to Abraham Maslow's notion of self-actualization and its focus on personal development and self-responsibility. The concept became popular among holistic practitioners and was incorporated with other Eastern psychotherapeutic approaches, one example being transpersonal psychology. Based in "Eastern wisdom," this school of psychology has spiritual dimensions and explores transforming the consciousness of self and society (Lowenberg, 1989). The adoption of such notions overlapped with other countercultural ideas and philosophies.

The holistic health movement encompasses various alternative medical systems and therapies. Holism embraces "parapsychology, folk medicine, herbalism, nutritional therapies, homeopathy, yoga, massage, meditation, and the martial arts." Various practitioner groups are involved and these include an array of "lay alternative practitioners, psychic or spiritual healers, New Agers, holistic MDs, as well as chiropractors, osteopathic physicians, and naturopaths" (Baer, Hays, McClendon, McMoldrick, & Vespucci, 1998, p. 1495).

The New Age movement was part of the 1960s counterculture (Voas & Bruce, 2007) and has been termed an "American phenomenon" (York, 1995). Influenced by both the influx and adoption of Eastern philosophical ideas and practices, "New Age" philosophy revolves around the idea of a "new planetary culture." Proponents claim that this comes about through the attainment of "inner peace, wellness, unity, self-actualization, and the attainment of a higher level of consciousness." This phenomenon first emerged on the West coast of the US and Canada, eventually spreading to countries worldwide (Baer et al., 1998, p. 1496).

"New Age" healing emphasizes spirituality, self-care, and personal transformation. It questions institutional authority while focusing on individual responsibility (McGuire, 1993). In a nine-month ethnographic study of urban healing touch groups, Engebretson (1996) found that "New Age" practitioners valued "spirituality, group connection, egalitarianism, and intuitiveness" and used these forms of CAM in conjunction with biomedicine for "spiritual and general well-being" (p. 540). Numerous techniques have been associated with "New Age" healing. These range from "centering, channeling, astral projection, guided visualization, iridology, reflexology, chromotherapy, rebirthing, shiatsu, and healing with the power of pyramids and crystals" (Baer et al., 1998, p. 1496).

The notion of "New Age" has been widely used within the context of CAM and broadly captures overlapping religious and healing practices (Kaptchuk & Eisenberg, 2001; Low, 2004; McClean, 2005; York, 1995). Such approaches are frequently associated with health consumption in the so-called "spiritual marketplace" (Bowman, 1999). Some sociologists have cautioned that the "New Age" label has been used too widely and indiscriminately, thereby rendering practically every form of holistic healing as "New Age" (Bowman, 1999).

For example, some practices, such as Reiki, did not originate in the US and are therefore not a result of the "New Age" movement. Accordingly, practitioners of holistic healing may or may not identify with "New Ageism."

Sociologists have continued to point out that conventional medicine tends to label particular CAM approaches, such as energy medicine or spiritual healing, as "**quackery**" (see Foltz, 1994; Low, 2004). Quacks give the false impression that they are acting scientifically yet believe sincerely in their approach (Wardwell, 1994). The idea that such depictions are part of the political strategies of more powerful groups is further exemplified in Jonas's (2002) portrayal of energy healing practices as "frontier therapies" that "challenge our conceptual and paradigmatic assumptions about the nature of biological or scientific reality" (p. 34). Such characterizations tend to perpetuate the subordination of CAM practitioners while maintaining the dominance of the medical profession (McGuire, 1988).

The Changing Face of Non-Conventional Healing Practices: 1990–Present

There is evidence to indicate that the relations between biomedicine and CAM have softened over time. For example, a study on the coverage on CAM in five US medical journals showed that the medical profession condemned CAM during the 1960s and 1970s, but by the 1990s attempts to disparage alternatives had been largely abandoned (Winnick, 2005). Although the biomedical community appears to be more tolerant of CAM, struggles and tensions continue to exist and support for CAM varies among groups, regions, and countries.

In seminal work on CAM in Ontario, Kelner et al. (2004) examined the medical profession's receptiveness to the professionalization of CAM practitioners such as chiropractors, naturopaths, acupuncturists, homeopaths, and Reiki practitioners. As part of the study, researchers interviewed ten leaders from medicine, nursing, physiotherapy, clinical nutrition, and public health. Overall, the health care professionals did not endorse professionalization, and were unsympathetic toward CAM groups. These negative attitudes were especially directed towards naturopaths, homeopaths, and Reiki practitioners. Interestingly, nurses in particular seemed more interested in taking over CAM practices than referring patients to CAM providers. All ten leaders were against including CAM practitioners in the provincial government's health insurance scheme and all were resistant to the notion of any government funding for CAM groups.

Research patterns indicate that physicians tend to distance themselves from CAM practitioners. Although doctors may support the use of some forms of CAM, relatively few adopt CAM therapies professionally. When this endorsement does occur, it generally extends into only a few select practices (Hollenberg, 2006; Kelner et al., 2004). In Verhoef and Sutherland's (1995) survey of 200 general practitioners in Alberta and British Columbia, more than half supported the use of acupuncture, chiropractic services, and hypnosis but only 16 per cent of the participants were trained in and practised forms of CAM. Referral patterns also varied according to age and sex. More recently, a national survey of 13,088 physicians conducted by Hirschkorn, Andersen, and Bourgeault (2009) showed that doctors in British Columbia are more receptive to offering CAM services than physicians in other provinces. Despite these attitudes, organizational settings such as medical schools and hospitals may discourage physicians from doing so. A lack of professional knowledge can also prevent access to CAM. For example, health care professionals in a tertiary care centre in Nova Scotia supported the use of select therapies, but their lack of CAM knowledge deterred them from conversing with patients about these options (Brown et al., 2007).

In general, there is greater acceptance of CAM within the UK and Europe than in North America (Winnick, 2005). The extent of this acceptance, though, varies between and among groups of health professionals. For instance, some research supports the idea that family physicians and other allied health professionals are more receptive to CAM than specialists. Kolstad et al. (2004) examined the use and effects of CAM by a group of oncology health workers in Norway. The sample included 828 Norwegian oncologists, nurses, clerks, and therapeutic radiographers. The findings showed that few oncologists had tried CAM to treat their own health problems compared to the other health care worker groups, who were more likely to use CAM when ill.

Although UK physicians are generally more accepting of CAM practices than their Canadian counterparts, they show relatively greater interest in adopting or co-opting these CAM therapies. Adams (2004) conducted interviews with 25 general practitioners in Edinburgh and Glasgow who used acupuncture, homeopathy, hypnotherapy, and neurolinguistic programming. He found that the doctors exerted medical dominance by both denigrating lay therapists and appropriating their practices.

Professional relations are also central to the adoption of CAM within health occupations. Adams & Tovey (2001) found that nurses in the UK have been intricately involved in adopting CAM practices but, similar to physicians, are selective in the therapies that they choose. Nurses tend to favour aromatherapy, reflexology, and massage over chiropractic care and acupuncture. Shuval's (2006) study of nurses working in both biomedical and CAM settings in Israel produced similar results. She argues that doctors and nurses adopt different sets of therapies, suggesting that traditional divisions of labour persist despite some reconfiguration in "conventional" health professional scopes of practice. She argues that the adoption of CAM practices by nurses does not challenge biomedicine and that nurses are constrained by a medical profession that keeps "the boundaries of biomedicine closed" (p. 1784).

The situation for non–health professional CAM practitioners, commonly referred to as lay practitioners, appears even more precarious. Tovey & Adams (2002) argue that the appropriation of CAM therapies by physicians and nurses within their professional scope of practice may jeopardize lay practitioners' long-term viability as CAM providers.

Alternatively, the viability of CAM within contemporary health care is not solely dependent on the biomedical community's acceptance of CAM. CAM is uniquely suited to fill gaps in existing health care services. In rural and remote communities in Ontario, for example, access to biomedical health care is limited; individuals are more likely to seek the help of naturopathic doctors, chiropractic doctors, registered midwives, and traditional Aboriginal healers (Hollenberg et al., 2013). It appears that these providers are currently playing a significant role in health care provision by offering holistic care in underserviced areas. Additionally, in Vokey LeBlanc's (2010) research on 50 energy healers located in Atlantic Canada and Ontario, she found that healers provided service largely to medically compromised people. Practitioners were most welcomed in mainstream spaces where cutting-edge biomedical acute care tends not to tread. Services were commonly provided to palliative care patients, those living with stigmatizing conditions such as HIV/AIDS, the elderly in nursing homes, women in abusive situations, or those struggling with mental health issues and relationship problems.

Use of CAM: Prevalence and Utilization Patterns

Similar to other nations, Canadians use CAM to prevent illness, maintain health and well-being, and treat chronic illness (Esmail, 2007; Kelner & Wellman, 1997a; Low, 2004). In most industrialized countries, prevalence varies between 30 and 75 per cent, and the overall response by the public to CAM is positive (Andrews, Adams, Segrott, & Lui, 2012). A recent review of CAM use in 10 Westernized countries (Austria, Australia, Canada, Denmark, Germany, Great Britain, Italy, South Korea, Switzerland, and the United States) revealed an overall prevalence of 32 per cent, with use in Canada estimated at 16 per cent (Frass et al., 2012). Earlier studies show that over 70 per cent of Canadians have used some form of CAM at least once and more than one half of Canadians used alternative therapies in 2006 (Esmail, 2007, p. 4).

There are well-documented utilization trends showing that out-of-pocket spending on CAM has increased in industrialized countries (Bodeker, Kronenberg, & Buford, 2007; de Bruyn, 2002; Eisenberg et al., 1998; Esmail, 2007). Despite reports that the rapid growth in the CAM industry has reached a plateau (Esmail, 2007; Tindle, Davis, Phillips, & Eisenberg, 2005; Kelner, 2005), there are strong indications that the commercialization of CAM continues to thrive (Andrews & Boon, 2005). The estimated total out-of-pocket spending on alternative medicine in Canada in the latter half of 2005 and first half of 2006 was $7.84 billion (Esmail, 2007, p. 5). Utilization also varies regionally across the country. Use is highest among Westerners and lowest among Atlantic Canadians.

Overall patterns indicate that typical CAM users are middle-aged, affluent, well-educated, white women with poorer health status (Adams, Easthope, & Sibritt 2003; Andrews et al., 2012; Astin, 1998; Kelner & Wellman, 1997b; Wiles & Rosenberg, 2001). The use of CAM is high among people living with chronic illness conditions, especially those with allergies, back and neck problems, and arthritis. Furthermore, up to 93 per cent of people experiencing cancer use some form of CAM (Esmail, 2007). The most popular forms of CAM used by Canadians reflect these chronic health issues: massage, prayer, chiropractic medicine, relaxation techniques, and herbal therapies are all widely used choices (Esmail, 2007, p. 4).

Other research findings point to some interesting variations. Some US studies indicate that there are no racial or gender differences in the use of alternative medicine (Astin, 1998). Canadian findings suggest that CAM use is not necessarily confined to the better educated and financially privileged, as many people might assume (Andrews & Boon, 2005). Specific patient populations, such as those with prostate cancer (White & Verhoef, 2006) and HIV/AIDS, report high CAM use patterns among men (Pawluch, Cain, & Gillett, 2000; Foote-Ardah, 2003; Gillett, Pawluch, & Cain, 2002). Some research suggests that younger, retired, and perhaps more affluent older people use CAM (Andrews, 2002), but utilization is also high among children and youth with chronic illnesses (Adams, Kemper, & Vohra, 2012). These differences reinforce the underlying complexities associated with CAM use as well as inconsistencies in study designs and methodologies.

CASE STUDY

Integrative Oncology

People diagnosed with cancer have expressed the desire for more holistic treatments beyond surgery and chemotherapy. Indeed, use of CAM among cancer patients is more common than for people diagnosed with other illnesses (Cassileth & Vickers, 2005). At the same time, people are reluctant to abandon traditional treatments. The field of "integrative oncology" represents a meeting point between CAM and biomedicine.

Those who practise integrative oncology insist that "we do not promote alternative care; rather, we are pushing for greater integration with the current model of care" (Seely, 2014, p. 46). Integrative oncology usually involves treatments that are largely accepted by bio-medicine, such as dietary changes, relaxation, and exercise, alongside other more contentious interventions such as energy field manipulation and reflexology. Practitioners of integrative oncology argue that it provides symptom relief rather than treating the cancer itself. They argue that it can help facilitate biomedical cancer treatment by making chemotherapy more bearable and relieving some of the psychological distress associated with cancer.

Some hospitals and cancer clinics within the US have opened centres for integrative oncology within the hospital itself. Canada has also recently witnessed a dramatic expansion in integrative oncology. For example, the Ottawa Integrative Cancer Centre, a regional arm of the Canadian College of Naturopathic Medicine, opened up in 2011. The centre sees more than 10,000 patients per year. Its staff members aim to provide a whole body and whole person approach to cancer treatment and prevention. They offer massage therapy; mind–body therapies, including yoga and hypno-visualization; and forms of psycho-social counselling.

Despite its popularity with some members of the public, practitioners of integrative oncology have been subject to criticism, especially from within traditional biomedicine. Critics argue that integrative oncology raises false hopes, lacks scientific evidence, and wastes both time and resources, and maintain that some techniques, such as intravenous vitamin injections, might actually be harmful to patients (Gorski, 2014). Supporters, meanwhile, see such criticisms as a product of biomedicine's fear that it may lose its monopoly on treatment.

Of course, other biomedical physicians support some use of some CAM techniques, seeing it as complementary rather than competitive. All in all, the case of integrative oncology demonstrates the complexity of labelling something as "purely" CAM or "purely" biomedicine: practitioners on both sides of the debate support many of the practice's central tenets such as reducing stress, improving diet, and getting more exercise.

Why People Are Attracted to CAM

The concepts of "push" and "pull" have been used to frame the reasons that people are attracted to CAM (Astin, 1998; Foote-Ardah, 2003). Generally speaking, people are often pushed toward CAM because they are dissatisfied with conventional medicine (Astin, 1998), displeased with medical encounters, and/or unhappy with the doctor–patient relationship (Siahpush, 1999). People are also pulled toward CAM because treatments are compatible with their world views and personal health beliefs (see Astin, 1998; Siahpush, 1999).

The rise in popularity of CAM has also been attributed to wider socio-political changes (Sharma, 2000; Sointu, 2006a), sometimes framed in terms of postmodern values (Coulter & Willis, 2004; 2007) and postmodern consumer behaviour (Saks, 2001). According to Siahpush (1999), postmodernism includes a rejection of scientific authority, disillusionment with conventional medicine, problems within the doctor–patient relationship, a consumerist attitude, belief in self-responsibility, a heterogeneous social network, and psychological need (Siahpush, 1999). Postmodernism has also been described as an era in which consumption is pervasive (Bury, 1997), and collective meaning is replaced by individualism (Annandale & Clark, 2000). For example, in an ethnographic study of spiritual healers in the UK, McClean (2005) concluded that the current emphasis on taking personal responsibility for health illustrates "the subjectification and personalization of public life." In other words, preoccupation with oneself is characteristic of individualism (p. 628).

Although not theoretically linked to a "postmodernism," other studies suggest that some CAM users hold "an alternative world view." Pawluch et al. (2000) demonstrate this in their study of individuals with HIV/AIDS. Their alternative therapy ideology involved accepting that HIV/AIDS is a chronic illness condition; making responsible decisions and being committed to and proactive about health; maintaining a holistic understanding of health that encompasses physical, mental, emotional, and spiritual wellbeing; and remaining open to trying available therapies. Similarly, in Low's (2004) study of CAM

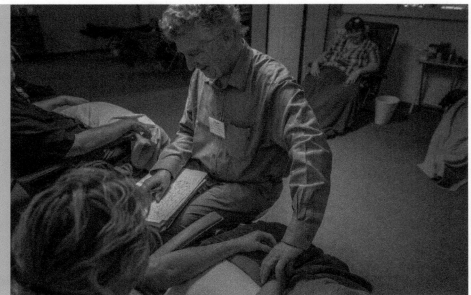

© ZUMA Press Inc/Alamy

The community acupuncture model, in which clients can access affordable acupuncture treatments by receiving treatment in a shared space rather than a one-on-one practitioner–client environment, eschews many of the conventions of allopathic medicine.

users, participants valued an approach to health and healing that encompassed holism, balance, and personal control. She argued that this view influenced participants' reasons for accessing therapy, their client–practitioner relationships, and the specific kinds of therapy that they used.

Additionally, in their review of 94 CAM studies, Bishop, Yardley, and Lewith (2007) note that users commonly value natural, holistic approaches and view themselves as "unconventional" and "spiritual." Other literature suggests that complementary therapies are related to spirituality only in that this notion is part of broader value systems that embrace holism (Astin, 1998; McClean, 2005; Low, 2004). Still other sociologists argue that both pragmatism and one's belief systems influence decisions about CAM use (Sharma, 1992). Recent research on older people's use of CAM tends to support this view. Older people are inclined to seek out CAM as a way to gain control over health and the aging process. More specifically, CAM users are generally seeking to manage chronic health issues (Fries, 2014; Hurd Clarke, & Bennet, 2012). The holistic philosophy associated with CAM provides compassionate alternatives to the increasingly techno-scientific and potentially harmful effects associated with biomedical care (Fries, 2014).

Ultimately, there are likely important differences among groups of CAM users and numerous avenues to CAM treatments (Bishop et al., 2007). This reinforces the idea that users are heterogeneous in their world views and share common beliefs with non-users (Fadlon, 2004; Pawluch, et al. 2000).

The Experience of CAM

Research on the experience of CAM provides insight into the meanings that people attach to therapies that offer potential tools for healing holistically and to their healing effects (McGuire, 1988). Quite often it is a chronic illness condition that sparks the impetus for a healing quest. Numerous studies show that chronic illness encompasses a wide spectrum of conflicting and contradictory events that are fraught with tensions and uncertainty (Charmaz, 1999). Within this context, involvement in CAM cannot be divorced from the meanings attached to suffering, as "[s]uffering involves more than coping. Suffering calls for attempts to control one's life as well as to cope with it. It gives rise to actions as well as feelings. It shapes new stories and moral meanings. Suffering poses existential problems of identity and continuity of self" (Charmaz 1999, p. 364).

Empirical studies demonstrate that CAM therapies and treatments hold both positive and negative implications for the relief of suffering. Some research shows that people find their encounters with CAM "empowering" because they receive "recognition" for their life concerns and validation for their experiences and values (Sointu, 2006b). Additionally, CAM approaches have transformative potentials that entail changes in perceptions of health and illness and/or perceived changes in personal health (Low, 2004; Pawluch et al., 2000; Sointu, 2006b). Sointu (2006a) argues that use of CAM practices "allow for experiences of profound change, interpreted and even experienced as the responsibility of the person, seen as a means of self-fulfillment, and understood in terms of interconnectedness of the mind, the body and even the spirit" (pp. 218–19). Similarly, Low (2004) found that through CAM, participants sought to transform themselves by creating a "new sense of self which they perceive as healthy" (p. 93). Through the process of healing, some adopt a "healer identity" which comes about through use of and training in various healing modalities. In some cases, users become so enamoured with CAM that they decide to train as practitioners. Others noted changes in their personalities—having more confidence or being less worried—and some explained that their value systems and priorities concerning health changed in a positive way.

In contrast, not all CAM therapeutic encounters are positive. In an Australian study of cancer patients, Broom (2009) found that, despite the liberating and positive effects that participants experienced with CAM, there was a tendency towards overreaction to the imperative of "positive thinking." He argued that this was detrimental to some patients who were already compromised by their illness situations. His findings counter other studies that reinforce shared responsibility and shared decision-making within the CAM therapeutic relationship, especially with respect to "psycho-social" aspects and "lifestyle change" (Kelner, 2000).

While risk of harm exists within any therapeutic encounter, the impact of ridicule from those who oppose CAM also holds potential negative consequences. Low (2004, 2005) explains that CAM users are frequently labelled deviant. Despite the positive effects from the therapeutic interventions, study participants often felt stigmatized because of their participation in CAM and used a variety of strategies to alleviate the impact. For example, they avoided certain therapies, practitioners, or therapeutic environments that they perceived lacked legitimacy. Likewise, Sointu (2006b) concluded that CAM use is not "culturally valued" and that this places people in a position of "inferiority, exclusion, and invisibility;" she refers to this marginalization as "biomedical misrecognition" (p. 498).

Interestingly, other studies indicate that people with HIV use CAM as a strategy to reduce the stigmatizing effects of their illnesses. Through the use of CAM they were able to gain a greater sense of control over their life situations (Foote-Ardah, 2003; Pawluch et al., 2000). In Vokey LeBlanc's (2010) research on energy healing, although participants experienced both empowerment and stigma for their involvement in Reiki therapies, the intrinsic rewards that participants reaped from their involvements tended to counter the opposition they encountered. Through their involvement, participants chip away at pervasive myths and misconceptions about CAM therapies.

Undoubtedly, the CAM experience is shaped through social and situational context. Many avoid revealing their use of CAM in circumstances where they may meet disapproval; a case in point is in interactions with health professionals who are not receptive to CAM, but this also occurs among work colleagues, friends, and acquaintances. Not all users experience positive therapeutic encounters or find all forms of therapy beneficial (Vokey LeBlanc, 2010). Overall, there is a need for more studies on the experiences of CAM use by people with chronic illness.

Chapter Summary

Through a sociological lens, this chapter has looked at CAM within the context of conventional medicine. The chapter first considered the social construction of various definitions and classifications of CAM, reinforcing the idea that social meanings are produced within particular historical, social, and cultural contexts which reflect the interests and social locations of various groups. The polarization of CAM is further reinforced by politically charged definitions that tend to exclude CAM from mainstream biomedicine. According to some scholars, these exclusionary definitions aim to marginalize systems of healing and therapies that threaten biomedical philosophy and practice. More recently "integrative health care" attempts to bring CAM and biomedicine together in a more egalitarian and collaborative system of care. Most research suggests that such a relationship between biomedical health professionals and CAM practitioners does not exist. Despite the advancements of some CAM practitioner groups in gaining professional health status, biomedicine continues to hold a dominant position within mainstream health care.

The chapter reinforces that two key concepts are fundamental to CAM: holism and vitalism. Holism refers to the idea that an individual must be considered as a whole physically, psychologically, spiritually, and within the context of his or her environment. Since this approach views disease as a result of imbalance among the physical, psychological, social, and spiritual dimensions of the person, healing occurs through the process of rebalancing or creating harmony among these elements. In practice, the combined goals of holistic healing are to treat the entire person, to locate the underlying cause of the illness, and to facilitate the body's own healing response through an individualized plan of care. CAM systems also hold moral assumptions such as the belief in "the goodness of nature" and one's responsibility to act in a way that ensures "good health." It is also assumed that the therapeutic relationship is inherently beneficial and serves as a catalyst for self-healing. The trustworthiness of holistic practice and the scientific effectiveness of a holistic approach are contested by opponents of CAM.

Vitalism is a term that refers to the idea that life is contingent on a source of cosmic energy or a specific life force. Current terms for this life force energy include "subtle energy" or "bio-field energy," yet the existence of such energy has not been proven scientifically. Western biomedicine largely dismisses the concept of a "life force." This principle continues to spark debate over what constitutes a conventionally acceptable form of medicine and to what extent a healing system, therapy, or practitioner group is dismissed within conventional health care.

Historically, in Westernized societies, biomedicine has held a dominant position within mainstream health care. Allopathic medicine gained a superior and controlling position within health care by establishing its superior professional status. While some CAM groups have taken this route to gain social legitimacy, the majority have not. The most successful CAM practitioners are those who have transformed their practices to conform to conventional medical and health professional standards.

Other historical and culturally specific events paved the way for the re-emergence of CAM. In North America, the health and countercultural movements of the 1960s precipitated greater exposure to and public acceptance of CAM. It was during this era that CAM practices, previously eclipsed by biomedicine, (re)emerged. The "New Age" label became quite popular during this period and was used quite indiscriminately to describe practically every form of holistic healing. This provided biomedical scholars with another way to brand alternate forms of healing as "quackery."

Currently, although the relations between biomedicine and CAM appear less inflammatory than in the past, tensions remain between the two. With respect to health professionals, there are numerous factors that influence attitudes toward the practice of CAM. Residence, age, gender, exposure to knowledge and training in CAM, and organizational restrictions within hospitals and medical schools can all influence a health care provider's likelihood of accepting CAM as a valid practice. There are also concerns that health professionals, in the process of appropriating CAM therapies, will negatively impact the long-term viability of CAM practices. It is unclear how our evolving, pluralistic health care system will influence the interface between CAM and biomedicine. Considering current gaps in conventional health care provision and the overall demand for health care services, CAM providers will likely continue to be part of contemporary health care provision.

People use CAM to manage health and to deal with chronic illness. Although the general patterns show that use is highest among more affluent and well-educated white women, other studies suggest that CAM is a more widespread and intricate part of the fabric of health care in Canada. People are attracted to CAM for a variety of reasons. Conceptually these have typically been framed within a "postmodern" thesis, an "alternative" world view, and "push and pull" factors. Motivations to pursue CAM treatments range from dissatisfaction with biomedicine and problems within the doctor–patient relationship, to the desire to find more personal and meaningful ways to manage health and illness. In today's consumer society, people are encouraged to take responsibility for their own health and to be proactive in making choices about managing health and illness. These traits, while part of the holistic approach to healing, are not unique to CAM users.

People report both positive and negative experiences with using CAM. Research shows that the CAM experience is situational. Commonly, individuals assert that the therapeutic experience is empowering and, in some cases, transformational. For others, the therapeutic encounter can be less than satisfying. In any therapeutic relationship there are risks and responsibilities; the extent to which these may be exploited within CAM remains unclear. CAM users may feel stigmatized through their involvement with CAM, while others may use CAM as a way to overcome the stigma attached to specific diseases. Finally, although CAM continues to be marginalized within biomedicine, CAM continues to be an intricate part of contemporary health care that is largely driven by public demand. How the practice of CAM systems and therapies will continue to evolve in the future remains uncertain.

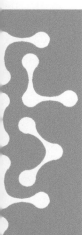

STUDY QUESTIONS

1. Should CAM practices and treatments be covered within publicly funded health care systems?
2. What is meant by the terms *vitalism* and *holism*? How do these concepts differ from biomedicine?
3. Why has use of CAM increased in recent years?
4. What is quackery? What might a social constructionist approach to health say about it?
5. What barriers might inhibit the growth of CAM?

SUGGESTED READINGS

Callahan D. (Ed.). (2007). *The role of complementary and alternative medicine: Accommodating pluralism.* Washington: Georgetown University Press.

Lee-Treweek G., Heller T., Spurr S., MacQueen H., & Kantz J. (Eds). (2005). *Perspectives on complementary and alternative medicine.* Abingdon: Routledge Taylor & Francis.

Schneirov, M. & Geczik, J. (2003). *A diagnosis for our times: Alternative health, from lifeworld to politics.* Albany: State University Press of New York.

SUGGESTED WEB RESOURCES

Health Canada. Natural Health Products: www.hc-sc.gc.ca/dhp-mps/prodnatur/about-apropos/index-eng.php

Canadian Association of Naturopathic Doctors: www.cand.ca/What_is_Naturopathic_Medicine.78.0.html

ABC News: How integrative oncology helps cancer patients: www.youtube.com/watch?v=bJ7wSXPKl-k

GLOSSARY

Alternative medicine Approaches to health care outside of the current widely accepted biomedical framework.

Complementary medicine Works in conjunction with biomedicine, rather than in opposition to it.

Complementary and alternative medicine (CAM) A wide array of healing practices. Most are outside of typical biomedical practices and may have an ancient or indigenous history.

Integrative medicine An approach to medicine that consolidates biomedicine and CAM.

Medical pluralism The existence of a diversity of medical perspectives.

Placebo effect Noticeable effects of treatment that occur when participant is given a placebo (for example, an inert sugar pill) and told it will be effective.

Professionalization The process through which practitioners adhere to a set of legal requirements to create a uniformly regulated standard of quality. This allows professions to assert their legitimacy and competence amid other vocations.

Quackery Giving the false, unfounded impression of using a scientific method and rationale.

Vitalism The concept that human life is a result of a universal or spiritual energy force.

REFERENCES

Adams, D., Kemper, K., & Vohra, S. (2012). Complementary and alternative medicine use among infants, children and, adolescents. In J. Adams, G.J. Andrews, J. Barnes, A. Broom, & P. Magin (Eds), *Traditional, complementary and integrative medicine: An international reader* (pp. 44–52). Hampshire: Palgrave MacMillan.

Adams, J. (2004). Demarkating the medical/nonmedical border: Occupational boundary-work within the GP's accounts of their integrative practices. In P. Tovey, G. Easthope, & J. Adams (Eds), *The mainstreaming of complementary and alternative medicine: Studies in social context* (pp. 140–57). New York: Routledge Taylor & Francis Group.

———— & Tovey, P. (2001). Nurses' use of professional distancing in the appropriation of CAM: A text analysis. *Complementary Therapies in Medicine*, *9*(3), 136–40.

————, Easthope, G., & Sibbrit, D. (2003). Exploring the relationship between women's health and use of complementary and alternative medicine. *Complementary Therapies in Medicine*, *11*, 156–58.

Andrews, G. J. (2002). Private complementary medicine and older people: Service use and user empowerment. *Ageing & Society*, *22*, 343–68.

———— & Boon, H. (2005). CAM in Canada: Places, practices, research. *Complementary Therapies in Clinical Practice*, *11*, 21–7.

————, Adams J., Segrott J., & Wai Lui, C. (2012). The profile of complementary and alternative medicine users and reasons for complementary and alternative medicine use. In J. Adams, G.J. Andrews, J. Barnes, A. Broom & P. Magin (Eds), *Traditional, complementary and integrative medicine: An international reader* (pp. 11–15). Hampshire: Palgrave MacMillan.

Annandale, E. & Clark, J. (2000). Gender, postmodernism and health. In W.J. Gabe & M. Calnan (Eds), *Health, medicine and society: Key theories, future agendas* (pp. 51–66). London: Routledge.

Armstrong, P. (2002). The context for health-care reform in Canada. In P. Armstrong, C. Amaratunga, J. Bernier, K. Grant, A. Pederson, & K. Wilson (Eds), *Exposing privatization: Women and healthcare reform in Canada* (pp. 11–48). Wilson, Aurora: Garamond Press.

Astin, J. A. (1998). Why patients use alternative medicine: Results of a national study. *Journal of the American Medical Association*, *279*(19), 1548–53.

Baer, H. A. (2008). The emergence of integrative medicine in Australia: The growing interest of biomedicine and nursing in complementary medicine in a southern developed society. *Medical Anthropology Quarterly*, *22*(1), 52–66.

————, Hays, J., McClendon, N., McMoldrick, N., & Vespucci R. (1998). The holistic health movement in the San Franscisco Bay area: Some preliminary observations. *Social Science & Medicine*, *47*(10), 1495–1501.

Barry, C. (2012). The role of evidence in alternative medicine: Contrasting biomedical and anthropological approaches. In J. Adams, G.J. Andrews, J.

Barnes, A. Broom, & P. Magin (Eds), *Traditional, complementary and integrative medicine: An international reader.* (pp. 187–95). Hampshire: Palgrave MacMillan.

Benoit, C. (1991). *Midwives in passage. Canadian Review of Sociology*, *30*(1), 139–140.

Bishop, F., Yardley, L., & Lewith, G. T. (2007). A systematic review of beliefs involved in the use of complementary and alternative medicine. *Journal of Health Psychology*, *12*(6), 851–67.

Bodeker, G., Kronenberg F., & Burford, G. (2007). Policy and public health perspectives on traditional, complementary and alternative medicine: An overview. In G. Bodeker & G. Burford (Eds), *Traditional, complementary and alternative medicine: Policy and public health perspectives* (pp. 9–38). London: Imperial College Press.

Boon, H. (1998). Canadian naturopathic practitioners: Holistic and scientific world views. *Social Science & Medicine*, *46*(9), 1213–25.

————, Kelner, M., Wellman, B., & Welsh, S. (2004). Responses of established healthcare to the professionalization of complementary and alternative medicine in Ontario. *Social Science & Medicine*, *59*(5), 915–30.

————, Verhoef, M., O'Hara, D., Finday, B., & Majid, N. (2004). Integrative healthcare: Arriving at a working definition. *Alternative Therapies in Health and Medicine*, *10*(5), 48–56.

Bourgeault, I. L. (2000). Delivering the "new" Canadian midwifery: The impact of midwifery on integration into the Ontario healthcare system. *Sociology of Health & Illness*, *22*(2), 172–96.

Bowman, M. (1999). Healing in the spiritual marketplace: Consumers, courses and credentialism. *Social Compass*, *46*, 181–89.

Broom, A. (2009). I'd forgotten about me in all of this: Discourses of self-healing, positivity and vulnerability in cancer patients' experiences of complementary and alternative medicine. *Journal of Sociology*, *45*(1), 71–87.

Brown, J., Cooper, E., Frankton, L., Steeves Wall, M., Gillis-Ring,J., Barter, W., McCabe, A., & Frenandez, C. (2007). Complementary and alternative therapies: Survey of knowledge and attitudes of health professionals at a tertiary pediatric/women's care facility. *Complementary Therapies in Clinical Practice*, *13*(3), 194–200.

Bury, M. C. (1997). *Health and illness in a changing society*. London: Routledge.

Cant, S. L. & Sharma, U. (1999). *A new medical pluralism? Doctors, patients, and the state.* London: UCL Press Limited.

Canter, P. H. (2008). Vitalism and other pseudo-science in alternative medicine: The retreat from science. In E. Ernst (Ed.), *Healing hype or harm: A critical analysis of complementary or alternative medicine* (pp. 152–61). Devon: Imprint Academic.

Cassileth, B. R. & Vickers, A. J. (2005). High prevalence of complementary and alternative medicine use among cancer patients: Implications for research and clinical care. *Journal of Clinical Oncology, 23*(12), 2590–92.

Charlton, B. G. (2008). Healing but not curing: Alternative medical therapies as valid new age spiritual healing practices. In E. Ernst (Ed.), *Healing hype or harm: A critical analysis of complementary or alternative medicine* (pp. 68–77). Devon: Imprint Academic.

Charmaz, K. (1999). Stories of suffering: Subjective tales and research narratives. *Qualitative Health Research, 9*(3), 362–82.

Clarke, J. N. (2012). *Health, illness and medicine in Canada* (6thed.). Toronto: Oxford University Press.

Coburn, D. (2001). Health, healthcare, and neo-liberalism. In P. Armstrong, H. Armstrong, & D. Coburn (Eds), *Unhealthy times political economy perspectives on health and care* (pp. 45–65). Toronto: Oxford University Press.

———— & Biggs, C. L. (1986). Limits to medical dominance: The case of chiropractic. *Social Science & Medicine, 22,* 1035–46.

Conrad, P. & Barker, K. K. (2010). The social construction of illness: Key insights and policy implications. *Journal of Health & Social Behavior, 51*(S), S67–S79.

Coulter, I. (2004). Integration and paradigm clash. In P. Tovey, G. Easthope, & J. Adams (Eds), *The mainstreaming of complementary and alternative medicine: Studies in social context* (pp. 103–22). London, New York: Routledge Taylor & Francis Group.

———— (2012). Evidence-based complementary and alternative medicine: Promises and problems. In J. Adams, G.J. Andrews, J. Barnes, A. Broom, & P. Magin (Eds), *Traditional, complementary and integrative medicine: An international reader* (pp. 204–11). Hampshire: Palgrave MacMillan.

———— & Willis, E. (2004). The rise and rise of complementary and alternative medicine: A sociological perspective. *Medical Journal of Australia, 180,* 587–89.

———— & Willis, E. (2007). Explaining the growth of complementary and alternative medicine. *Health Sociology Review, 16*(3–4), 214–25.

Crellin, J., Anderson, R., & Connor, J. (1997). *Alternative healthcare in Canada: Nineteenth and twentieth century perspectives.* Toronto: Canadian Scholars' Press Inc.

de Bruyn, T. (2002). *A summary of national data on complementary and alternative healthcare- current status and future development: A discussion paper.* Ottawa: Health Canada.

Eisenberg, D., Roger, D., Ettner, S., Appel, S., Wilkey, S., VanRompay, M., & Kessler, R. (1998). Trends in alternative medicine use in the United States, 1990–1997: Results of a follow-up national survey. *Journal of the American Medical Association, 280,* 1569–75.

Engebretson, J. (1996). Urban healers: An experiential description of American healing touch groups. *Qualitative Health Research, 6*(4), 526–41.

Ernst, E. (2008). *Healing, hype or harm: A critical analysis of complementary or alternative medicine.* Exeter: Societas.

Esmail, N. (2007). Complementary and alternative medicine in Canada: Trends in use and public attitudes, 1997–2006. *Fraser Institute, 87,* 1–53.

Fadlon, J. (2004). Meridians, chakras and psycho-neuro-immunology: The dematerializing body and the domestication of alternative medicine. *Body & Society, 10*(4), 69–86.

Foote-Ardah, C. E. (2003). The meaning of complementary and alternative medicine practices among people with HIV in the United States: Strategies for managing everyday life. *Sociology of Health and Illness, 25*(5), 481–500.

Frass, M., Strassl, R. P., Friehs, H., Mullner, M., Kundi, M., & Kaye, A. D. (2012). Use and acceptance of complementary and alternative medicine among the general population and medical personnel: A systematic review. *The Ochsner Journal, 12,* 45–56.

Foltz, T. G. (1994). *Kahuna healer: Learning to see with ki.* New York & London: Garland Publishing Inc.

Freidson, E. (1970). *Profession of medicine: A study of the sociology of applied knowledge.* Chicago: University of Chicago Press.

Fries, C. J. (2011). Moving beyond biomedicine: Medical pluralism. In A. Segall & C. J. Fries (Eds), *Pursuing health and wellness: Healthy societies, healthy people* (pp. 312–334). Don Mills, Ontario: Oxford University Press.

————— (2014). Older adults' use of complementary and alternative medical therapies to resist bio-medicalization of aging. *Journal of Aging Studies, 28*, 1–10.

Furnham, A. & Vincent C. (2000). Reasons for using CAM. In M. Kelner & B. Wellman (Eds), *Complementary and alternative medicine: Challenge and change* (pp. 61–78). The Netherlands: Harwood Academic Publishers.

Gabe, J. & Calnan, M. (2000). Healthcare and consumption. In S. J. Williams, J. Gabe, & M. Calnan (Eds), *Health, medicine and society: Key theories, Future agendas* (pp. 255–73). London: Routledge.

Gillett, J., Pawluch, D., & Cain, R. (2002). How people with HIV/AIDS manage and assess their use of complementary therapies: A qualitative analysis. *Journal of the Association of Nurses in AIDS Care, 13*, 17–27.

Glik, D. C. (1990). The re-definition of the situation: The social construction of spiritual healing experiences. *Sociology of Health and Illness, 12*(2), 151–68.

Gorski, D. H. (2014). Integrative oncology: Really the best of both worlds? *Nature Reviews Cancer, 14*, 692–700.

Greenhalgh, T., Howick, J., & Maskrey, N. (2014). Evidence based medicine: A movement in crisis? *BMJ : British Medical Journal, 348*, g3725.

Hirschkorn, K. (2005). *The regulation and professionalization of herbal medicine.* Ph.D. dissertation, Department of Sociology, McMaster University.

—————, Andersen R., & Bourgeault, I. L. (2009). Canadian family physicians and complementary/alternative medicine: The role of practice setting, medical training, and province of practice. *Canadian Review of Sociology, 46*(2), 143–59.

Hollenberg, D. (2006). Uncharted ground: Patterns of professional interaction among complementary/alternative and biomedical practitioners in integrative healthcare settings. *Social Science & Medicine, 62*(3), 731–44.

—————, Lytle, M., Walji, R., & Cooley, K. (2013). Addressing provider shortage in underserviced areas: The role of traditional, complementary and alternative medicine (TCAM) providers in Canadian rural healthcare. *European Journal of Integrative Medicine, 5*, 15–26.

Hurd Clarke, L. & Bennet, E. V. (2012). Constructing the moral body: Self-care among older adults with multiple chronic conditions. *Health 17*(3), 1–18.

Illich, I. (1976). *Limits to medicine-medical nemesis: The expropriation of health.* London: Penguin.

Jonas, W. B. (2002). Policy, the public, and priorities in alternative medicine research. *The Annals of the American Academy, 583*, 29–43.

Kaptchuk, T. J. & Eisenberg, D. M. (2001). Varieties of healing 2: A taxonomy of unconventional healing practices. *Annals of Internal Medicine, 135*, 196–204.

Kelner, M. (2000). The therapeutic relationship under fire. In M. Kelner & B. Wellman (Eds), *Complementary and alternative medicine: Challenge and change* (pp. 79–97). Amsterdam: Harwood Academic Publishers.

————— (2005). The status of CAM: Where are we now? How I became interested in CAM and how it changed my life. Keynote speech for ACHRN conference, University of Nottingham, Nottingham, England.

————— & Wellman, B. (1997a). Healthcare and consumer choice: Medical and alternative therapies. *Social Science & Medicine, 45*, 203–12.

————— & Wellman, B. (1997b). Who seeks alternative healthcare? A profile of users of five modes of treatment. *The Journal of Alternative and Complementary Medicine, 3*, 127– 40.

————— & Wellman, B. (2000). Introduction. In M. Kelner & B. Wellman (Eds), *Complementary and alternative medicine: Challenge and change* (pp. 1–24). Amsterdam: Harwood Academic Publishers.

—————, Boon, H., Wellman, B., & Welsh, S. (2002). Complementary and alternative groups contemplate the need for effectiveness, safety and cost-effectiveness research. *Complementary Therapies in Medicine, 10*(4), 235–39.

—————, Wellman, B., Boon, H., & Welsh, S. (2004). Responses of established healthcare to the professionalization of complementary and alternative medicine in Ontario. *Social Science and Medicine, 59*, 915–30.

Kolstad, A., Risberg, T., Bremnes, Y., Wilsgaard, T., Holte, H., Klepp, O., Mella, O., & Wist, E. (2004). Use of complementary and alternative therapies: A national multicentre study among health professionals in Norway. *Support Care Cancer, 12*(5), 312–18.

Lee-Treweek, G. & Stone, J. (2005). Critical issues in the therapeutic relationship. In T. Heller, G. Lee-Treweek, J. Kantz, J. Stone, & S. Spurr (Eds), *Perspectives on complementary and alternative medicine* (pp. 231–55). Abingdon: Routledge Taylor & Francis.

Low, J. (2004). *Using alternative therapies: A qualitative analysis.* Toronto: Canadian Scholars Press Inc.

———— (2005). Avoiding the other: A technique of stigma management among people who use alternative therapies. In D. Pawluch, W. Shaffir, & C. Miall (Eds), *Doing Ethnography: Studying everyday life* (pp. 273–85). Toronto: Canadian Scholars Press.

Lowenberg, J. S. (1989). *Caring and responsibility: The crossroads between holistic practice and traditional medicine.* Philadelphia: University of Pennsylvania Press.

McAlister F. A., van Diepen, S., Padwal, R. S., Johnson, J. A., & Majumdar, S. R. (2007). How evidence-based are the recommendations in evidence-based guidelines? *PLoS Medicine* 4(8): e250.

McGuire, M. (1988). *Ritual healing in suburban America.* London: Rutgers University Press.

———— (1993). Health and spirituality as contemporary concerns. *The Annals of the American Academy, 57,* 144–54.

McClean, S. (2005). The illness is part of the person: Discourses of blame, individual responsibility and individuation at a centre for spiritual healing in the north of England. *Sociology of Health & Illness, 27*(5), 628–48.

Micozzi, M. S. (2006). *Fundamentals of complementary and alternative medicine* (3rd ed.). St. Louis: Saunders Elsevier.

O'Connor, B. B. (2000). Conceptions of the body in CAM. In M. Kelner & B. Wellman (Eds), *Complementary and Alternative Medicine: Challenge and Change* (pp. 39–60). The Netherlands: Harwood Academic.

Pawluch, D., Cain, R., & Gillett, J. (2000). Lay constructions of HIV and complementary therapy use. *Social Science and Medicine, 51,* 251–64.

Porcino, A. J., Boon, H. S., Page, S. A., & Verhoef, M. J. (2011). Meaning and challenges in the practice of multiple therapeutic massage modalities: A combined methods study. *BMC Complementary and Alternative Medicine, 11*(75), 1–11.

Saks, M. (2001). Alternative medicine and the healthcare division of labour: Present trends and future prospects. *Current Sociology, 49*(3), 119–34.

Seely, D. (2014). Moving Towards Integrative Oncology as a System of Cancer Care. *Ottawa Life,* April, 46.

Sharma, U. (1992). *Complementary medicine today: Practitioners and patients.* London: Routledge.

———— (2000). Medical pluralism and the future of CAM. In M. Kelner & B. Wellman (Eds), *Complementary and alternative medicine: Challenge and change* (pp. 211–22). The Netherlands: Harwood Academic.

———— & Black, P. (2001). Look good, feel better: Beauty therapy as emotional labour. *Sociology,* 35(4): 913–31.

Shuval, J. (2006). Nurses in alternative healthcare: Integrating medical paradigms. *Social Science & Medicine, 63*(7), 1784–95.

Siahpush, M. (1999). A critical review of the sociology of alternative medicine: Research on users, practitioners, and the orthodoxy. *Health and Place,* 4(2), 159–78.

Sointu, E. (2006a). Healing bodies, feeling bodies: Embodiment and alternative and complementary health practices. *Social Theory and Health,* 4, 203–20.

———— (2006b). Recognition and the creation of wellbeing. *Sociology, 40*(3), 493–510.

Stone, J. & Katz, J. (2005a). Can complementary and alternative medicine be classified? In T. Heller, G. Lee-Treweek, J. Kantz, J. Stone, & S. Spurr (Eds), *Perspectives on complementary and alternative medicine* (pp. 33–57). Abingdon: Routledge Taylor & Francis.

———— (2005b). The therapeutic relationship and complementary and alternative medicine. In T. Heller, G. Lee-Treweek, J. Kantz, J. Stone, & S. Spurr (Eds), *Perspectives on complementary and alternative medicine* (pp. 205–30). Abingdon: Routledge Taylor & Francis.

Tataryn, D. J. (2002). Paradigms of health and disease: A framework for classifying and understanding alternative and complementary therapies. *The Journal of Alternative and Complementary Medicine, 8*(6), 877–92.

Tindle, H. A., Davis, R. B., Phillips, R. S., & Eisenberg D. M. (2005). Trends in the use of complementary and alternative medicine by US adults: 1997–2002. *Alternative Therapies in Health and Medicine, 11*(1), 1–42.

Tovey, P. & Adams, J. (2001). Primary care as intersecting social worlds. *Social Science & Medicine,* 52, 695–706.

————. (2002). Towards a sociology of CAM and nursing. *Complementary Therapies in Nursing and Midwifery, 8*(1), 12–16.

Verhoef, M. & Sutherland. L. (1995). Alternative medicine and general practitioners: Opinions and behavior. *Canadian Family Physician, 41,* 1005–11.

Verhoef, M. J., Boon, H., & Mutasingwa, D. R. (2006). The scope of naturopathic medicine in Canada:

An emerging profession. *Social Science and Medicine, 63*(2), 409–17.

Voas, D. & Bruce, S. (2007). The spiritual revolution: Another false dawn for the sacred. In K. Flanagan & P. Jupp (Eds), *A sociology of spirituality* (pp. 41–63). Hampshire: Ashgate Publishing Company.

Vokey LeBlanc, Y. (2010). *Contemporary healing: A social worlds analysis of Reiki in practice.* (doctoral dissertation). McMaster University, Hamilton, Ontario, Canada.

Wardwell, W. (1994). Alternative medicine in the United States. S*ocial Science and Medicine, 38*(8), 1061–68.

White, M. & Verohef, M. (2006). Cancer as part of the journey: The role of spirituality in the decision to decline conventional prostate cancer treatment and to use complementary and alternative medicine. *Integrative Cancer Therapies, 5*(2), 117–22.

Wiles, J. & Rosenberg, M. W. (2001). Gentle caring experience: Seeking alternative healthcare in Canada. *Health & Place, 7,* 209–24.

Winnick, T. A. (2005). From quackery to complementary medicine: The American medical profession confronts alternative therapies. *Social Problems, 52*(1), 38–121.

York, M. (1995). *The emerging network: A sociology of the new age and neo-pagan movements.* Lanham, Maryland: Rowman & Littlefield Publication Inc.

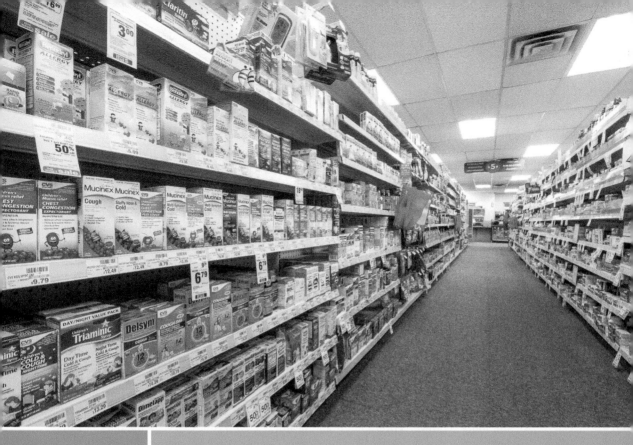

12

Consumerism, Health, and Health Care

Mat Savelli

LEARNING OBJECTIVES

In this chapter, students will learn

- how consumerism has informed discussions of health
- the transformation of the "passive patient" into the "active and informed consumer"
- how market liberalization and globalization have contributed to the marketization of health care
- about debates on the rise of consumerism and marketization in health

Introduction

When individuals fall ill or otherwise seek medical intervention, how do we classify them? Are they *patients,* whose primary responsibility is to submit to the physician's authority and follow her directions as closely as possible? Or perhaps we might describe these individuals as *clients* who, acknowledging their own lack of expertise, effectively "hire" the physician to provide medical knowledge and instruction. Increasingly, however, such individuals are described as *consumers*—people who may work in partnership with health care providers but ultimately take charge of their own health-related decisions. In this conception, consumers are informed about their condition, proactive about their health, and feel empowered to choose the treatment option that best meets their needs. This chapter examines the concept of **consumerism** and how it challenges historical and stereotypical understandings of how people approach the issue of health improvement.

Roots of Consumerism

Whether health-seeking individuals ought to be considered consumers rather than patients has been debated since the late 1960s. This discourse reflects a series of cultural and socio-political trends that have altered the relationship between individuals and professional structures of power and expertise, such as education and medicine. During this period, the notion that "the trained expert knows best" has come under attack. Individuals have become considerably more empowered in their dealings with specialists of all stripes. In the early years, the movement to redefine patients as active consumers was led by grassroots activists; by the 1990s, however, governments and health-related businesses were the ones pushing that notion (Tomes, 2006).

One major factor in this shift has been the increasing dominance of free-market capitalism and the emergence of neoliberalism (Tousijn, 2006). As explained by Applbaum (2006), adherents of these ideologies make fundamental assumptions about human behaviour that have helped to shape the idea of the medical consumer. First is the idea that human beings possess a virtually limitless number of pains and discomforts, which are matched only by their desire for products and services to remedy these ills. Second, by offering people a variety of choices, the free market is the best possible avenue to fulfill these desires. Finally, the competitive nature of the market ensures that individuals are offered the best possible services and products at the lowest possible cost.

Applied to health care, this philosophy holds that individual consumers should be able to access a range of services by choosing between different treatment modalities and health care providers. In addition, it suggests that health and health care are goods that might be (or even should be) purchasable. In response, many governments have acted upon these beliefs by introducing competitive mechanisms into state-sponsored health care programs and by increasing the range of services that individuals must pay to access. Within Canada, for example, health-related services such as dentistry, optometry, and ambulance use are not fully covered by the publicly funded system. At the same time, governments have encouraged health care organizations to strengthen the individual's autonomy vis-à-vis medical professionals and to enshrine a host of other patients' rights, such as informed consent. Taken as a whole, these changes have aimed to transform individuals from passive recipients of medical intervention into active participants in the process of protecting and promoting their own health.

Yet the transformation from patient to consumer should not be viewed as an exclusively state- or elite-driven activity. Individuals and organized groups have played a central role in this development. In recent decades, coordinated patient groups and advocacy organizations (frequently representing people diagnosed with the same condition) have fought to ensure individuals' freedom to make decisions about their own health and potential treatments. In the United States, for example, the National Alliance on Mental Illness (NAMI) has long advocated that individuals hospitalized for mental illness should not have their right to transparent, consensual treatment waived. Such groups also serve as vital sources of information, providing their members with knowledge and the latest news about their condition and its potential treatments, thereby empowering the individual to make informed decisions regarding their care.

The advent of the internet has also dramatically altered the ways in which individuals access information regarding their health (Hardey, 1999; 2001). It has allowed existing patient groups to make their knowledge and perspectives much more accessible, and at the same time, social media, forums, and listservs allow people from geographically dispersed areas to share information, ask one another questions, and provide mutual support. Interactive websites, meanwhile, offer individuals the opportunity to track their symptoms, read about potential diagnoses, and explore the full array of possible treatments. By facilitating the creation of new communities and providing a limitless supply of information, the internet has helped to create a phenomenon known as the **informed consumer** or the **expert patient**.

The Informed Consumer

As stated previously, the mantras of choice and the free market have underpinned the consumer movement. In order for individuals to navigate the plethora of options available to them in a rational manner, it is considered vital that they be maximally informed about the benefits, drawbacks, risks, and costs of any potential health intervention that they seek out. It is little use asking someone with an injured knee to choose between surgery and physiotherapy, for example, unless they understand that surgery's instant results (but potential long-term stiffness and pain) must be measured against physiotherapy's slower and potentially less effective (but also less dangerous) approach. When the variables of cost, insurance options, waiting lists, and potential surgeons and physiotherapists are added into the equation, it is clear that consumers must obtain a wealth of information if they are to make well-informed choices. As we discussed earlier, a host of sources aim to offer this knowledge to consumers.

The goal of arming consumers with information is not simply to help them make informed decisions; knowledge also helps to empower consumers and reduce the power inequalities between patients and health care providers. Traditionally, the relationship between patient and practitioner has been characterized as a one-way conversation rather than a dialogue between two equal participants. For critics, this inherent power inequality can help explain some of the worst abuses of medical care over the twentieth century, such as the use of lobotomies in psychiatric care. Embedded in the notion of the informed consumer is the idea that the patient should possess the requisite knowledge to meet the health care provider on a more even playing field. Although individuals have long possessed their own expertise (relating to their experience of illness, for example), the power differential between doctor and patient can only be evened out by reframing the medical encounter as a meeting between two experts (Tuckett, Boulton, Olson, & Williams, 1985). Ultimately, the informed consumer is one who, by virtue of their experience and knowledge of their condition, feels comfortable working in partnership with a health care provider rather than acting as a subordinate. Together, the pair can pursue the common goal of improving the patient's health.

Although political and socio-cultural changes have facilitated this shift in the power dynamic, the changing nature of health (and its threats) has also been key. Previously, people tended to seek medical intervention primarily during acute health crises, such as broken bones and infectious disease. Through the implementation of public health measures and technological changes in medicine, the need for emergency health interventions has declined. Health care provision is now overwhelmingly focused on managing long-term issues such as diabetes, hypertension, and mental illness. Such conditions tend to require regular supervision and periodic changes in treatment. As Charles, Gafni, and Whelan (1997) have pointed out, the relationship between patient and practitioner in this scenario tends to be long in duration; the traditional hierarchical model may fail to give individuals a sense of ownership over their condition.

The Consumerist Approach to Accessing and Assessing Care

Shifting its focus from acute to chronic health problems has also helped transform health care provision into a buyer's market (Reeder, 1972). While health emergencies might favour the physician's training, experience, and quick thinking, chronic conditions provide consumers with the opportunity to research their ailments and shop around for potential treatments. As a consequence, patients have become considerably empowered because physicians cannot afford to be dismissive of their concerns. Should one practitioner frown upon an individual's desire to become more involved in their own treatment, consumers with chronic (and not immediately life-threatening) health problems can always choose to seek out an alternative provider.

The role of the health care provider is also transforming. As discussed in Chapter Eleven, people are increasingly turning to complementary or alternative medicine (CAM). These systems, which include naturopathy and homeopathy, have become important players in the world of consumerist health care. Alternative treatments may be attractive to individuals for a variety of reasons including lower cost, fear of side effects from mainstream medical treatment, and the belief that biomedical treatment may be ineffective. With the aim of offering consumers increased choice (and often in the hopes of saving money), government health care programmes, employer-sponsored benefits schemes, and health insurance policies have started to cover a wider range of treatments outside of the traditional biomedical sphere (Clarke, Doel & Segrott, 2004). As a consequence, people may seek out acupunctural treatment to alleviate back pain or might consult a naturopath for an alternative to expensive, side-effect-producing drug regimens.

In this competitive market, practitioners must strive to retain consumers or face losing them to other health care providers. Consequently, gauging consumer satisfaction is an important component of modern medical provision. Health care providers and researchers have deployed both qualitative and quantitative tools to measure the extent to which consumers are satisfied with their services. These tools have become an important barometer that helps shape future decisions regarding clinic organization and the overall direction of care. Even in health care systems where physicians are salaried (rather than paid per patient visit), governments have started rewarding hospitals and clinics that boast high consumer satisfaction, while punishing those deemed to be "failing" consumers. In this regard, consumer power has clearly increased at the expense of the health care provider.

Provider-designed satisfaction surveys are only one of the ways in which consumers can express their opinion of the services provided by practitioners. In recent years, social media platforms have become powerful tools for sharing opinions on virtually every aspect of health care provision. For example, consumer communities can rate and slate the performance of MDs, hospitals, insurance companies, pharmaceuticals, and care facilities. Thus, people have increasingly started to rely upon the opinions of fellow consumers when weighing up decisions like whether to ask for a specific medication or seek out treatment with a particular specialist. By sourcing information from patients themselves, yet another layer of information is available to consumers when making choices about the direction of their care.

Criticisms of the Informed Consumer

Although proponents of the concept of the informed consumer are quick to point out its advantages, the idea is not without its critics. For example, with the proliferation of websites dedicated to health matters, consumers are increasingly turning to the internet for information. On

CASE STUDY

PatientsLikeMe

The internet has been a central component of the consumerist movement in health, especially with reference to the idea of the expert patient. One website that exemplifies this point is www.patientslikeme.com. PatientsLikeMe is similar to other social networking websites, allowing users to fill out profiles with personal information such age, gender, ethnicity, education, and so on. Yet it also asks users to complete medical histories (listing past diagnoses and treatments) and post up-to-date information on their symptoms and care.

Connecting users with other people who share their specific health conditions, the site offers users the option to follow one another, tracking the development of their illness and its treatment. Users can also browse through forums to learn what other consumers think about specific physicians, hospitals, and treatments. For example, site members can complete and access surveys on specific medications, finding out if fellow users found the drug useful and whether they experienced side effects.

In addition to individual users, the website can be utilized by pharmaceutical companies and health care providers. Companies use the website to recruit subjects for clinical trials, providing individuals with the option of accessing experimental treatments before they are approved for widespread use. Additionally, users can opt to make their profile visible to caregivers and health care providers, granting their physicians, nurses, and other carers access to their daily fluctuations in symptoms and perspectives on treatment. Finally, site members can choose to donate their data "for you, for others, for good," providing researchers with access to an individual's personal information.

the whole, websites are not monitored for quality; nor is the issue of authorship always clear (Fox & Ward, 2006). As a consequence, information that may appear unbiased may in fact derive from sources with specific (usually commercial) interests in promoting certain points of view. Thus, while an individual may feel that they are consulting objective medical data to determine how to best manage their condition, their "expertise" may derive from inaccurate or skewed sources.

As a consequence, many physicians remain somewhat hesitant and skeptical about the notion of the expert patient. As explained by Shaw and Baker (2004), some medical providers fear that informed consumers, with their frequent questions and suggestions, represent a far heavier caseload. Arriving for consultation with a series of potentially difficult, baseless, or time-consuming queries, these patients may contribute little to their own care and actually limit the time available to other patients. Other physicians may appreciate the knowledge that patients have acquired in pursuit of their own care but worry that these individuals are also the most likely to demand untested and costly treatments. For such health care providers, the informed consumer might also be termed the "frustrating patient."

As mentioned previously, many government bodies, health care organizations, and insurance companies have poured time and funding into promoting the notion of the informed consumer. By providing training courses for those with chronic illnesses and by offering reduced insurance premiums for individuals who demonstrate greater attentiveness to their overall health, these groups have striven to incentivize the development of expert patients. Often, governments and insurance companies aim to empower people with the assumption that such consumers will prove less costly in the long run. Whether these efforts have been successful, however, is a matter of substantial debate. As Deborah Lupton (2007) has argued, the creation of a knowledgeable and confident consumer who meets the physician on a level playing field may occur in some instances, but many individuals, particularly older people and those with less education, may still defer to medical authorities. More skeptical individuals, meanwhile, might become so dismissive of physician expertise that the medical encounter is one characterized by deep distrust rather than the productive partnership envisioned by advocates of consumerism.

It is also worth noting that many individuals feel overwhelmed and incapable of handling the complex information that accompanies many health problems (Henwood, Wyatt, Hart, & Smith, 2007). These individuals may not actually want increased responsibility for their own care, preferring to place their trust in the experience and wisdom of a physician. Medical professionals undergo many years of training to develop their expertise; it may be unrealistic to expect people without such training to feel confident taking charge of their complex health issues. Perhaps this point can explain why, as research by Deber, Kraetschmer, Urowitz, and Sharpe (2005) has shown, many individuals prefer the term *patient* to either *client* or *consumer* when describing themselves.

Health Care Providers' Response to Consumerism

Although individuals may take on only some characteristics of the informed consumer, providers of medical services have nonetheless responded to the increasing consumerism of the health care landscape. Recall that government regulators have sought to introduce competitive mechanisms into publicly funded health care systems such as those in Canada and the United Kingdom. In the United States, where health care has traditionally been seen as an individual responsibility (rather than a collective right), legal changes through the Affordable Care Act have also sought to create greater competition among providers and insurance companies. Whether these changes reduce overall health care costs remains to be seen; regardless, it is clear that providers are responding to increased **marketization** with a series of strategies to ensure they remain attractive to consumers in an arena of competition and choice.

In many regards, hospitals, clinics, and individual providers have attempted to replicate the tactics of traditionally profit-driven businesses as they seek to attract and retain patients. This is true even within publicly funded systems. On the one hand, providers have made serious efforts to borrow strategies from the hospitality industry to improve patient satisfaction. Ford and Fottler (2000) documented a number of instances in which hospitals and clinics adapted strategies from hotels and restaurants in the hopes of providing a better overall "total healthcare experience," rather than merely focusing on improving clinical outcomes. For example, hospitals typically demand that patients turn up on the morning of their surgery, but some hospitals have begun to offer multi-night packages that include a stay in lavishly decorated rooms, gourmet meals, and a nurse who may attend to the consumer's needs as attentively as a waiter. Many clinics have also started training all staff, from custodians to physicians, in so-called "best practice" customer service techniques. In their efforts to foster

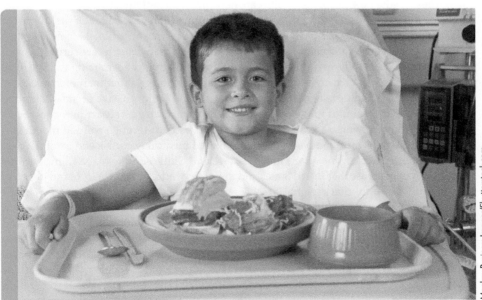

Monkey Business Images/Shutterstock.com

Heavily marketized hospitals have borrowed strategies from the hospitality industry to improve patient satisfaction. Hospital meals are an area of the patient experience that can be influenced by a consumerist approach and by health care providers' interest in increasing their competitiveness and in courting patients.

a clinic-wide culture of customer service, these programmes instruct staff in techniques such as complaint resolution, overall attentiveness, and the use of "key phrases" to enhance consumer satisfaction. Along similar lines, hospital programs to improve staff satisfaction proceed from the mantra that happier workers create happier environments.

The physical environment of the so-called "**healthscape**"—the actual space of the hospital or clinic—has also received substantial attention from hospital managers in their efforts to promote consumer satisfaction. While functional, the sterile, traditional hospital design, with its minimal decoration and use of bland colours, did little to influence the wellbeing of patients. As a result, medical institutions are increasingly being refitted in the hopes of creating comfortable and convenient environments for consumers. Hospital managers might order brighter paint for surgical recovery rooms or ask that staff dress in scrubs only during procedures, thereby decreasing the "institutional" feeling of the environment. Other commonly implemented conveniences include allowing consumers to wear underwear under hospital gowns, offering valet parking, and providing entertainment (like wifi or tablets) between consultations with staff.

Altering the consumer experience within the clinic doors is only one aspect of health care providers' efforts to remain competitive. Although widely believed to be important in retaining pre-existing consumers, these sorts of changes do little to attract new "customers." As previously discussed, mainstream news media, websites, and social media have all become important facets in shaping consumer decisions on where to seek out health care (Hardey, 2008). These media rank hospitals, health care networks, and individual practitioners according to a wide array of criteria. Yet these sources of information are outside of the control of the clinic or provider; beyond trying to provide the best service possible, there is little they can do to influence this information. In light of this reality, many health care service providers and organizations rely upon the more traditional medium of advertising to maximize consumer awareness and, increasingly, to project a specific image about their practice.

In this regard, branding, slogans, and public relations techniques have become central to the competitive strategies of many major providers. Such strategies attract new consumers but also help shape the message disseminated by past patients through word of mouth and social media. Perhaps most famously, a combination of medical expertise and careful image management has seen organizations like the Cleveland Clinic and the Mayo Clinic become household names across the United States and the wider world. In fact, their "brand identity" is sufficiently powerful that regional "franchises" have been established across the United States and in other major world cities such as Abu Dhabi. The pressure on hospitals to adapt to the logic of brand management is sufficiently intense that the lines between public and private health care spaces are becoming blurred (Brown & Barnett, 2004). Another example of such branding is the Hospital for Sick Children in Toronto, which is far better known across Canada by its "SickKids" moniker. Even though most individuals will never utilize services or receive treatment at SickKids or the Mayo Clinic, their level of brand recognition ensures a constant supply of patients and funds. Of course, not every hospital or practitioner achieves such a level of fame, but branding strategies and public relations staff are employed by health care providers of all sizes.

In an era in which health services are becoming more sensitive to the demands of consumers and the achievement of customer satisfaction, the language of brand management can provide an extra competitive edge. The fact that health care providers are actively devising brand identities, a concept strongly linked to fostering consumer loyalty across the business world, indicates the extent to which market forces are dramatically reshaping the health provision landscape.

Controversies Regarding Health Care Marketization

For critics, the wholesale adoption of language and practices traditionally associated with the world of business is indicative of a new reality in which health is viewed as a **commodity** that can be bought and sold. These criticisms are not new; as early as 1980, Relman warned of a "new medical-industrial complex" (p. 963) in light of a proliferation of private, for-profit hospitals. Such a situation contrasts sharply with the notion of health (or at least health care) as a fundamental right to be enjoyed equally by all people, regardless of economic or health status. Thus, while consumerism seeks to empower patients, its focus on **individualism** also poses a challenge to health care systems in places like Canada and the United Kingdom where health care has come to be conceptualized as a collective right. Put simply, there is a tension between consumerism's emphasis on maximal choice (whereby individuals choose what to treat, when to treat, and how to treat it) and publicly funded health care systems' need to organize and ration the provision of treatments.

The links between the rise of consumerism and the idea of health as a commodity are perhaps best exemplified through an examination of people's changing relationship with pharmaceutical medications. Since the 1970s, the increasing prevalence of consumerist discourse in health has gone hand in hand with a dramatic upswing in drug prescriptions. Previously, most drug prescriptions were written on an ad hoc basis as treatments focused primarily on acute medical problems—think, for example, of antibiotics used to combat an infection. From the 1970s onwards, however, increasing numbers of individuals possessed prescriptions for chronic conditions such as diabetes, hypertension, mental illness, and high cholesterol. As mentioned previously, this trend reflects broad changes in people's health statuses as chronic illnesses have overtaken acute medical emergencies as the dominant reason for seeking medical care.

What counts as a chronic medical condition, however, has been substantially influenced by the consumerist narrative; in particular, individuals have more power to shape definitions of health and wellbeing. Through the process of medicalization, many facets of people's lives that would not previously have been described as issues in need of medical intervention have become reconceptualised as health-related problems. While the medical profession and pharmaceutical companies undoubtedly contribute to this process, the medicalization of normal bodily changes like balding, acne, and erectile dysfunction is possible only because large numbers of consumers are willing to *buy* these issues as health problems. The word *buy* is chosen deliberately; the medicalization of these types of issues has largely followed the availability of purchasable pharmaceutical interventions.

Frequently called "lifestyle" drugs, these medications are the source of much debate. Because they treat conditions that are non–life threatening, critics dismiss such prescriptions as needless drains on physicians' time and health resources. For their defenders, however, such drugs are reflective of the success of consumerism: these medications offer individuals the option of defining and dealing with pain and distress on their own terms. Rather than waiting for a physician to decide what should (and should not) be the subject of a medical intervention, the lifestyle drugs (and their associated conditions) give consumers the right to choose what they see as a health problem.

A major factor in the boom in pharmaceutical consumption is the fact that consumers are far more knowledgeable about a wide range of medications than in the past. Many drugs, such as Lipitor, Ritalin, and Viagra, have become household names, acquiring such a familiarity that they are routinely mentioned in popular films and television series. Consequently, people tend to be familiar not only with drug names but also the conditions they are meant to treat.

How has such recognition come to pass? In the North American context, perhaps the most significant factor is **direct-to-consumer (DTC) advertising**. Historically, governments have limited pharmaceutical advertisements solely to media that overwhelmingly cater to prescribers, such as medical journals. This limitation is based on a few key precepts: First, health is a matter of substantial insecurity for many individuals; these laws aimed to prevent commercial enterprises from capitalizing on these insecurities. Second, lawmakers felt that determining the benefits, risks, and potential complications of a pharmaceutical treatment was a complex process that required the expertise of a trained physician. Through the lens of health consumerism, however, both of these arguments have been described as paternalistic, characteristic of a "doctor knows best" attitude that limits patient knowledge, choice, and autonomy.

Direct-to-consumer advertising attempts to remedy this power imbalance between physicians and consumers. In recent decades, pharmaceutical companies in the United States have launched massive marketing campaigns aimed squarely at the consumer, bypassing the physician. Consumers have been bombarded by television commercials, magazine advertisements, and radio announcements promoting new drugs. Yet these advertisements do not merely advertise drugs: they also convey information about the conditions that these medications are meant to treat. In this way, DTC advertising plays an important role in medicalization. Although DTC marketing is not legal in Canada, these adverts do reach Canadian consumers, since the majority of the Canadian population lives within close enough proximity of the United States to receive American television and radio. Through this avenue and other "loopholes," Canadian consumers demonstrate heightened awareness of new medications available on the market (Mintzes, 2006).

Beyond traditional media like print and television, the internet serves as a powerful vehicle for disseminating knowledge about new and pre-existing pharmaceutical treatments. "Disease awareness" websites, frequently sponsored and hosted by pharmaceutical companies, provide consumers with on-demand information about their potential condition and, naturally, available drug treatments. Other sources of knowledge include patient group websites, social media, and other online forums, all of which allow consumers to share stories and information on their experience with different medications. Beyond knowledge about the drugs themselves, however, users of these sites also provide one another with information on how to access these medications. For example, the proliferation of online pharmacies (many of which do not require a legal prescription) allow drugs to be sold as consumer goods in the truest sense of the word. On the advice of their peers, consumers may select their preferred medication and, with just a few clicks, expect it to arrive at their door days later.

The overall effect of DTC advertising is controversial and advocates of consumerism do not always agree on whether these practices benefit or harm consumers. Supporters of DTC suggest that such advertisements provide consumers with knowledge about their condition and potential treatments; consequently, individuals can feel more confident when speaking to their physician. One way to view this situation is that patients are empowered vis-à-vis their physicians, but critics of DTC (and there are many—only a handful of countries around the world permit it) suggest that DTC reduces physicians to little more than drug dispensers. Fearing patient dissatisfaction (and its public expression, which might hurt their status in the health care marketplace), physicians are more likely to give into consumer demands, even when the desired medication may not be appropriate (Mintzes et al., 2003). Thus, DTC encourages people who lack the requisite medical expertise to believe they know as well as a physician whether a given treatment is valuable (Applbaum, 2006). Additionally, DTC drives up the cost of drugs (since advertising is expensive) and creates a heavy burden on publicly funded health care systems where prescription drug costs are partially or fully subsidized. Even when consumers pay for the medication themselves, the expense of a visit to the prescribing physician is usually drawn from the public purse (Donohue, Cevasco & Rosenthal, 2007).

Finally, DTC may increase the likelihood of iatrogenic harm. For example, after an intensive marketing campaign, tremendous consumer demand helped propel Vioxx (an anti-inflammatory medication) into becoming one of the most popular drugs of the early 2000s (Green, 2006). A few years later, Vioxx had to be recalled and pulled from the market when it emerged that the drug substantially increased the likelihood of heart disease. Further investigation revealed that many of those who suffered heart trouble had likely not needed the medication in the first place. Consumer-focused advertisements had evidently played a substantial role in motivating individuals to "ask [their] doctor about Vioxx," thus increasing the prescription rate. The issue of DTC advertising demonstrates that determining exactly what is best for consumers is not always a straightforward process.

Medical and Health Tourism

An intrinsic component of the shift towards free market capitalism has been the strengthening of the global marketplace. Although goods, people, and services have crossed national borders for hundreds of years, recent decades have witnessed an unprecedented growth in the level of economic interconnectivity and interdependence (see Chapter Seven for more). Health and medicine have naturally been affected by these changes. The practices of medical and health tourism serve as intersection points for the rise of economic globalization and health consumerism.

In the simplest sense, **medical tourism** refers to the act of crossing national borders in order to access health care treatments. Historically, North America and Western Europe were the principal destinations, as wealthy consumers from other parts of the world sought out rare and costly treatments that were not available within their own countries. Contemporary medical tourism differs greatly from this model; most of today's medical tourists are middle class and depart from Western countries in search of cheaper care elsewhere (Hopkins, Labonté, Rybbeksm & Packer, 2010; Pafford, 2009). South Asia, Latin America, and Eastern Europe have all become common destinations for West Europeans and North Americans seeking out treatments ranging from minor dental work and breast augmentation to complex heart surgery and cancer care. Although the exact numbers are difficult to pin down, it is clear that increasing numbers of consumers travel each year for health and medical tourism.

How has this reversal come about? Like most market interactions, the answer involves factors on both the supply and demand sides. From the demand perspective, health care costs in the Western world continue to spiral as governments abandon (or weaken) welfare initiatives, such as publicly provided medical care. In places where most medical costs are still covered, limited budgets and an undersupply of practitioners have led to ballooning waiting lists. Faced with the unappetizing choice of spending tremendous amounts of money out of pocket or enduring years on waiting lists, many individuals are opting to explore cheaper and quicker treatment options in the rest of the world. This point is especially true of elective surgeries such as knee replacements, liposuction, or rhinoplasty. On the supply side, clinics and hospitals in destination countries have seized this market opportunity by equipping themselves with advanced medical technologies. When combined with highly skilled (and frequently Western-trained) practitioners operating at a fraction of the cost, it is little surprise that these countries have been successful in attracting consumers. Finally, changes in the nature of the market itself have been key: lower-cost air travel and the internet have made it much easier for care providers to connect with customers.

Attracting consumers has not been a simple task. As Connell (2006) points out, countries in Latin America, South Asia, and Eastern Europe have all had to overcome stereotyped images of their medical staff and facilities as backward and unhygienic. Hospitals and clinics have employed a wide variety of strategies to combat this stigma. For example, many health care providers have sought to replicate Western clinics by fostering a brand identity. Both the Asian Heart Institute (in Mumbai, India) and Bumrungrad International Hospital (in Bangkok, Thailand) have successfully carved out key niches in the medical tourism market through the use of wide-ranging public relations strategies. Other clinics, such as the Cleveland Clinic Abu Dhabi, pay to license the names of Western institutions to lend an air of familiarity. For hospitals that lack name-brand recognition, alternative strategies include offering luxurious package deals to attract consumers. Taking advantage of their location in "exotic" and frequently tropical locales, these hospital networks team up with local tourism agencies so that patients can combine treatments like corrective eye surgery with a safari or a trip to the beach. Even after flights, hotels, and other expenses are combined, individual consumers still reap drastic savings compared to the cost of treatment in their home countries. Government agencies have also gotten involved; recognizing the potential economic benefits of a strong medical tourism sector, they may offer tax incentives to clinics attracting foreign clientele, build up travel infrastructure, or include medical treatment as part of official tourism information.

Government agencies and businesses in destination countries are not the only ones to get involved in medical tourism. In Britain, for example, the National Health Service (NHS) has sent patients abroad for care to try and reduce their waiting list for certain treatments. Similarly, American insurance companies have found it far cheaper to send their clients abroad. Some insurers offer incentivized policies (such as no deductible) for individuals willing to receive their treatment overseas (Horowitz, 2007). Meanwhile, new businesses in Canada, such as Timely Medical Alternatives and Surgical Tourism Canada, act as brokers who connect Canadian consumers with hospital networks abroad. In this regard, the health care industry is simply following the trend set by other sectors that have long outsourced

CASE STUDY

Bumrungrad International Hospital

Located in Thailand's capital city, Bangkok's Bumrungrad International Hospital was founded in 1980 and has become one of the largest hospitals in Asia. In addition to servicing domestic clients, Bumrungrad has become a symbol of international medical tourism. Offering inpatient and outpatient treatment in dozens of technologically advanced specialist clinics, the hospital employs more than 150 interpreters to meet the linguistic needs of their 400,000 annual foreign clients. The hospital offers a diverse range of services ranging from breast lifts to stem-cell transplantation, often done at a fraction of the cost demanded elsewhere.

Following the consumerist trend in health care, Bumrungrad offers its clients numerous opportunities to personalize their visit. Inpatients can choose among "Single Deluxe rooms," "Premier Atrium Deluxe rooms," and "Premier Royal Suites," which cost nearly $1000 per night. The whole hospital is equipped with wifi access and clients may rent laptops and tablets. In its quest to maximize patient satisfaction, the hospital also offers services such as chauffeured airport transfer, private nurses, and the choice of Western, Asian, or Middle Eastern menus.

As an exemplar of the interconnections between health, commerce, and globalization, Bumrungrad Hospital is a publicly traded company on the Stock Exchange of Thailand, with domestic and foreign banks and insurance companies among its major shareholders. The company had a turnover of nearly $500 million in 2013.

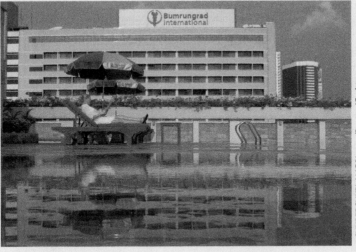

© SUKREE SUKPLANG/X90021/Reuters/Corbis

At Bumrungrad International Hospital, medical tourists can access a range of services and comforts that might be more difficult to access in their home countries. What kinds of advantages and problems can the rise of medical tourism present for the countries that cater to large numbers of medical tourists?

to the developing world in order to reduce costs and seek out new market opportunities (Turner, 2007).

On the whole, medical tourism embodies some of the most important tenets of the consumerist movement. By being able to seek out care abroad, individuals gain greater choice in treatments and may be able to access services on demand. The customer-driven model of such institutions ensures that the consumer's wishes are a priority. Yet many critics of medical tourism suggest that the trend toward foreign health care is not without its costs. For consumers, the potential problems begin with their search for care. Most individuals seek information about foreign care on the internet, and these websites are typically run by agencies and brokerages rather than medical experts. Accordingly, the information listed on such sites may not be medically accurate. At the same time, tourist agencies are not bound by professional medical ethics; rather, they seek to maximize profit by convincing consumers of the need for and viability of treatment without necessarily detailing the risk of side effects and other complications (Lunt, Hardey, & Mannion, 2010). Once an individual arrives in the foreign destination for care, they may face a medical culture distinct from their own. Host medical institutions and personnel may not be bound by the same legal or ethical requirements to provide informed consent or financial compensation for malpractice.

For destination countries, and in particular for their populations, medical tourism presents a host of potential problems. The very economic dislocation that makes seeking out health care in these countries so financially attractive may in fact worsen on account of Western medical tourists. For example, host governments spend large sums of money improving travel infrastructure and advertising medical services abroad; some critics suggest that the money might be better spent providing services to relieve widespread poverty and improve health care for local populations. Supporters argue that the money gained through medical tourism will trickle down to all members of society, but critics fear that such funds will remain in the hands of the elite (foreign-trained physicians and members of the government) rather than reach the poor. As a consequence, health inequalities look likely to continue (or worsen) as local physicians face the choice of taking on a local patient for a fraction of the sum that they could make by instead catering to foreign consumers. Thus, while the brain drain of physicians and other medical practitioners to rich, Western countries might be stemmed by the chance to earn more at home, a sort of "internal brain drain" may occur as larger numbers of medical professionals abandon the public sector for lucrative private work. In sum, by focusing on serving the needs of Western consumers, medical tourism might prevent local patients from accessing care.

Chapter Summary

The last few decades have witnessed a shift in how people accessing health care are conceptualized. Rather than passive patients depending on the expertise of medical professionals, individuals are increasingly described as consumers of health care services. The notion of the medical consumer implies someone who is knowledgeable, rational, proactive about health, and willing to work in partnership with (rather than be subordinate to) physicians.

Many governments, inspired by political and economic policies favouring liberalism and the free market, have sought to facilitate the creation of medical consumers. They have passed laws and created policies to foster competition within the medical marketplace. Such policies aim to create greater consumer choices at a lower cost. Along with patient lobbying organizations and internet groups, they have promoted certain consumer rights to help empower individuals vis-à-vis their health care providers.

A key element of this empowerment has been the proliferation of choice; individuals are increasingly able to pick and choose their treatments from a diverse group of providers, including non-traditional biomedical alternatives. Against this backdrop of increased competition, health care providers must seek to promote customer satisfaction, turning to a host of new tools to measure and improve the consumer experience. Providers must now rely on sophisticated marketing techniques, innovative services, and branding strategies to try and attract new consumers.

The rise of consumerism has coincided with a dramatic increase in the use of pharmaceutical medications, especially for chronic conditions. New drugs that blur the lines between medicine and consumer goods have become important elements of the health landscape. Additionally, direct-to-consumer advertising has challenged the health care provider's traditional role as an intermediary, allowing people to develop a more personal knowledge regarding their treatment options. These changes in the role of pharmaceuticals have been both celebrated and vilified as consequences of the shift that sees health as something purchasable.

Finally, medical tourism is a phenomenon that demonstrates the global implications of the shift towards consumerism in health. Increasingly, individuals from wealthier countries are visiting foreign countries in order to access medical services at a fraction of the cost charged in their home countries. Employing many of the same marketing techniques utilized by their Western counterparts, hospitals and clinics in South Asia, Eastern Europe, and Latin America have broadened the scope of competition within global health care provision. But while these options may represent additional choice for wealthy consumers, they also present a series of potentially negative consequences for both foreign and domestic patients.

Although the rise of consumerism in health has split opinion, few would argue with the point that it has produced some clear benefits, a few significant drawbacks, and a fresh challenge to traditional medical dominance. As a consequence, consumerism has fundamentally reshaped the medical system and how individual people manage their health.

STUDY QUESTIONS

1. How would you characterize the difference between a health consumer and a patient?
2. How can we best account for the rise of health consumerism?
3. Are prescription medications consumer goods?
4. Consider the arguments for and against medical tourism. Who benefits and who suffers as a consequence of the expansion of medical tourism?
5. Why do some critics see the rise of the informed consumer/expert patient as a threat?

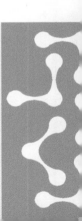

SUGGESTED READINGS

Bookman, M. Z. & Bookman, K. R. (2007). *Medical tourism in developing countries.* New York: Palgrave Macmillan.

Chambre, S. M. & Goldner, M. (Eds) (2008). Patients, consumers, and civil society. Special issue of *Advances in Medical Sociology.*

Donohue, J. (2006). A history of drug advertising: The evolving roles of consumers and consumer protection. *Milbank Quarterly, 84*(4), 659–99.

SUGGESTED WEB RESOURCES

Patients Beyond Borders: www.patientsbeyondborders.com

Dave deBronkart's TEDx Talk: Meet e-Patient Dave: www.ted.com/ talksdave_debronkart_meet_e_patient_dave

Medical Tourism India in Numbers: www.youtube.com/watch?v=k2f9owU-EH4

GLOSSARY

Commodity Something that can be purchased and sold.

Consumerism An ideology in which an individual consumes goods and services to fulfill their own interests. Consumers have the freedom to make informed, rational choices.

Direct-to-consumer (DTC) advertising Pharmaceutical advertising that is aimed directly at the consumer (as opposed to advertising to the prescribing physician).

Healthscapes The tangible aspects of the health care system. Examples include hospitals, clinics, or the physical layout of a health care organization.

Individualism Stresses that the individual is more important than the collective group.

Informed consumer (expert patient) A consumer who knows the risks, benefits, and costs of what they are acquiring or purchasing (in this case, health care). The expert patient, then, can be thought of as a hyper-informed consumer.

Marketization The process in which previously public services become increasingly like private businesses, facilitating competition between firms vying to attract consumers.

Medical tourism International travel for the sake of acquiring medical treatment.

REFERENCES

Applbaum, K. (2006). Pharmaceutical marketing and the invention of the medical consumer. *PLoS Medicine, 3*(4), e189.

Brown, L. & Barnett, J. R. (2004). Is the corporate transformation of hospitals creating a new hybrid health care space? A case study of the impact of co-location of public and private hospitals in Australia. *Social Science & Medicine, 58*(2), 427–44.

Charles, C., Gafni, A., & Whelan, T. (1997). Shared decision-making in the medical encounter: What does it mean? (or it takes at least two to tango). *Social Science & Medicine, 44*(5), 681–92.

Clarke, D. B., Doel, M. A., & Segrott, J. (2004). No alternative? The regulation and professionalization of complementary and alternative medicine in the United Kingdom. *Health & Place, 10*(4), 329–38.

Connell, J. (2006). Medical tourism: Sea, sun, sand and ... surgery. *Tourism Management, 27*(6), 1093–1100.

Deber, R. B., Kraetschmer, N., Urowitz, S., & Sharpe, N. (2005). Patient, consumer, client, or customer: what do people want to be called? *Health Expectations, 8*(4), 345–51.

Donohue, J., Cevasco, M., & Rosenthal, M. (2007). A decade of direct-to-consumer advertising of pre-scription drugs. *New England Journal of Medicine, 357,* 673–81.

Ford, R. C. & Fottler, M. D. (2000). Creating custom-er-focused healthcare organizations. *Healthcare Management Review, 25*(4), 18–33.

Fox, N. J. & Ward, K. J. (2006). Health identities: From expert patient to resisting consumer. *Health, 10*(4), 461–79.

———— & O'Rourke, A. J. (2005). The "expert patient": Empowerment or medical dominance? The case of weight loss, pharmaceutical drugs and the Internet. *Social Science & Medicine, 60*(6), 1299–1309.

Green, R. M. (2006). Direct-to-consumer advertising and pharmaceutical ethics: The case of Vioxx. *Hofstra Law Review, 35,* 749–59.

Hardey, M. (1999). Doctor in the house: The Internet as a source of lay health knowledge and the chal-lenge to expertise. *Sociology of Health & Illness, 21*(6), 820–35.

———— (2001). "E-health": The internet and the transformation of patients into consumers and producers of health knowledge. *Information, Communication & Society, 4*(3), 388–405.

———— (2008). Public health and Web 2.0. *The Journal of the Royal Society for the Promotion of Health, 128*(4), 181–89.

Henwood, F., Wyatt, S., Hart, A., & Smith, J. (2003). "Ignorance is bliss sometimes": Constraints on the emergence of the "informed patient" in the changing landscapes of health information. *Sociology of Health & Illness, 25,* 589–607.

Hopkins, L., Labonté, R., Runnels, V., & Packer, C. (2010). Medical tourism today: What is the state of existing knowledge? *Journal of Public Health Policy, 31*(2), 185–98.

Horowitz, M. D. (2007). Financial savings in medical tourism. *Medical Tourism Magazine, 1,* 14–15.

Lunt, N., Hardey, M., & Mannion, R. (2010). Nip, tuck and click: Medical tourism and the emergence of web-based health information. *The Open Medical Informatics Journal, 4,* 1–11.

Lupton, D. (1997). Consumerism, reflexivity, and the medical encounter. *Social Science & Medicine, 45*(3), 373–81.

Mold, A. (2010). Patient groups and the construction of the patient-consumer in Britain: An historical overview. *Journal of Social Policy, 39*(4), 505–21.

Mintzes, B. (2006). Direct-to-consumer advertis-ing of prescription drugs in Canada. *Health Council of Canada.* Accessible online: www.healthcouncilcanada.ca/tree/2.38-hcc_dtc-advertising_200601_e_v6.pdf

————, Kravitz, R. L., Bassett, K., Lexchin, J., Kazanjian, A., Evans, R. G., ... Marion, S. A. (2003). How does direct-to-consumer advertising (DTCA) affect prescribing? A survey in primary care environ-ments with and without legal DTCA. *Canadian Medical Association Journal, 169*(5), 405–12.

Pafford, B. (2009). The third wave—medical tourism in the 21st century. *Southern Medical Journal, 102*(8), 810–13.

Reeder, L. G. (1972). The patient–client as consumer. Some reflections on the changing professional–client relationships. *Journal of Health and Social Behaviour, 13,* 406–12.

Relman, A. (1980). The new medical-industrial com-plex. *New England Journal of Medicine, 303*(17), 963–70.

Shaw, J. & Baker, M (2004). "Expert patient"—dream or nightmare? *British Medical Journal, 328*(7442), 723–4.

Tomes, N. (2006). Tomes, N. (2006). Patients or health care consumers? Why the history of contested terms matters. In R. Stevens, C. Rosenberg, & L. Burns (Eds), *History & Health Policy in the United States: Putting the Past Back In* (pp. 83–110). New Brunswick: Rutgers University Press.

Tousijn, W. (2006). Beyond decline: Consumerism, managerialism and the need for a new medical professionalism. *Health Sociology Review, 15*(5), 469–80.

Tuckett, D., Boulton, M., Olson, C., & Williams, A. (1985). *Meetings between experts: An approach to sharing ideas in medical consultations.* London: Tavistock.

Turner, L. (2007). First world healthcare at third world prices: Globalization, bioethics and medical tour-ism. *BioSocieties, 2*(3), 303–25.

Part IV

Future Challenges and Directions

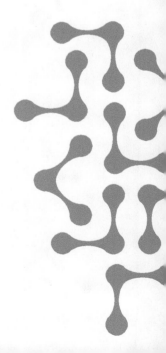

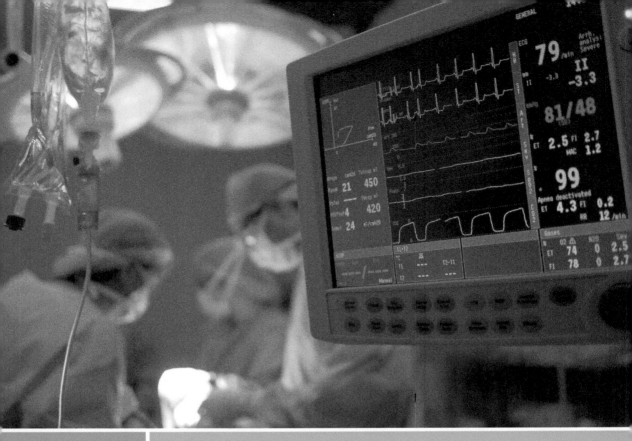

13

Technology

Joshua Evans

LEARNING OBJECTIVES

In this chapter, students will learn

- how to assess the evolving role of technology in health and health care
- technology's central place in shaping how we experience, understand, and treat health and illness
- the ways in which certain types of illness, disease, and risk for illness are made visible through the use of technology
- the role of technology in redefining what is means to be "normal" in the context of health

Introduction

We undoubtedly live a technologically textured life (Ihde, 1990). Our very existence as a species is inseparable from the technology we have surrounded ourselves with. In this regard, technology has been central to understandings of human evolution. We can characterize entire epochs, such as the Stone Age, and societies, like Industrial Society, through their defining technological artifacts (Wyatt, 2008). In these cases, **technology** is generally viewed as a material artifact, or tool, that extends or enhances human existence in the world. Technology encompasses the material artifacts that we use in our everyday lives. This way of thinking about technology, as an artificial tool or prosthesis, places it firmly in the non-human world, opposing it to natural, living substances. Opposing technology to life, including our own, establishes a fundamental dichotomy between technology and society, and between technology and nature.

The field of biomedicine in particular, and the experience of health more broadly, is no exception to the pervasiveness of technology and this type of dichotomous thinking. Technology is an inescapable element of contemporary healthscapes (Clarke, 2010) and greatly influences the way we experience illness and interpret our health. Medical technologies are "the various devices, instruments, and therapies used for diagnostic, therapeutic, rehabilitative, preventive, or experimental purposes as well as the practice and procedures associated with them" (Hogle, 2008, p. 841). This definition encompasses an endless list of materials and practices, from "the most mundane band-aids and pencils to sophisticated machines such as MRIs and artificial hearts, from virtually neutral infusion pumps to highly symbolic procedures and devices such as the drug Viagra or genetic tests" (Timmermans & Berg, 2003, p. 99). From diagnosing disease and replacing bodily functions to compiling information about individuals and populations, medical technologies now saturate the human experience from birth to death (Hogle, 2008).

Consider, for a moment, the following scenario—a routine physical assessment with a primary care physician. The setting is a basic examination room equipped with an examination table, chair, desk, and computer, and many other material artifacts. The assessment would most likely begin with the physician accessing the patient's electronic medical record on a desktop computer or tablet before listening to the heart and lungs with a stethoscope, measuring blood pressure with a sphygmomanometer, and examining the ears with an otoscope. The physician might then send the patient to a medical laboratory for blood analysis. There, a technician draws blood using a syringe and flask to be used in further diagnostic equipment such as centrifuges, Petri dishes, gas chromatographs, and colorimeters. Perhaps the physician also sends the patient for a chest X-ray at another medical laboratory, one also equipped with computerized tomography (CT) scanners and magnetic resonance imaging (MRI) machines. A week later, upon reviewing the results, the physician recommends a diuretic for the patient to treat high blood pressure.

This common scenario encompasses a sizeable list of medical devices and technical procedures, in both the examination room and the medical laboratory. It reminds us that contemporary medical practice, which depends heavily on sophisticated diagnostic and therapeutic devices, can accurately be described as **technomedicine** (Rose, 2007). Importantly, the scenario also invites us to consider technology's role in the development of a **medical gaze** (Foucault, 1973). First introduced by philosopher and historian Michel Foucault, the medical gaze is the mode of perception, and the knowledge foundation, of modern, scientific biomedicine. Foucault believed that the emergence of biomedicine was not simply the result of specific scientific breakthroughs by leading researchers but rather the consequence of a series of subtle shifts. By the nineteenth century, medicine had switched its focus from listening to patients' accounts of illness (an indirect way of searching for disease) to locating objective signs of the disease in the three-dimensional space of the human body. Using new types of scientific tools, such as stethoscopes, physicians were able to "bypass" the patient to get directly at the disease. Thus, individuals and their bodies, at least from the perspective of clinical medicine, became separate entities. Physicians became "experts" at dealing with human bodies, although not necessarily experts at dealing with human beings. The medical gaze, to be precise, is not simply the physician's act of looking but rather the wider philosophy that promotes this way of understanding illness. The medical gaze we are familiar with today evolved through several important historical and geographical developments. As this chapter explores, the modern medical gaze is inextricably entangled with the ongoing application and development of medical technology.

Medical technologies of various kinds, from the "low-tech" to the "high-tech," are integral components of contemporary biomedicine. This chapter critically examines medical technologies, paying particular attention to their role in increasing the visibility of disease and risk in individuals and the population. A central focus of this chapter is the way in which medical technologies, as elements of the medical gaze, influence the formation of medical knowledge. In particular, medical technologies influence what we believe is normal and what is pathological, what constitutes a healthy and an unhealthy body, and increasingly, how the body might be enhanced and optimized.

The chapter begins by reviewing the way in which medical technologies have been critically examined by social scientists. We must pay particular attention to the ways in which medical technologies are used and how they shape our social interactions. Some technologies, such as those used in genetic testing or organ replacement surgery, are more than "equipment." They represent the interaction of countless facets of the medical system including devices, professionals, buildings, goals, biomedical knowledge, and assumptions about human beings (Mol, 2002; Rose, 2007). The "medical gaze," therefore, can be approached itself as a socio-technical assemblage (Rose, 2007; Abi-Rached & Rose, 2010). Approaching the medical gaze in such a way allows us to see how technological interventions have changed our perception of health, medicine, and human beings themselves.

Critical Engagements with Medical Technologies

Social science perspectives on health, technology, and society have developed along several different pathways over the past 25 years (Casper and Morrison, 2010; Timmermans & Berg, 2003). As Timmermans and Berg (2003) note, medical sociologists have developed three primary perspectives for looking at medical technology:

1. **Technological determinism**—a cynical approach. Technological determinists understand technology as a dominant social force with its own internal logic. In this view, technology restricts the autonomy of caregivers and silences the ill. For instance, a person's feelings and experience of their own illness often matters less to physicians than the "objective information" revealed by an X-ray machine. As a consequence,

technological determinists believe that technology deepens and extends the medical dominance of society. Two assumptions underlie technological determinism: that technological developments occur independently of society and that technological change drives social change (Wyatt, 2008). Furthermore, technological determinists view medical technology as an instrument of medicalization (Zola, 1972). For example, critics suggest that problems such as baldness or social anxiety became medicalized *after* the invention of the technologies used to treat these conditions. Thus, medicalization promotes a so-called "medical-industrial complex"—the idea that industry can use technology to gain undue influence in medicine (Reiser, 1978). For example, it has been suggested that pharmaceuticals and gene therapies, both important medical technologies, have elevated the power of pharmaceutical and biotechnology companies beyond that of physicians. While medical doctors were once the primary purveyors of new medical knowledge, these businesses now dictate new disease categories and interventions (Conrad, 2005).

2. **Social essentialism**—a somewhat less antagonistic stance towards technology. Social essentialists view technology as a passive, blank slate whose meaning is socially constructed (Timmermans & Berg, 2003). In this perspective, technologies are merely tools that acquire meaning through the way they are utilized. In that sense, those who use a technology influence how society perceives it. In this sense they are material artifacts that "function as sociological catalysts: they are tools that generate interactions or social meanings but do not act, affect, or evolve in themselves" (Timmermans & Berg, 2003, p. 101). Scholarship on modern hospitals, a quintessential medical technology, argues that the social significance of a hospital is directly determined by the priorities of the institution and its workers. As such, these organizations reflect the dominant understandings of health and illness at a given time (Curtis, Gesler, Fabian, & Priebe, 2007; Risse, 1999; Kearns, Ross Barnett, Newman 2003). Today, for example, a focus on "patient-centred" health care guides the basic design and operating principles of new hospital spaces (Bromley, 2012).

3. **Technology-in-practice**—Timmermans and Berg (2003) argue that technological determinism and social essentialism either overestimate or underestimate the role of medical technologies in social settings. The third approach, referred to as technology-in-practice, instead understands medical technology as one "actor" among many in a diverse network of patients, physicians, standards, and practices that together constitute particular forms of diagnoses, treatments, and care. Whereas deterministic approaches see medical technologies as innately powerful, and essentialist approaches see their power as socially constructed, the "technology-in-practice" approach claims their importance is best understood by situating them in relation to practices (Mol, 2002). Doing so reveals them as "central mediators in the construction and reproduction of novel worlds—including patient identities, professional identities, and the overall organization of health care work" (Timmermans & Berg, 2003, p. 108). For example, seemingly mundane technologies, such as the patient-centred medical record, have been fundamental in establishing the identity of ill individuals as "patients" (Berg & Harterink, 2004).

These three ways of understanding technology are distinct lenses for critically examining human–technology relationships in health and health care. Scholars have utilized these

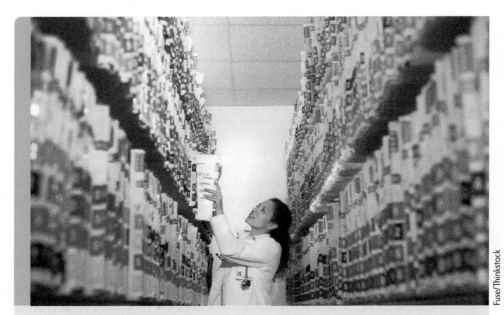

Fuse/Thinkstock

The patient record is a relatively simple form of technology that allows medical professionals and institutions to keep histories of their clients' medical lives.

perspectives for examining the impact of technologies on health care practice; for assessing how medical technologies reconceptualize and reconfigure human bodies; and for considering how technologies relate to health social movements (Casper & Morrison, 2010).

Transforming Health Care Practice

Human–technology interactions influence health care practices, creating new forms and locations of care. Many medical technologies have been transformational in creating new categories of patienthood and personhood (Schillmeier & Domenech, 2010). For example, people hoping to address the health problems associated with aging have created technologies that redefine both the experience of aging as well as the process of caring for elder people. Such technologies include telecare, a health care service offered via telephone and internet communication tools, and "smart homes" that are equipped with sensors and other technologies that enhance independence and quality of life (Milligan, Mort, & Roberts, 2010). On the one hand, some praise this technology for shifting professional health care into the home—physicians, nurses, and other types of carers can monitor a person remotely, perhaps saving individuals from exhausting and time-consuming trips to the hospital. On the other hand, critics question whether these technologies might subject individuals to undue surveillance and control (Mort et al., 2013). Beyond eldercare technologies, concerns have emerged around the role of technologies in clinical encounters between patients and doctors. The influence of technology on all aspects of the health care system has led to a reframing of patient and practitioner in technological terms, resulting in a sort of **technogovernance** that redistributes the responsibilities of both patient and practitioner (May, Rapley, Moreira, Finch, & Heaven, 2006).

Reconfiguring the Human Body

Beyond technogovernance of the health care process itself, medical technologies can impact bodily experiences. Technology can help individuals conform to normative ideas of a healthy, able body. It also has the power to completely transform what we consider "normal." Medical technologies have long been used to replace bodily functions. For example, people have been using false teeth for thousands of years (Crubzy, Murail, Girard, & Bernadou, 1998). Today the list of available replacement body parts available is extensive, including a wide range of devices such as artificial hearts, artificial respiration machines, artificial retinas, cochlear implants, and artificial limbs, to name only a few (Hogle, 2008). Medical technologies are often presented as a "technological fix" for various types of physical, and even mental, impairment. Assistive technologies range from "low-tech" devices, such as wheelchairs, to "high-tech" apparatuses like insulin pumps. Beyond these assistive devices, pharmacological technologies, such as antipsychotic drugs, allow individuals to function differently in their day-to-day lives and to participate in mainstream social activities.

However, those living a technologically assisted life often see medical technology as both a positive and a negative presence in their lives, one that is irrevocably linked to their personal identity and social relationships (Kirk, 2010). Assistive technologies, especially those that are visible, can be stigmatizing by acting as a symbol of impairment, disease, or deviancy. In this sense, assistive technologies are central to the construction of (dis)ability itself—their very use implies an attempt to return a person to "normal" functioning. In doing so, they problematize the state of being impaired (Moser, 2006). Hence, assistive and prosthetic technologies indirectly alienate their users from the rest of society by reproducing a hierarchical ordering of bodily difference. In this regard, technologies are utilized to "elevate" impaired people closer to "normal" bodies.

When it comes to bodily differences, medical technologies are also pivotal in the transformation of what it means to be normal. Technoscientific innovations in the fields of genetic science, molecular biology, and nanotechnology are challenging the very boundaries between nature and culture, human and non-human. These technologies have disrupted our notions about the body and life itself (Clarke, Shim, Mano, Fosket, & Fishman, 2010). When medicine and technoscience meet, life itself may be transformed. Some medical technologies, such as neural and genetic enhancements, go beyond simply repairing or restoring the body. They aim to improve bodily function beyond what is normal or necessary for life. Such technologies push critics to question whether this is a new form of eugenics (Rose, 2007). These technologies also raise practical and ethical questions regarding the limits of the body and life itself (Shildrick, 2010). As Haraway (1991) has argued, we stand at the dawn of the era of cyborg bodies. An expanding range of biomedical enhancements aim to optimize human life forms, and human bodies are being reshaped and reconfigured in the process.

Health Social Movements

A third focus of studies on technology and health has drawn attention to the role of technology in social movements organized around diseases, access to care, and health inequities (Casper & Morrison, 2010). Medical technologies, like diagnostic devices, surgical therapies,

CASE STUDY

Seasonale

Seasonale (levenorgestrel/ethinyl estradiol) is a pharmaceutical pill that acts as an oral con-
traceptive. It was launched in 2003 and, like other birth control pills, it affects how the body
regulates sex hormones. What sets Seasonale apart from conventional contraceptives is the
fact that women are advised to take the pill consecutively for three months, only then taking a
week of placebo pills to bring about menses. In effect, this means that women taking Seasonale
menstruate only four times per year, instead of the average of twelve.

Seasonale has dramatically split opinion. On the one hand, the drug company that produces the pill and many of its users argue that Seasonale and similar medical technologies act as
agents of female empowerment. Women now have an unparalleled ability to control their lives.
Indeed, after the pill was launched, the Seasonale website offered users a personal planner to
"plan events like vacations, business travel, romantic encounters, and family reunions based on
your inactive [placebo] pill dates." In short, supporters of the medication see it as something
that frees women from the bondage of their period.

Seasonale is not without its critics. Feminist scholars note that the framing of Seasonale as a
solution to the "problems of womanhood" stigmatizes women's bodies as inherently problematic (Mamo & Fosket, 2009; Woods, 2013). Rather than seeing menstruation as a natural process
for female bodies, technologies like Seasonale promote the notion that menses is an unnatural
state that needs to be stamped out. Moreover, by transforming menstruation from a monthly to
a scheduled quarterly event, critics suggest that drugs like Seasonale fundamentally reshape
what it means to be a female human being. After all, in many cultures, menses has acted as
a central marker in the transition from girlhood to womanhood. How long, these critics ask,
before menstruation will be eliminated altogether?

and pharmaceutical interventions, have often inspired social activism. One significant and
recent example of such a movement is the global fight for universal access to antiretroviral
drugs for HIV/AIDS. These types of health movements have generated new forms of **biological citizenship**, as individuals build local and transnational communities of support to
engage in biomedical activism (Rose & Novas, 2004). In many cases, these individual and
collective identities are constructed through technoscientific means involving biomedical
information and technologies. These practices give rise to what Clarke et al. (2003) have
called technoscientific identities, wherein biomedical classifications are deeply integrated
into one's sense of self.

In this context, medical technologies are inextricably entangled with both individual personhood and technoscientific apparatuses. The development of technoscientific identities
can, on one hand, be seen as a result of technology's ability to stabilize lived experiences in
the face of biomedical risk and uncertainty (Sulik, 2009). Some medical technologies, on the
other hand, can lead to more, rather than less, diagnostic uncertainty. For example, genetic
technologies used for newborn screening can produce uncertain results or positive results
for diseases about which little is known. As a result, people may be "patients-in-waiting"
before they are even born (Timmermans & Buchbinder, 2010).

TABLE 13.1	Critical Engagements with Medical Technology		
	Impact of technology in and on practice	Reconfigurations of human bodies	Technologies and embodied health movements
Technological Determinist	How have technological innovations reorganized the goals and application of biomedicine?	How do technologies threaten civil liberties and even the very existence of some groups in society?	How have technological innovations provided the basis for new health movements?
Social Essentialist	How do doctors, nurses and patients respond to new technologies?	How are assistive and enhancement technologies understood in relation to identity?	What kinds of collective identities form around technologies?
Technology-in-Practice	How do technologies shift contexts or practices of care?	How do technologies mediate processes of embodiment?	How do technologies make possible new health movements?

Source: Adapted from Timmermans & Berg (2003); Casper & Morrison (2010).

It is not possible to fully address the breadth and depth of critical engagement with medical technology in one book chapter. The overview provided here also has admittedly deterministic leanings, stressing technology as an active actor through concepts such as "technogovernance," "cyborg bodies," and "technoscientific identities." As mentioned previously, however, there are many ways to engage with the topic of technology. Table 13.1 above provides a summary of the differing theoretical approaches to the study of technology and health.

Technomedicine and the Mutating Medical Gaze

While medicine once focused on curing diseases, it now also focuses on ameliorating health risks and optimizing our wellbeing. This is a process that Clarke et al. (2003) have labelled biomedicalization. Focusing our attention on the confluence of technology and social relations in contemporary biomedicine reveals how our medical gaze has shifted, altering the ways in which we understand health.

As mentioned in the introduction to this chapter, contemporary biomedicine is distinguishable as a particular way of seeing illness in the body. The concept of disease as a pathological disturbance within the physical body is a hallmark of Western biomedicine. Foucault (1973) described the emergence of "anatomo-clinical medicine" in early eighteenth-century France as a new mode of perception related to the spatialization of illness. This spatialization was threefold (see Philo, 2000). First, a primary spatialization of illness occurred in the two-dimensional form of classificatory tables of disease. These disease classifications provided a way of seeing the relations among diseases based on the similarity of their symptoms and signs. A secondary spatialization occurred as physicians began to locate abnormalities or "lesions" within the three-dimensional space of the body. Finally, a third spatialization occurred with the reorganization of hospitals as teaching and healing institutions.

The categorical spatialization of illness has persevered up until today. Classification systems persist in such forms as the World Health Organization's International Classification of Disease (ICD) and the American Psychiatric Association's *Diagnostic and Statistical Manual of Mental Disorders* (DSM). In the physical body, spatializations of illness are widely reflected in the proliferation of imaging technologies such as X-ray machines, computerized tomography (CT) scanning, and magnetic resonance imaging (MRI). These allow physicians to peer deeper into the innermost recesses of the human body. Beyond this, hospital design and a provider's approach to care are all influenced by spatializations of health within a broader society.

One example of a clinical medical technology that has stood the test of time is the stethoscope. This instrument was present at the birth of the clinic in the nineteenth century. Before the stethoscope, doctors relied on patients' subjective descriptions of their symptoms. With the advent of this device, health care shifted its focus to signs that a doctor could objectively detect in the body, thereby shifting the medical gaze. Importantly, the introduction of the stethoscope brought the physician and patient into a new diagnostic ensemble (Schubert, 2011). This diagnostic ensemble encompasses a body-focused relationship between the physician and patient, one in which instruments such as the stethoscope mediate the physician's examination of the body and diagnosis of disease. Yet the stethoscope is only one instrument among many that are used to "objectively" observe signs of disease in the body. The introduction of additional diagnostic devices, such as X-ray devices, CT scanners, MRI machines, and genetic tests, equips physicians with additional body-focused ways of making a diagnosis. Yet in spite of these new technologies, diagnostic data is still filtered through the practical judgment of physicians. As such, the human side of the ensemble is just as necessary as the technical aspects of health care (see Timmermans & Buchbinder, 2012).

In addition to focusing on a patient's "objective" symptoms, medicine in the twentieth century began to monitor the health of the population as a whole (Armstrong, 1995). In principle, this **surveillance gaze** submitted the entire population to close medical observation. The focus of this shift was not about diagnosing individuals as explicitly "healthy" or "sick" but rather about placing people along a continuum of healthfulness (or risk of illness). With this starting point, bodies are viewed through the lens of their future disease potential, and individuals are imagined in "risk categories" (Brown & Duncan, 2002). Imaging the continuum of health and illness has brought into question the dichotomous division of people into purely "healthy" or "sick"—we are all simultaneously healthy and sick.

This has involved exporting medical surveillance outside of the clinic and hospital into everyday life through targeted health promotion activities like community disease screenings. These types of programs allow the health care profession to continue defining "normality"—those outside the (usually statistical) boundaries of "normal" are deemed "at risk" or "ill," even when they might not feel unwell. For example, community screenings for high blood pressure (hypertension) involve testing large numbers of individuals against statistical norms. Those who attend such screenings are then placed along the spectrum of risk and told that they are "normal and healthy," "at risk," or "ill." As part of the surveillance gaze, each of those categories comes with instructions on what to do next: "continue your healthy lifestyle," "reduce sodium in your diet," or "start drug treatment."

As Armstrong (1995) details, one mundane yet pervasive surveillance technology is the height and weight growth chart that models the growth trajectory of an "average" person. Now, technology is far more advanced. Screening technologies, such as genomic medicine, allow health care providers to screen individuals for early signs of disease. However, these screening practices are themselves quite complex and can significantly influence individuals' experience of their body and sense of self. This effect is particularly notable as the field of health promotion is increasingly reliant on pervasive computer technology and social media to observe the health patterns of populations (Lupton, 2012).

CASE STUDY

The Quantified Self

The quantified self is a popular movement that seeks to intertwine technologies that generate data, especially as it relates to health, into people's daily lives. These technologies provide individuals with the ability to measure their daily "performance" across multiple parameters including sleep, food consumption, mood, and exercise. Through technologically assisted self-surveillance, "quantified selfers" or "biohackers" typically aim to utilize these technologies to improve their own health and maximize efficiency. In some cases, people use wearable sensors to track changes in the body like skin temperature and heart rate. These sensors can also measure a person's activity levels, the number of steps they take per day, or the number of calories they burn. Other tracking tools, such as apps for handheld devices, allow users to input their own information, such as the amount of time they spend daydreaming or how many cups of coffee they consume daily.

A multitude of iPhone apps exist to track a person's sleep patterns. Once installed, app users place their phones on their bed while they sleep; the app measures their movement throughout the night to determine how often they alternate between the phases of the sleep cycle. Not only does this provide data on how frequently the person tossed and turned, but it can also be used to set alarms to wake the person up during "ideal" periods when their sleep is lightest. Ironically, this process supposedly allows them to wake up "more naturally."

Whether the quantified self truly improves an individual's health is a matter of debate. Supporters see the movement as the ultimate way to know oneself, thereby facilitating the best possibility of improving health and changing behaviours. Only by producing scientific data can individuals understand the root causes of their problems and the best ways to improve their health. Critics, on the other hand, argue that much of the data is meaningless; the health goals promoted by such apps and programs ignore individual variability by equating health with statistical averages. Moreover, they question whether the anxiety that comes with constant surveillance could outweigh the possible health benefits of using these apps. Significant worry can also result from a fear of being unable to improve oneself in spite of this technology.

Regardless, the quantified self movement reflects the ways in which health-related technology can impact a person's identity and sense of self.

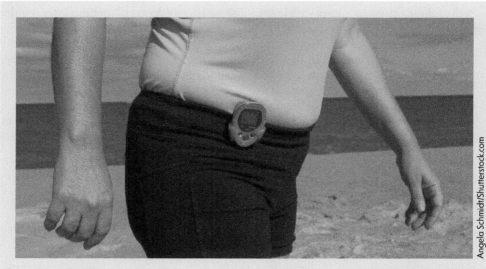

Angela Schmidt/Shutterstock.com

Devices like pedometers allow people to measure and track themselves against tangible standards. Unlike patient records, which are managed by institutions, tools like this can be ways of performing self-surveillance. How do medical technologies reflect the values of modern medical culture, discussed in Chapter Eight?

Technological enhancements to clinical medicine and the normalizing power of medical classification have fostered a third mutation in medical perception: the **molecular gaze**. Life is increasingly conceptualized on a molecular scale, and improving medical technology allows us to address disease on this scale. While the clinical gaze focuses on limbs, organs, and circulatory systems, and the surveillance gaze addresses the idea of health norms and risk across the population, the molecular gaze operates at the genetic and cellular level of the human body (Rose, 2007). Biology is no longer destiny but is open to re-engineering.

The molecular gaze has emerged at the confluence of technoscience and health care services, involving biomedical professionals, life scientists, venture capitalists, government regulators, and consumers. Major interests of this confluence include the pursuit of bodily enhancements and biosecurity (Clarke et al., 2010). The human brain, for example, has emerged as a rather profitable site of intervention. A new array of neurotechnologies, such as psychopharmaceutical drugs, has been introduced into diagnostic and normalizing ensembles (Abi-Rached & Rose, 2012). The molecular gaze's aim of preventing illness and optimizing health has greatly influenced the field of biomedicine, giving rise to new ways of living (Adams, Murphy, & Clarke, 2009).

Chapter Summary

In summary, this chapter has outlined some of the critical perspectives on health, society, and technology, paying particular attention to recent shifts and transformations in the many fields of biomedicine. The chapter emphasized that medical technologies cannot be approached as isolated materials with innate properties. They also cannot be considered blank slates. Their significance comes from their relationship with various "socio-technical" ensembles. Medical technologies are thus best understood by paying particular attention to the types of encounters and experiences they help enact and the types of ensembles they are a part of.

In addition, the chapter has tried to demonstrate how one cannot properly examine medical technology without acknowledging how it overlaps with a broader and more fundamental medical gaze. Technologies are not only consequences of this gaze but are constitutive elements of it. In this sense, medical technologies are never neutral, nor are they completely detached or severed from human judgment. This view challenges the notion that life and technology are two separate entities. Technology is a fundamental mediator of life and, as such, takes on pronounced significance in fields such as medicine and in people's everyday experiences. Whether viewed as an independent social force, a socially constructed artifact, or a practice in and of itself, technology is undeniably important in shaping health care practices and understandings of health.

STUDY QUESTIONS

1. What does the term *technomedicine* mean? Would you agree that modern health care can be characterized as such?
2. Compare and contrast the attitudes of people adhering to the technological determinist, social essentialist, and technology-in-practice viewpoints.
3. Where is the line drawn between technological enhancement and "normal" medicine?
4. How might medical technology challenge what it means to be human?
5. What role should the government play in regulating health-related technology?

SUGGESTED READINGS

Fukuyama, F. (2003). Our posthuman future: Consequences of the biotechnology revolution. New York: St Martin's Press

Lupton, D. (2013). The digitally engaged patient: Self-monitoring and self-care in the digital health era. *Social Theory & Health*, *11*(3), 256–70.

Rose, N. (2003). Neurochemical selves. *Society*, 41(1), 46–59.

SUGGESTED WEB RESOURCES

Assistive Technologies (Science Museum, UK): www.sciencemuseum.org.uk/broughttolife/themes/ technologies/assistivetechnologies.aspx

Quantified Self: Guide to Self-Tracking Tools: http://quantifiedself.com/guide/tag/health

Root Wolpe, P. It's Time to Question Bio-Engineering. TED Talk: www.ted.com/talks/ paul_root_wolpe_it_s_time_to_question_bio_engineering?language=en

GLOSSARY

Biological citizenship A sense of belonging within a group of individuals with a shared biological trait, regardless of geographical location. These groups may engage in biomedical activism. For example, HIV-positive individuals could advocate for improved access to antiretroviral drugs for their condition.

Medical gaze A term introduced by French scholar Michel Foucault. It describes a philosophy of health and illness that focuses on objective physical symptoms instead of patients' subjective experiences. Technologies such as the stethoscope contribute to the medical gaze by allowing doctors to observe such symptoms without any patient input, thus "bypassing" the patient.

Molecular gaze Observing health at a microscopic, molecular level.

Social essentialism A sociological perspective stating that the characteristics of an object are determined by social perception and society as a whole. For technology, this means that we as humans determine the moral value of technology according to how we use it.

Surveillance gaze Observing the entire population medically to dictate what constitutes normal health, and categorizing individuals accordingly.

Technogovernance The notion that technology shapes the entirety of the patient–carer relationship.

Technological determinism A sociological perspective on technology. Views technology as a dominant, independent, uncontrollable force in society, with its own free will and logic.

Technology The material artifacts we use to improve our everyday lives or the world around us.

Technomedicine The practice of medicine that is heavily dependent on technological devices and advancements (see Rose, 2007).

Technology-in-practice A sociological perspective on technology, arguing that technology's moral value comes from its context. Technology in the health care field, for example, is only one aspect of a broader network of the health care system, and its value comes in the value of its position in this framework.

REFERENCES

Abi-Rached, J. M. & Rose, N. (2010). The birth of the neuromolecular gaze. *History of the Human Sciences*, *23*(1), 11–36.

Adams, V., Murphy, M., & Clarke, A. E. (2009). Anticipation: Technoscience, life, affect, temporality. *Subjectivity*, *28*(1), 246–65.

Armstrong, D. (1995). The rise of surveillance medicine. *Sociology of Health & Illness*, *17*(3), 393–404.

Berg, M. & Harterink, P. (2004). Embodying the patient: Records and bodies in early twentieth-century US medical practice. *Body & Society*, *10*(2–3), 13–41.

Bromley, E. (2012). Building patient-centeredness: Hospital design as an interpretive act. *Social Science & Medicine*, *75*(6), 1057–66.

Brown, T. & Duncan, C. (2002). Placing geographies of public health. *Area*, *34*(4), 361–369.

Casper, M. J. & Morrison, D. R. (2010). Medical sociology and technology critical engagements. *Journal of Health and Social Behavior*, *51*(1 Suppl), S120–S132.

Clarke, A. E. (2010). From the rise of medicine to biomedicalization: US healthscapes and iconography c.1890–present. In A. E. Clarke, L. Mamo, J. R. Fosket, J. R. Fisher, & J. K. Shim (Eds.), *Biomedicalization: Technoscience and transformations of health and illness in the US* (pp. 104–46). Durham: Duke University Press.

———, Shim, J. K., Mano, L., Fosket, J. R., & Fishman, J. R. (2003). Biomedicalization: Technoscientific transformations of health, illness, and US biomedicine. *American Sociological Review, 68*, 161–94.

Conrad, P. (2005). The shifting engines of medicalization. *Journal of Health and Social Behavior*, *46*(1), 3–14.

Crubzy, E., Murail, P., Girard, L., & Bernadou, J. P. (1998). False teeth of the Roman world. *Nature, 391*(6662), 29–30.

Curtis, S., Gesler, W., Fabian, K., Francis, S., & Priebe, S. (2007). Therapeutic landscapes in hospital design: A qualitative assessment by staff and service users of the design of a new mental health inpatient unit. *Environment and Planning C, 25*(4), 519–610.

Foucault, M. (1973). *The birth of the clinic: An archeology of medical perception.* London: Routledge.

Haraway, D.J. (1991). *Simians, cyborgs, and women: The reinvention of nature.* London: Routledge.

Hogle, L. F. (2008). Emerging medical technologies. In E. J. Hackett, O. Amsterdamska, M. E. Lynch, & J. Wajcman, (Eds.), *The new handbook of science and technology studies* (pp. 841–874). Cambridge: MIT Press.

Ihde, D. (1990). *Technology and the lifeworld: From garden to Earth.* Bloomington: Indiana University Press.

Kearns, R. A., Ross Barnett, J., & Newman, D. (2003). Placing private health care: Reading Ascot Hospital in the landscape of contemporary Auckland. *Social Science & Medicine, 56*(11), 2303–15.

Kirk, S. (2010). How children and young people construct and negotiate living with medical technology. *Social Science & Medicine, 71*(10), 1796–1803.

Lupton, D. (2012). M-health and health promotion: The digital cyborg and surveillance society. *Social Theory & Health, 10*(3), 229–44.

Mamo, L. & Fosket, J. R. (2014). Scripting the body: Pharmaceuticals and the (re) making of menstruation. *Signs, 40*(1), 925–49.

May, C., Rapley, T., Moreira, T., Finch, T., & Heaven, B. (2006). Technogovernance: Evidence, subjectivity, and the clinical encounter in primary care medicine. *Social Science & Medicine, 62*(4), 1022–30.

Milligan, C., Mort, M., & Roberts, C. (2010). Cracks in the door? Technology and the shifting topology of care. In M. Schillmeier & M. Domenech (Eds.), *New technologies and emerging spaces of care dwelling: Bodies, technologies and home* (pp. 19–38). Farnham: Ashgate.

Mol, A. (2002). *The body multiple: Ontology in medical practice.* Durham: Duke University Press.

Mort, M., Roberts, C., & Callen, B. (2013). Ageing with telecare: Care or coercion in austerity? *Sociology of Health & Illness, 35*(6), 799–812.

Moser, I. (2006). Disability and the promises of technology: Technology, subjectivity and embodiment within an order of the normal. *Information, Communication & Society, 9*(3), 373–95.

Philo, C. (2000). Foucault's geography. In M. Crang & N. Thrift (Eds.), *Thinking space* (pp. 205–38). London: Routledge.

Reiser, S. J. (1978). *Medicine and the reign of technology.* Cambridge: Cambridge University Press.

———. (1981). *Medicine and the reign of technology.* Cambridge: Cambridge University Press.

Risse, G. B. (1999). *Mending bodies, saving souls: A history of hospitals.* Oxford: Oxford University Press.

Rose, N. (2007). *The politics of life itself: Biomedicine, power, and subjectivity in the twenty-first century.* Princeton: Princeton University Press.

——— & Novas, C. (2004). *Biological citizenship.* Hoboken: Blackwell Publishing.

Schillmeier, M. & Domènech, M. (eds.) (2010). *New medical technologies and emergent spaces of care.* Farnham: Ashgate.

Schubert, C. (2011). Making sure: A comparative micro-analysis of diagnostic instruments in medical practice. *Social Science & Medicine, 73*(6), 851–57.

Shildrick, M. (2010). Some reflections on the sociocultural and bioscientific limits of bodily integrity. *Body & Society, 16*(3), 11–22.

Sulik, G. A. (2009). Managing biomedical uncertainty: The technoscientific illness identity. *Sociology of Health & Illness, 31*(7), 1059–76.

Timmermans, S. & Berg, M. (2003). The practice of medical technology. *Sociology of Health & Illness, 25*(3), 97–114.

Timmermans, S. & Buchbinder, M. (2010). Patients-in-waiting: Living between sickness and health in the genomics era. *Journal of Health and Social Behavior, 51*(4), 408–23.

Woods, C. S. (2013). Repunctuated feminism: marketing menstrual suppression through the rhetoric of choice. *Women's Studies in Communication, 36*(3), 267–87.

Wyatt, S. (2008). Technological determinism is dead; Long live technological determinism. In R. Scharff & V. Dusek (Eds), *Philosophy of technology: The technological condition* (pp. 165–180). Cambridge: MIT Press.

Zola, I. K. (1972). Medicine as an institution of social control. *Sociological Review, 20,* 487–504.

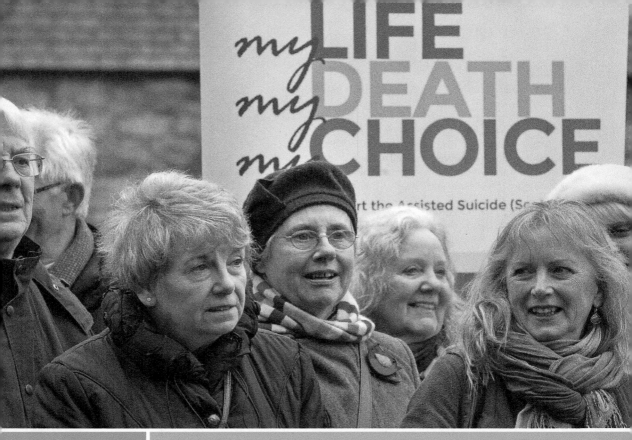

14

Ethical Issues in Health and Health Care

Elizabeth Peter, James Gillett, and Mat Savelli

LEARNING OBJECTIVES

In the following chapter, students will learn

- how ethics relates to health and health care
- the key ethical challenges facing individuals, health care providers, and policy makers
- how ethical concerns in health and health care are addressed

What Are the Key Ethical Challenges in Health and Health Care?

In January 2015, the Supreme Court of Canada overturned a 1993 ruling that prevented Canadians with "grievous and irremediable medical conditions" from ending their life with the assistance of a physician. Before this landmark case, physician-assisted suicide was unlawful in Canada (Payton, 2015). Legislation of physician-assisted suicide varies greatly from location to location. In countries like the Netherlands and Belgium, provisions exist that enable people who are suffering from medical conditions to arrange to end their lives. In the United States, laws on physician-assisted suicide are decentralized and therefore vary considerably between states. The practice is legal in Oregon, Washington, and Vermont (see Bernat & Beresford, 2014) but illegal in most remaining states. As a result of the ruling in Canada, the government is required to develop a set of guidelines to determine the parameters and processes around physician-assisted suicide.

Physician-assisted suicide is an excellent example of the sorts of ethical challenges in modern health care. On the one hand, some citizens argue that honouring the so-called "right to die" misrepresents the lives of people living with severe disabilities and could lead to a serious misuse of end of life directives. Conversely, citizens living with debilitating conditions argue that they deserve the right to freely decide to end their life under the counsel of a physician (Deschepper, Distelmans, & Bilsen, 2014). Later in the chapter we will examine this challenge in more detail. In the meantime, the right to die movement and the issue of physician-assisted suicide can help students understand the nature of ethical challenge's in health and health care.

The first step is to understand what is meant by **ethics**. Often, people think of ethics as the difference between right and wrong. They may associate the concept with moral or religious values. A simple definition is hard to articulate easily. Velasquez, Andre, Shanks, and Meyer (2010) identify two components of ethics that are helpful in framing the concept. First, ethics involves "well-founded standards of right and wrong that prescribe what humans ought to do, usually in terms of rights, obligations, benefits to society, fairness, or specific virtues" (Velasquez et al., 2010). Standards of right and wrong situated in a societal context and enforced by the rule of law are accompanied by a second component. Ethics, according to Velasquez and colleagues (2010), also involves continuous reflection of our own morality and that of broader social institutions.

The concept of ethics as a dynamic set of moral standards which provide a guide to determining what is right and wrong works well in the abstract. However, issues that arise in a pluralistic and complex society often do not have clear or simple standards of right and wrong. Rather, what is right or wrong in regards to a particular issue is contested; different groups have their own perspectives on what is "correct." This is especially true for issues relating to health care. In the case of physician-assisted suicide, for example, all invested parties do not necessarily share a common perspective. Some people are advocates for the right to die, whereas others are concerned that this right will jeopardize the lives of people with disabilities. Another factor that makes ethics complex relates to the availability of resources. Ideally, everyone should have access to new medical technologies and the best possible health care; in reality, however, the resources available to provide that care are limited. Thus, difficult decisions need to be made about the most ethical use of health care resources: some people are going to be placed on waiting lists or may even be denied access to treatments or care.

Ethical challenges, then, arise when the right course of action is not necessarily clear. Such situations require careful consideration and dialogue in order to determine the best course of action. In the case of assisted suicide, individuals and groups are now offering a legitimate argument for why assisted suicide ought to be allowed under specific conditions. Whereas once the idea of the right to die was considered unethical, this standard is being questioned and challenged. In many industrialized societies, values and beliefs relating to end of life care are shifting; assisted suicide is an ethical challenge that citizens are increasingly taking under consideration.

The study of ethics in health care is typically called bioethics or health care ethics. The term *bioethics* has been defined by Reich as "the systematic study of human conduct in the area of the life sciences and health care, insofar as this conduct is examined in the light of moral values and principles" (Jennings, 2014, xv). Scholars in bioethics use many different methods in their work, including philosophical perspectives, empirical data, theological beliefs, and legal sanctions, in order to examine the complexity of ethical issues in health care and the life sciences. Critical approaches have also become common in bioethics, with some scholars explicitly labelling their approach as critical bioethics (Hedgecoe, 2004). Other critical scholars may categorize their work under the umbrella of feminist bioethics (Lindemann, 2014). These critical approaches blur the boundaries between ethics and politics, investigating power differences and their impact on everyday ethics and bioethics scholarship. They also critique the dominant conceptualization in ethical theory that views people as autonomous, equal, and rational; critical scholars understand individuals as socially connected, vulnerable, and interdependent. In addition, critical approaches question the conceptualization of ethical knowledge as idyllic and derived from reason, not real life experience. As such, critical approaches emphasize the use of empirical approaches to understand bioethical issues (Liaschenko & Peter, 2006).

What are the current key ethical challenges in health care? This question was posed to bioethicists in an article by Jonathan Breslin and his colleagues (Breslin et al., 2005). They identified ten ethical challenges facing citizens in most Western industrial nations:

- Conflicts over treatment decisions
- Determining essential services
- The lack of services for vulnerable populations
- A shortage of health care workers to provide care
- Medical error
- Decisions about end of life care
- The ability to give informed consent prior to receiving care
- The risks and benefits of participation in medical research
- Determining who can make health care decisions on behalf of another
- The emergence of new medical technologies

The list reflects the perspective that bioethicists bring to questions regarding health and health care. If one was to ask patients, politicians, or health care professionals for their list, it would likely be different. Such is the challenging nature of ethical dilemmas: what we consider to be ethically important varies according to a wide range of actors in a pluralistic society. Given this diversity of perspectives, bioethicists are in a unique position to consider the central ethical challenges in health and health care today. Since their occupation is to explore, study, and support the resolution of ethical issues, they are in a privileged position to influence society's understanding of, and response to, ethical issues.

Treatment Decisions

In describing a case study of an older man involved in a car accident, Kulvatunyou and Heard (2004) highlight ethical challenges that can arise when patients and doctors disagree on a course of treatment. In this example, doctors provided treatment to a Jehovah's Witness who, because of his religious beliefs, refused a blood transfusion. Religious beliefs are one common reason patients alter or refuse a particular course of medical care, even if health care providers believe it is "in their best interest" (Koenig, 2004). Bioethicists identified such disagreements between patients and health care professionals over treatment decisions as a primary ethical challenge (Breslin et al., 2005). Refusing to accept a potentially life-saving treatment because of religious beliefs is an extreme example of a disagreement. Beyond this example, there are less serious (but still significant) tensions that can arise between patients, families, and health care professionals when determining a course of treatment.

It is not uncommon for patients or their families to advocate for treatment that a physician deems unnecessary, irrelevant, or potentially harmful. Increasing use of complementary and alternative medicine, for instance, can create such an ethical challenge. In such cases, patients may seek to incorporate treatment modalities that an allopathic physician views as harmful or unnecessary (Adams, Cohen, Eisenberg, & Jonsen, 2002). Conversely, there are instances in which physicians may advocate strongly for a treatment approach that the patient is uncomfortable or unsure about. Decisions regarding cancer medications, for example, can be difficult. These drugs are toxic and may worsen a patient's quality of life even though they may be effective in treating the disease. Patients and physicians in this situation face difficult decisions about the best course of action. Among health care providers, physicians especially exercise considerable medical, moral, and legal authority. They may exert pressure on patients to adopt a course of treatment that they do not wish to follow. Accordingly, a patient may not comply with the doctor's plan or may not fully share in making treatment decisions (Guenter, Gillett, Cain, Pawluch, Travers, 2010).

The physician–patient relationship can be seriously jeopardized if the two are unable to find common ethical grounds upon which to base treatment decisions. Accordingly, the relationship may be rife with tension and conflict, potentially decreasing a patient's quality of care or fostering a hostile work environment. Current debates over the over use of antibiotics, vaccines, and prescription drugs in general hint at the broader public health implications of ethical struggles over treatment decisions.

In the article cited at the beginning of this section about the Jehovah's Witness in the car accident, Kulvatunyou and Heard (2004) sought to outline a course of treatment that would be acceptable to the patient while also conforming to medical practices. This type of scholarship makes it clear that finding an ethical standard that includes all stakeholders is a priority. A mutually acceptable common ground may not always be possible, but attempting to resolve the issue in such a way is an important step forward in effectively addressing the ethical challenges of making treatment decisions.

Access to Health Care and Waiting Lists

One of the pillars of the public health care system in Canada, and in many public health care systems, is universal access to care (Madore, 2005). The extent to which the health care system successfully meets this principle and the factors which limit access, especially to those who require care the most, is an ongoing topic of debate. An assumption underlying public health care systems is that all citizens will have reasonable access to care; in practice, however, that may not be the case, particularly when resources are scarce. Wilson and Rosenberg (2004) conducted a study on perceptions of health care availability in Canada. They asked people about their perceptions of current health care availability, then provided statistics on the realities of health care accessibility. Despite the fact that Canadians are not confident in the availability of health care, most Canadians valued the idea of accessibility and experienced relatively few barriers to care. Limits to health care access were generally connected to structural forms of disadvantage, like socio-economic status, age, and illness. It is important to recognize that, while Canadians are universally entitled to care, this care is narrowly defined as hospital and physician services. As Chapter Nine discussed, other forms of care, such as drugs, dental, and psychological care, for example, often require that people possess

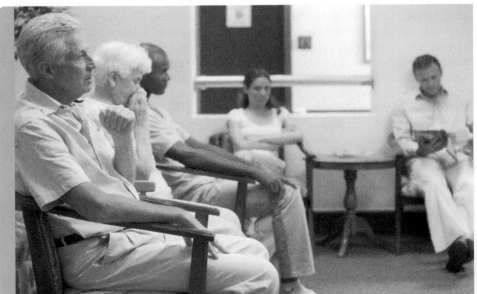

Monkey Business Images/Thinkstock

The issue of wait times is a well-known problem in Canadian health care. Why does waiting exist? What effects can long waits have on the provision of universal care?

private insurance or pay directly. Financial barriers can greatly limit accessibility. Similarly, in the United States, ethnicity and race are major social and cultural factors that create barriers to health care accessibility. Snowden and Yamada (2005), for instance, identify a direct relationship between cultural differences and differential opportunities to access care in the United States.

According to the panel of bioethicists guiding this chapter, the lack of accessibility among vulnerable populations represents a major ethical challenge in situations where universal access is implied and expected (Breslin et al., 2005). Goins and colleagues (2005) illustrate these challenges in more detail in their qualitative study of rural older adults' access to health care. Based on their experiences, elderly rural residents felt their lack of income and social isolation made it difficult to receive care. Beyond that, they also noted a lack of competent health care providers in rural settings.

Expanding from this study, there appear to be two contexts in which the availability of adequate care is compromised. First, the social circumstances in which an individual is living can create barriers to health care—this is especially true for vulnerable populations. In the case of mental illness, social stigma can compound existing factors that might act as a barrier to care (Eisenberg, Golbertstein, & Gollust, 2007). Corrigan (2004) notes that the negative associations that our culture links with mental illness limit opportunities for care and can discourage people from wanting or feeling like they should receive care. Secondly, there are cultural barriers that prevent or limit access to care for many individuals who could benefit from assistance.

It is ethically problematic when there are barriers preventing individuals taking advantage of health care that is meant to be accessible to everyone in society. Evidently, there are a number of barriers that place people in vulnerable positions in society at a disadvantage. This situation encourages us to consider what measures can be taken to address the challenges of unequal access to care. What compounds this question is that there are limited resources available for health care, and the availability of these resources may even be decreasing. Such issues are especially relevant to disadvantaged groups. What can be done? One strategy suggests that resources allocated to health care systems could concentrate more on chronic conditions rather than acute conditions, since chronic health issues are more prevalent among disadvantaged groups (Breslin et al., 2005). Giving those who face barriers to health care access opportunities to express their concerns is also important (Goins et al., 2005). Meanwhile, programs to raise awareness about the stigma of mental health may also improve conditions for access.

One of the main concerns about the accessibility debate is whether the perceived lack of accessibility is a sufficient justification for broad-based revisions to public health care. Consider the complex issue of "elective" surgeries. Should public health insurance cover the cost of breast augmentation? What about for women who have mastectomies to treat breast cancer? What about knee surgery to help someone overcome pain? Does the "rightness" of covering the cost depend on whether the person needs a good knee to make a living, like an athlete? What if that athlete makes millions of dollars per year? For any of these surgeries, it may be contentious for the cost to be covered through public health insurance; after all, they each "take away" personnel and resources from other individuals. At the same time, it is difficult to measure pain and suffering—what might seem like a frivolous issue for one person could be experienced very seriously by another. Bioethicists are thus heavily involved in debating issues regarding what types of treatments might be reasonably covered in a system that guarantees universal access to health care. Wilson and Rosenberg (2004) caution that is important to clearly define for the public what is meant by "reasonable" and "ethical" accessibility to care, considering need and geographic location. They contend that, as in any health care system, there are compromises that must be made regarding general access to care. However, it is crucial to ensure that these compromises not be used to justify the lack of available of services for those in situations of structural disadvantage.

Shortage of Health Care Workers

The shortage of health care workers is commonly identified as a primary barrier to accessing health care. Such an example can be found in the case of rural older adults. Certainty, the availably of physicians, nurses, and allied health professionals is key to ensuring that vulnerable populations have access to timely care and that waiting lists for procedures are reduced or given a rationale for their necessity. Nonetheless, there are ethical challenges linked specifically to making sufficient health care workers available across a population. In many Western nations, this issue takes the form of ensuring an adequate distribution of workers across different jurisdictions. Governance structures can limit or enable the training and movement of providers. For instance, in Canada, specific health care professionals may be licensed to practise in one province but not in another, since institutions like education and medical care are governed and organized provincially. These limitations exist despite the fact that each province must follow the five guiding principles of the Canada Health Act, of which accessibility is one (Asanin & Wilson, 2008).

Another challenge relates to a global shortage of health care workers. The increasing migration of individuals, often from low-income to middle- and high-income nations, raises the ethical issue of hiring foreign, as opposed to locally trained, workers. Hiring foreign workers might be an effective way of overcoming worker shortages and ensuring that all Canadians (regardless of geographic location) have access to physicians and nurses with minimal wait times. But on the other side of the argument is the fact that this migration may be creating a critical shortage of health care providers across much of the low-income world, including parts of Africa, South America, and Southeast Asia. This process, described in the case study below, has significantly impeded the provision of lifesaving health services, such as immunization, HIV prevention, and the treatment of AIDS in those regions (Taylor, Hwenda, Larson, & Daulaire, 2011). Pond and McPake (2006) argue that addressing the critical shortage of health care workers in low-income countries requires greater cooperation and dialogue among nations about the international movement of highly trained professionals from low-income to high-income nations. Moreover, such practices must be combined with policies that encourage greater stability and security in the working conditions of health care workers in countries facing critical shortages.

In Canada, the main challenge regarding ethical access to health care relates to **primary care physicians** (Breslin et al., 2005). While the growth in the number of physicians in the country is rising faster than the population, these doctors are unequally distributed throughout the country. As such, many Canadians still do not have access to primary care physicians. This creates a situation in which many Canadians, particularly in rural and remote areas, do not have access to primary care (Canadian Health Services Research Foundation, 2012).

CASE STUDY

"Brain Drain" in Sub-Saharan Africa

Recent decades have witnessed an increasing debate regarding the international migration of health care workers. This issue affects most countries in the world, in one form or another. From the perspective of health ethics, this migration raises a series of difficult questions involving not only the migrating individuals themselves, but the governments and health care systems of their "home" and "destination" countries as well.

Sub-Saharan Africa is one of the areas most affected by outflowing medical migration. Countries in the region have been greatly affected by the legacy of colonialism, political instability, and economic disruption. As a result of these factors, the burdens of poverty and disease have deepened. To further complicate the matter, most countries in this region experience a critical shortage of physicians, nurses, and other health care workers (Mills et al., 2011).

Thus, it is hardly surprising that the emigration of large numbers of Sub-Saharan medical workers to wealthy Western countries like Canada and the United States has raised some ethical flags. These countries dedicate substantial time and scarce financial resources in order to train physicians and nurses; with a much greater disease burden in their home countries, does it really make sense for those individuals to move to rich countries where their services might be less needed? After all, Sub-Saharan hospitals and clinics themselves are facing tremendous staff shortages. The problem of wealthy countries "poaching" doctors from poorer ones is indicative of a broader "brain drain," where many of the best-educated individuals are leaving Sub-Saharan Africa behind for more lucrative careers elsewhere. Outward medical migration has cost the region roughly $2 billion, whereas Canada has saved almost $400 million by hiring doctors from Sub-Saharan Africa (Mills et al., 2011).

At the same time, however, the individuals who are migrating make the point that they should not be forced to stay against their will or to be held accountable for the "failings" of their country. If they are actively being recruited for a lucrative or prestigious position in a foreign country, should they not have the right to leave? Like health care professionals anywhere in the world, they would argue that they worked hard for their degrees and have therefore earned the right to move wherever they see fit. Finally, many perceive the opportunity to move abroad (especially to former colonial powers) as a chance to "make a better life" for their family (Castles, 2000). Should anyone be able to deny them that?

The ethics of medical migration becomes even more difficult to navigate when international aid and financial policies are taken into account. For example, much of the poverty that increases the rate of disease and encourages outmigration can arguably be traced to the policies of the very countries benefitting from doctor migration, whether through the legacy of colonialism or the cuts in public health care services demanded by Western-dominated international financial institutions like the IMF and World Bank. As mentioned in Chapter Seven, these organizations typically insist that economically unstable countries must decrease their spending on public health if they wish to receive aid. Frequently, these demands exacerbate existing health problems in these countries (Tankwanchi et al., 2013). Thus, the issue of medical migration involves complex ethical questions for governments and health care workers around the world—all of which has a serious impact on individuals who need care, especially in low-income countries.

In most public health care systems, the bulk of care is provided at the primary care level. Patients can access the services of a medical specialist on the basis of a referral from a primary care practitioner. If citizens are unable to enroll with a family physician or a nurse practitioner, not only are they not being provided with adequate access to care, but unnecessary burdens are then placed on other aspects of the health care system. For example, people without primary care are forced to go to walk-in clinics or emergency rooms when they experience health problems. As a result, care that should be provided in the community instead takes place in hospitals. Neither of these venues can provide the same level of care, despite costing the health care system far more (Wellstood, Wilson, & Eylse, 2005). As Wang and Luo (2005) note, poor access to providers has effects along two lines: spatial, in that the distribution of providers is lower across regions that are underserved, and social, in that there are not necessarily providers available to assist those who are marginalized or require a greater degree of care.

In health care systems that value access to quality care, a lack of trained health care providers is a serious ethical problem. It creates a cascade of challenges around how to ensure that there are available physicians and nurses to provide health care services, especially at the primary level. Ensuring that adequate health care employees are hired equalizes access to health care and avoids needlessly wasting the system's resources. To address such challenges

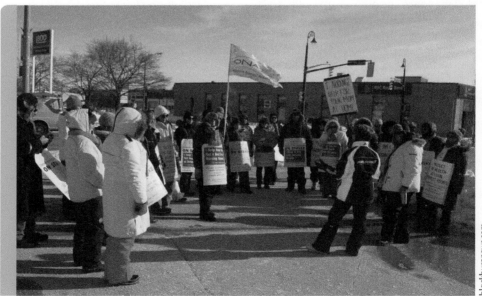

blackburnnews.com

Sarnia community care coordinators, who are members of the Ontario Nurses' Association, strike in January 2015 as part of rolling protests against low wage increases for coordinators working in community care access centres rather than in hospital settings. In a climate where shortages and unequal distributions of health care workers are much discussed, how can health systems incentivize their workers to work in community-based medicine?

in the Canadian context, strategies have aimed to make the primary care system "patient and family centred, accessible, effective, efficient, safe, coordinated and population–health oriented" (Aggarwal & Hutchison, 2012). Over the last ten years, multidisciplinary, inter-professional primary care teams have become increasingly common across Canada. More primary care providers, including family physicians, nurse practitioners, and midwives, are educated each year and are now employed in health care systems across the country. Regulations for non-physician providers have been reformed, and incentives are offered to family physicians who include nurse practitioners and other providers in their team practices. Yet despite the significant progress made since 2000, Canada lags behind many high-income countries in terms of timely access to primary care, particularly team-based, patient-centred care (Aggarwal & Hutchison, 2012). Substantial improvement is still needed if Canada is going to meet its ethical obligations regarding access to care.

Medical Error

Moving away from questions of access and the availability of care to ethical concerns regarding the nature of care itself, one of the most contentious recent issues to emerge is **medical error** (also termed **malpractice**). Regulated health care professionals are professionally and legally bound to adhere to specific standards of care when treating patients. Breaches of standards of care often stem from actions a health care professional should have taken, or actions they performed negligently. If an error results in harm to a patient, the health care professional is legally culpable (Keatings & Smith, 2010). Since health care workers can be sued for malpractice, providers may feel uneasy or distrustful in their interactions with patients (Studdert, Mello, & Brennan, 2004). In Canada, few injured patients sue their health care practitioners (Flood & Bryan, 2011). Still, this legal dimension alone presents ethical implications of medical error on a number of fronts, including when to disclose error to patients and the determination of what is considered an acceptable amount of error when a treatment or procedure causes harm.

Interest in discussing medical error is relatively recent (Breslin et al., 2005). For many generations the general assumption was that error happened only occasionally and was therefore not a component of regular medical practice. Generally speaking, health care is increasingly willing to examine its own practices. As a result, more attention is being drawn to medical error, how to address it, and how to develop strategies for limiting any problems that might arise when things go wrong.

A landmark study by Baker et al. (2004) revealed that 7.5 per cent of hospital admissions in Canada were associated with an **adverse event**, defined by the researchers as an "unintended injury or complication that results in disability at the time of discharge, death or prolonged hospital stay and that is caused by health care management rather than by the patient's underlying disease process" (p. 1679). Approximately 38 per cent of these adverse events were potentially preventable, pointing to the need to build a safer and more accountable health care system.

Ten years later, Baker (2014) reported on initiatives directed at the level of individual medical professionals and at care organizations to create a culture of safety within the health care system. The Canadian Patient Safety Institute (CPSI) was created to raise awareness and develop best practices to support patient safety. Progress has been made in challenging institutional norms that limited or delayed the disclosure of errors. Today, regulatory guidelines and practice norms require that health care professionals disclose any errors that may have harmed a patient (Baker, 2014). This change is ethically important because it helps foster transparency, accountability, and trust. It promotes a more equal partnership between patients, families, and their care providers. It also provides opportunities for carers to learn from their mistakes. A more public approach has also been developed by the CPSI through the creation of Patients for Patient Safety Canada, which encourages the public to become involved at the institutional and policy levels. While more progress is still needed, particularly by some health care organizations, there is a clear movement to build a safer health care system (Baker, 2014).

End of Life Care

A range of ethical challenges can emerge when making decisions regarding end of life care. Often it is assumed that **end of life decisions** only need to be made by older adults. However, the increasing prevalence of critical and debilitating illness, often in the form of cancer or autoimmune disorders among individuals of all ages, means that end of life decisions are an issue across the entire life course (Van der Heide et al., 2003). Moreover, such decisions are not merely up to the individual; rather, they often occur within the broader context of the patient, family, and health care team.

The involvement of caregivers, loved ones, and health care providers in making end of life decisions lends a level of ethical complexity to this issue. As a result, these decisions are often contentious, especially when aggressive measures are used to maintain someone's life (Peter, Mohammed & Simmonds, 2014). Death and dying are not widely discussed or easy to address in most cultures. This problem has been compounded by the medicalization of death, through which the lives of dying people are maintained by medical technology in ways previously unimagined. Prior to World War II, deaths were generally quicker, often as a result of an infectious disease. The advent of antibiotics, the respirator, and many new medical techniques has rapidly changed the nature of death, particularly in high-income countries. People tend to have prolonged deaths, and the decision to stop a life-prolonging treatment requires making difficult ethical decisions (Hardwig, 2006).

From the vantage point of bioethicists looking at ethical challenges in the Canadian context, two aspects to end of life care are most prominent (Breslin et al., 2005). The first surrounds the notion of competency. In cases of older adults with dementia, for instance, making decisions around end of life care requires a careful balance between taking the person's wishes into consideration while respecting the authority of their surrogate decision-maker. In such circumstances, judgment calls on issues like the level of pain relief and when to shift from curative to palliative care are as difficult as they are necessary (Sachs, Shega, & Cox-Hayley, 2004). Ideally, the process of making substitutive decisions will be made ahead of time and will involve the person who is critically ill. However, insufficient planning, medical emergencies, or the emotional shock of coming to terms with the end of life can complicate the surrogate role (Sudore & Fried, 2010). In some contexts, legislation identifies who has the authority to be the surrogate decision-maker; this may help in situations marked by conflict or differences of opinion (Breslin, et al, 2005). For families, the ethical difficulty of being in this situation can be traumatic and burdensome on social relations (Braun, Beyth, Ford, & McCullough, 2008).

Related to this first challenge is determining when the end of life should occur. This ethical issue is less about competency and is more a matter of self-determination. As mentioned earlier in this chapter, discussions about physician-assisted suicide are pushing social boundaries to allow people to end their own lives if they meet a set of legally established criteria. These criteria consider an adult's competency, consent, medical condition, suffering, and probable length of life (Carter v Canada, 2015). Increasingly, discussions about what it means to have a "good death" and the need to negotiate this process with health care providers, family, and friends is opening up new ground for many individuals who might find it difficult to consider end of life particularities (Kring, 2006). It can present health care professionals, patients, and family members with the ethical challenge of making the best possible decisions to prevent and relieve suffering, while maintaining life as long as they believe necessary.

Many attempts are being made to ease this process for all concerned. One step, as mentioned earlier, stresses the importance of planning. There are increasing resources available to health care providers and individuals that highlight the importance of developing a plan for end of life care (Sudore & Fried, 2010). A second step is the recognition by health care professionals that perspectives on the end of life and the burden on families and loved ones is socially and culturally variable (Kwak & Haley, 2005). Providers need to accept that there is generally no single model or experience that will apply equally to all people in all social contexts. And last, people working directly in this area, including those living with critical and terminal illnesses, are calling for a broader public discussion and debate about issues regarding end of life. Only through a wider public engagement, they argue, can death and dying be destigmatized (Izumi, Nagae, Sakura, & Imamura, 2012).

Participation in Medical Research

We usually think of health care in the form of medical services, whether at the primary care level, in hospital emergency rooms, or at complementary medical centres in the community. Involvement in medical research represents a rather different form of public participation in health care. Participants are regularly solicited to be involved in a variety of different kinds of research, often through surveys on patient satisfaction or enrollment in randomized clinical trials for new treatments. The ethics of human-focused medical research has provoked substantial debate for quite some time, although it has become especially prominent since the latter half of the twentieth century.

The notion of **informed consent** is a particularly crucial issue in health care (Breslin, et al., 2005). In the United States, the history of consent to medical research is contentious, in large part because of the Tuskegee syphilis experiment. Also discussed in Chapter Five, the Tuskegee story holds an important place in our evolving understanding of medical ethics. This experiment took place in Alabama between 1932 and 1972. Researchers divided local African American men into two groups, the first made up of men who had previously contracted syphilis and the second consisting of those who had not. Over the next forty years, researchers observed these men to see how the disease progressed. The subjects were

CASE STUDY

Alexis St Martin

An interesting early Canadian example of medical research and ethics is the nineteenth-century story of Alexis St Martin. As described by Rutkow (1998), St Martin was a hunter and voyageur who, after receiving a gunshot wound to the stomach, was enlisted in medical research by William Beaumont, a military surgeon posted nearby. The wound to St Martin's stomach healed incompletely so that it was possible to see into his stomach and observe the process of digestion. Over the next several years, Beaumont and St Martin engaged in research by placing different types of food into the stomach and observing the process of digestion. The early work of Beaumont was extremely important to the development of gastroenterology.

From a medical ethics point of view, this case is interesting in that it was one of the first times where written consent was obtained, as documented in Beaumont's journal. However, in the accounts of the relationship between the two men, it is unclear whether St Martin's continued involvement in the experiments was truly voluntary as we would understand it today (Green, 2010).

not told about the nature of the research (being told only that they were being treated for "bad blood"), nor were they asked to give consent for their participation (Freimuth et al., 2001). Moreover, the infected men were not treated, despite the discovery midway through the study that penicillin could effectively cure syphilis. As a consequence, some of the men died from syphilis and a number of their wives and children were also infected. Eventually the research was deemed unethical, sparking a movement to improve patient safety in medical research. Despite the improved ethical safeguards that resulted from this discovery, the Tuskegee trial fuelled the already high levels of distrust in medical science among the public and among marginalized groups (Freimuth et al., 2001).

In contemporary medical research there are better guidelines and policies to ensure the ethical treatment of participants, including the requirement that people give informed consent (Flory & Emanuel, 2004; TCPS2, 2014). Despite these improvements, however, we still know little about people's motives for participating in research and what they expect to gain from the process. Some preliminary work suggests that there are a number of motivations for research participation. People may hope that their involvement will improve the likelihood that they will survive or improve their health. Other reasons for participating could include patients being coerced into the study or the belief that acting as a research subject may provide society with some benefit. The wide range of vulnerabilities and motivations of participants needs to be taken into account when considering the ethics of research (Cox & McDonald, 2013).

In recent years, a number of patient groups have formed in response to perceived mistreatment during medical research; these groups are politically well organized and advocate for changes to the structure of medical research and the protection of medical research subjects. In the 1990s, for example, people with HIV/AIDS engaged in treatment activism directed at creating a more humane and ethical practice for evaluating experimental medications (Gillett, 2011). More recently, groups of paid participants in medical research trials have been organizing as self-proclaimed "guinea pigs" and demanding improvements to the way they are treated and compensated. Weinstein (2001) documents the work of Robert Helms, a guinea pig activist who cultivates counter or lay expertise among those who are participants in medical research, articulating an alternative account of medical bioethics and the current state of medical science. In short, Helms argues that defining bioethics cannot happen from above (the scientific and medical community); rather, the "guinea pigs" themselves must dictate the ethics of research. Activists such as Helms have an important voice, representing those who are marginalized within medical science and health care in general. Although sometimes controversial, they contribute a perspective that is not necessarily considered within institutional discourse—one that could be valuable in protecting the safety of those participating in medical research.

Chapter Summary

This chapter utilized the discussion of a panel of bioethicists at University of Toronto's Joint Centre for Bioethics to guide students through some key ethical challenges in contemporary Canadian health care. The challenges that the panel identified—informed consent in medical research, tensions in treatment decision-making, end of life care, medical error, the shortage of health care workers, and access to health care—are relevant to most health care systems in late industrial democratic societies. This list is not exhaustive; individuals and communities face a number of health-related ethical issues that merit substantial discussion and debate. This is particularly true when it comes to advancements in medical technologies. Medical science is moving forward very quickly; new medical technologies, especially those that can enhance human capacity, force bioethicists, health care providers, and lay people alike to tackle new ethical frontiers. Against this backdrop, many argue that scientific advancement is outpacing the ethical frameworks available to ensure that such technology is used properly and fairly in our current social, cultural, and political circumstances.

Looking across the distinct challenges that this chapter has identified, a number of common themes emerge. One is the importance of taking into consideration the risks that the current health care system poses to those who are most vulnerable. Power inequalities in society are reflected and reproduced in the health care system. These occur most often to those who have the fewest resources and least power to respond. Communities are beginning to organize politically to address these injustices and to change the structures of medical research and practice. In other situations, patient mobilization has failed to bring about broad, sweeping changes in health care. Ethical challenges are always present when it comes to questions of preserving life and preventing death. It is important to understand these challenges as being intertwined and set within specific social, historical, political, and cultural circumstances.

STUDY QUESTIONS

1. Why should we consider ethics in relation to health care?
2. Outline the ethical arguments for and against physician-assisted suicide.
3. How can ethics be used to assist vulnerable populations when it comes to health?
4. What is meant by the term *medical error* and why is it contentious?
5. Should Canada recruit foreign-trained health care professionals from low-income countries?

SUGGESTED READINGS

Boyd, K. (2015). The impossibility of informed consent? *Journal of Medical Ethics, 41*(1), 44–7.

Savulescu, J. (2015). Bioethics: Why philosophy is essential for progress. *Journal of Medical Ethics, 41*(1), 28–33.

Steinhauser, K. E., Christakis, N. A., Clipp, E. C., McNeilly, M., McIntyre, L., & Tulsky, J. A. (2000). Factors considered important at the end of life by patients, family, physicians, and other care providers. *Journal of the American Medical Association, 284*(19), 2476–82.

SUGGESTED WEB RESOURCES

Centre for Practical Bioethics: Case Studies: www.practicalbioethics.org/resources/case-studies

Talbot, M. (2012). Bioethics: An Introduction. Podcast series sponsored by the University of Oxford: http://podcasts.ox.ac.uk/series/bioethics-introduction

Boghuma Kabisen Titarji's TEDx Talk: Ethical Riddles in HIV Research: www.ted.com/talks/boghuma_kabisen_titanji_ethical_riddles_in_hiv_research

GLOSSARY

Adverse event An unintended injury or other negative consequence that results from an issue within the medical system.

End of life decisions Choices an individual must make regarding their medical treatment at the end of their life.

Ethics A dynamic decision-making framework that allows individuals to act in a way that aligns with their personal values, religious beliefs, or other important guiding principles.

Informed consent Providing all individuals who are being treated, or those participating in research studies, with all information that could possibly affect their wellbeing. This allows individuals to actively participate in a decision that could greatly affect them.

Medical error (malpractice) Physician error that breaches their legal contract with the patient. In such a circumstance, the physician is held culpable.

Primary care physicians Medical doctors who function as the first point of contact for a patient.

REFERENCES

Adams, K. E., Cohen, M. H., Eisenberg, D., & Jonsen, A. R. (2002). Ethical considerations of complementary and alternative medical therapies in conventional medical settings. *Annals of Internal Medicine, 137*(8), 660–64.

Aggarwal, M. & Hutchison, B. (2012). *Toward a primary care strategy for Canada.* Canadian Foundation for Healthcare Improvement.

Asanin, J. & Wilson, K. (2008). "I spent nine years looking for a doctor": Exploring access to health care among immigrants in Mississauga, Ontario, Canada. *Social Science & Medicine, 66*(6), 1271–83.

Baker, G. R. (2014). Governance, policy and system-level efforts to support safer healthcare. *Healthcare Quarterly, 17* (Special Issue), 21–6.

———, Norton, P. G., Flintoft, V., Blais, R., Brown, A., Cox, J., ... & Tamblyn, R. (2004). The Canadian Adverse Events Study: The incidence of adverse events among hospital patients in Canada. *Canadian Medical Association Journal, 170*(11), 1678–86.

Bernat, J. L. & Beresford, R. (2014). Assisted suicide and euthanasia. Ethical and legal issues. In Aminoff, Boller, & Swaab (Eds), *Handbook of clinical neurology* (Series 3, pp. 118–81). London: Elsevier.

Brandt, A. M. (1978). Racism and research: the case of the Tuskegee Syphilis Study. *Hastings Center Report, 8*(6), 21–9.

Braun, U. K., Beyth, R. J., Ford, M. E., & McCullough, L. B. (2008). Voices of African American, Caucasian, and Hispanic surrogates on the burdens of end-of-life decision making. *Journal of General Internal Medicine, 23*(3), 267–74.

Breslin, J. M., MacRae, S .K., Bell, J., Singer, P. A., & University of Toronto Joint Centre for Bioethics Clinical Ethics Group. (2005). Top ten health care ethics challenges facing the public: Views of Toronto bioethicists. *BMC Medical Ethics, 6*, E5.

Canadian Health Services Research Foundation (CHSRF) (2012). *Myth: Canada needs more doctors.*

Canadian Institutes of Health Research, Natural Sciences and Engineering Research Council of Canada, and Social Sciences and Humanities Research Council of Canada. (TCPS2) (2014). *Tri-Council policy statement: ethical conduct for research involving humans.*

Carter v. Canada (Attorney General), 2015 SCC 5.

Castles, S. (2000). International migration at the beginning of the twenty-first century: Global trends and issues. *International Social Science Journal, 52*(165), 269–81.

Corrigan, P. (2004). How stigma interferes with mental health care. *American Psychologist, 59*(7), 614.

Cox, S. M. & McDonald, M. (2013). Ethics is for human subjects too: participant perspectives on responsibility in health research. *Social Science & Medicine, 98*, 224–31.

Deschepper, R., Distelmans, W., & Bilsen, J. (2014). Requests for euthanasia/physician-assisted suicide on the basis of mental suffering: Vulnerable patients or vulnerable physicians? *JAMA Psychiatry, 71*(6), 617–18.

Eisenberg, D., Golberstein, E., & Gollust, S. E. (2007). Help-seeking and access to mental health care in a university student population. *Medical Care, 45*(7), 594–601.

Flory, J. & Emanuel, E. (2004). Interventions to improve research participants' understanding in informed consent for research: a systematic review. *Journal of the American Medical Association, 292*(13), 1593–1601.

Flood, C.M. & Bryan, B.T. (2011). Canadian medical malpractice law in 2011: Missing the mark on patient safety. *Chicago Kent Law Review, 86*(3), 1053–92.

Freimuth, V. S., Quinn, S. C., Thomas, S. B., Cole, G., Zook, E., & Duncan, T. (2001). African Americans' views on research and the Tuskegee Syphilis Study. *Social Science & Medicine, 52*(5), 797–808.

Gillett, J. (2011). *A grassroots history of the HIV/AIDS epidemic in North America.* Ann Arbor: Marquette Books.

Goins, R. T., Williams, K. A., Carter, M. W., Spencer, S. M., & Solovieva, T. (2005). Perceived barriers to health care access among rural older adults: A qualitative study. *The Journal of Rural Health, 21*(3), 206–13.

Green, A. (2010). Working ethics: William Beaumont, Alexis St Martin, and medical research in Antebellum America. *Bulletin of the History of Medicine, 84*(2), 193–216.

Guenter, D., Gillett, J., Cain, R., Pawluch, D., & Travers, R. (2010). What do people living with HIV/AIDS expect from their physicians? Professional expertise and the doctor–patient relationship. *Journal of the International Association of Physicians in AIDS Care, 9*(6), 341–45.

Hardwig, J. (2006). Medicalization and death. *APA Newsletter, 6*(1), 2–9.

Hedgecoe, A. M. (2004). Critical bioethics: Beyond the social science critique of applied ethics. *Bioethics, 18*(2), 120–43.

Izumi, S. S., Nagae, H., Sakurai, C., & Imamura, E. (2012). Defining end-of-life care from perspectives of nursing ethics. *Nursing Ethics, 19*(5), 608–18.

Jennings, B. (2014). Introduction. In Bruce Jennings (Ed.), *Bioethics*. (4th ed., Vol. 2., pp. xv–xxii) Farmington Hills, MI: Macmillan Reference USA.

Keatings, M. & Smith, O. (2010). *Ethical and legal issues in Canadian nursing* (3rd ed.). Toronto: Elsevier.

Koenig, H. G. (2004). Religion, spirituality, and medicine: Research findings and implications for clinical practice. *Southern Medical Journal, 97*(12), 1194–1200.

Kring, D. L. (2006). An exploration of the good death. *Advances in Nursing Science, 29*(3), E12–E24.

Kulvatunyou, N. & Heard, S. O. (2004). Care of the injured Jehovah's Witness patient: Case report and review of the literature. *Journal of Clinical Anesthesia, 16*(7), 548–53.

Kwak, J. & Haley, W. E. (2005). Current research findings on end-of-life decision making among racially or ethnically diverse groups. *The Gerontologist, 45*(5), 634–41.

Liaschenko, J. & Peter, E. (2006). Feminist ethics: A way of doing ethics. In A. Davis, V. Tschudin, & L. de Raeve (Eds), *Essentials of teaching and learning in nursing ethics: Content and methods* (pp. 181–90). London: Elsevier.

Lindemann, H. (2014). Feminism. In Bruce Jennings (ed.). *Bioethics* (4th ed. Vol. 2.) (pp. 1185–92). Farmington Hills, MI: Macmillan Reference USA.

Madore, O. (2005). *The Canada Health Act: Overview and options*. Library of Parliament, Parliamentary Information and Research Service.

Mills, E. J., Kanters, S., Hagopian, A., Bansback, N., Nachega, J., Alberton, M., Au-Yeung, C. G., Mtambo, A., Bougeaut, I., Luboga, S., Hogg, R. S., & Ford, N. (2011). The financial cost of doctors emigrating from sub-Saharan Africa: Human capital analysis. *British Medical Journal, 343*, 1–13.

Payton, L. (2015). Supreme Court says yes to doctor-assisted suicide in specific cases. CBC News. Retrieved from www.cbc.ca/news/politics/supreme-court-says-yes-to-doctor-assisted-suicide-in-specific-cases-1.2947487

Peter, E., Mohammed, S., & Simmonds, A. (2014) Narratives of aggressive care: Knowledge, time & responsibility. *Nursing Ethics, 21*(4), 461–72.

Pond, B. & McPake, B. (2006). The health migration crisis: the role of four Organisation for Economic Co-operation and Development countries. *The Lancet, 367*(9520), 1448–55.

Rutkow, I. M. (1998). Beaumont and St Martin: A blast from the past. *Archives of Surgery, 133*(11), 1259–59.

Sachs, G. A., Shega, J. W., & Cox-Hayley, D. (2004). Barriers to excellent end-of-life care for patients with dementia. *Journal of General Internal Medicine, 19*(10), 1057–63.

Snowden, L. R. & Yamada, A. M. (2005). Cultural differences in access to care. *Annual Review of Clinical Psychology, 1*, 143–66.

Studdert, D. M., Mello, M. M., & Brennan, T. A. (2004). Medical malpractice. *New England Journal of Medicine, 350*(3), 283.

Sudore, R. L. & Fried, T. R. (2010). Redefining the "planning" in advance care planning: Preparing for end-of-life decision making. *Annals of Internal Medicine, 153*(4), 256–61.

Tankwanchi, A. B. S., Özden, Ç., & Vermund, S. H. (2013). Physician emigration from sub-Saharan Africa to the United States: Analysis of the 2011 AMA physician masterfile. *PLoS Medicine, 10*(9), e1001513.

Taylor, A. L., Hwenda, L., Larsen, B. I., & Daulaire, N. (2011). *New England Journal of Medicine, 365*, 2348–51.

Van der Heide, A., Deliens, L., Faisst, K., Nilstun, T., Norup, M., Paci, E., … & van der Maas, P. J. (2003). End-of-life decision-making in six European countries: Descriptive study. *The Lancet, 362*(9381), 345–50.

Velasquez, M., Andre, C., Shanks, T., & Meyer, M. J. (2010). What is ethics. *Issues in Ethics, 1*(1), 1–2.

Wang, F. & Luo, W. (2005). Assessing spatial and non-spatial factors for healthcare access: Towards an integrated approach to defining health professional shortage areas. *Health & Place, 11*(2), 131–46.

Weinstein, M. (2001). A public culture for guinea pigs: US human research subjects after the Tuskegee study. *Science as Culture, 10*(2), 195–223.

Wellstood, K., Wilson, K., & Eyles, J. (2005). "Unless you went in with your head under your arm": Patient perceptions of emergency room visits. *Social Science & Medicine, 61*(11), 2363–73.

Wilson, K. & Rosenberg, M. W. (2004). Accessibility and the Canadian health care system: Squaring perceptions and realities. *Health Policy, 67*(2), 137–48.

Glossary

Adverse event an unintended injury or other negative consequence that results from an issue or problem within the medical system, usually during treatment.

Allopathic a type of medicine that focuses on diagnosing an illness and treating it using remedies that counter its symptoms. For example, an allopathic doctor would prescribe a painkiller for a headache.

Alternative medicine approaches to health care outside of the current widely accepted biomedical framework.

Behavioural approach views illness as a result of personal behaviours that can be modified.

Biological citizenship a sense of belonging within a group of individuals with a shared biological trait, regardless of geographical location. These groups may engage in biomedical activism. For example, individuals with HIV could advocate for improved access to antiretroviral drugs for their condition.

Biomedicine a system of healing that views illness as a biological manifestation affecting the individual. It relies upon ideas of mind–body dualism, physical reductionism, and specific etiology. It is considered the most legitimate form of healing by most Western governments and citizens.

Capitation a model of financing health care that pays providers a lump sum per patient to cover health care for a given period of time.

Class a component of one's identity, also known as socio-economic status. It is related to one's education, income, family background, and occupation.

Classic utilitarianism a political theory stating that all relationships are voluntary and, as such, the distribution of goods and services should do the most good for the greatest number of people.

Commodity something that can be purchased and sold.

Complementary and alternative medicine (CAM) a wide array of healing practices. Most are outside of typical biomedical practices and may have an ancient or indigenous history.

Complementary medicine works in conjunction with biomedicine, rather than in opposition to it.

Conceptual fields a method of studying a subject by incorporating the views of multiple disciplines in a holistic way (e.g., women's studies, social gerontology).

Constituency-based health movements these focus on health discrepancies between members of different demographics or constituencies, e.g., those of a certain race, gender, or sexuality.

Consumerism an ideology in which an individual consumes goods and services to fulfill their own interests. Consumers have the freedom to make informed, rational choices.

Contested illness an illness with inexplicable or uncertain medical symptoms. While patients experience the illness, it is unclear how or why. These illnesses may be a source of contention between patients and medical practitioners (e.g., fibromyalgia).

Co-payments the process in which patients pay for a portion of their services while insurers cover the remaining charges.

Critical health studies an approach to studying health that is characterized by "criticality." It is interested in challenging and analyzing current conceptions of health and health care. This involves questioning social, political, and economic practices; current norms and ideologies; and practices that marginalize or negatively affect individuals or groups.

Critical perspectives a way of studying a topic that addresses and analyzes the effects of institutional norms, models of thinking, power dynamics, and broader social influences on a given issue.

Cultural competency the ability to work with, and for, individuals from a number of cultural groups. There is no widely accepted working definition of this phrase.

Culture a widely defined, contested term. As culture is dynamic, there is no universal definition of the term. For the purposes of this text, culture is defined as the learned, shared, and transmitted behaviours that influence members of a given (culture sharing) group.

Direct-to-consumer (DTC) advertising pharmaceutical advertising that is aimed directly at the consumer (as opposed to advertising to the prescribing physician).

Disciplinarity   the notion that different disciplines, or fields of study, have unique ways of addressing an issue.

Embodied health movements bring together people who experience particular illnesses or diseases to advocate to increase awareness, raise funds, or alter policies.

End of life decisions   choices an individual must make regarding their medical treatment at the end of their life.

Ethics   a dynamic decision-making framework that allows individuals to act in a way that aligns with their personal values, religious beliefs, or other important guiding principles.

Evidence-based medicine an approach to biomedicine that statistically evaluates how patients respond to treatments and what interventions are most effective. Evidence-based medicine is an empirical approach to medicine that is based on scientific research, such as randomized controlled trials.

Folk health sector   encompasses healer-led medicine outside of the professionalized realm of biomedicine. Some examples include herbalists and spiritual healers.

Free market capitalism   an open economy in which vendors can buy and sell without any external interference such as government restrictions, international trade laws, or other taxes.

Gender   Unlike biological sex, gender has meaning beyond chromosomes; it involves complex social roles and expectations. Many societies divide gender along binary lines (men/women) but it should be noted that many individuals and societies recognize the existence of multiple gender identities.

Germ theory   Louis Pasteur's germ theory identified pathological organisms as the source of illness. It is one of the key contributing factors to the evolution of biomedicine.

Global humanitarianism addressing human rights violations and inequality on a global scale. Global humanitarian groups aim to ensure that the basic human rights of all individuals are met.

Globalization   the process by which countries, people, and corporations are brought into closer contact with one another. Through globalization, we can more easily travel and exchange ideas, money, and resources.

Health access movements   social movements that focus on ensuring adequate access to medical care for everyone in society.

Health field concept   a way to address health that addresses biology, the environment, lifestyle, and health care systems. The health field concept addresses factors beyond individual control.

Health promotion encouraging people to maintain and/or improve their personal health through public information campaigns.

Health sciences   the disciplines, typically scientific in nature, that work in conjunction with medicine. Examples include toxicology, genetics, occupational therapy, and pharmacy.

Health studies   addresses health, illness, and medicine through a social science, humanities, or interdisciplinary lens. Health studies researchers are interested in exploring issues related to health at the individual, cultural, economical, political, environmental and international levels.

Healthism   the idea that, through making proper lifestyle choices, one can be proactive in maintaining one's health or becoming healthier; an emphasis on an individual's responsibility for their health.

Healthscapes   the tangible aspects of the health care system. Examples include hospitals, clinics, or the physical layout of a health care organization.

Holism, holistic   relating to the system as a whole. Holism refers to the notion that health and disease can be understood only by approaching the individual as a whole—the physical body, mental state, social factors, the environment, and so on.

Iatrogenesis   harm or illness that results directly from medical treatment, such as the side effects of a prescription drug.

Individualism   stresses that the individual is more important than the collective group.

Informed consent   providing all individuals who are being treated, or those participating in research studies, with all information that could possibly affect their wellbeing. This allows individuals to actively participate in a decision that could greatly affect them.

Informed consumer (expert patient)   a consumer who knows the risks, benefits, and costs of what they are acquiring or purchasing (in this case, health care). The expert patient, then, can be thought of as a hyper-informed consumer.

Integrative medicine   an approach to medicine that consolidates biomedicine and CAM.

Interdisciplinarity   an approach to an issue in which a researcher draws on their personal experience with and knowledge of different disciplines (see Table 2.1 in Chapter Two).

Intersectionality the relationship between any and all of one's social identities. Posits that one's social identity is a result of the relationship between *all* of their various identities (gender, sexuality, race, class, etc.). None of these should be neglected.

Labelling theory the sociological concept that deviance is not an inherent quality but a label of society. In this sense, something is not "other" until society perceives and claims it is so.

Libertarianism a political ideology that emphasizes individual rights and argues for minimal state intervention into the lives of individuals.

Licensing using a system of formalized credentials to determine who can practise a given profession. For example, doctors must pass certification exams and complete medical school.

Machine metaphor a way of viewing the body, assuming that the body is but the sum of all of its "components" and "parts"—in a sense, the body is a machine made of individual mechanisms.

Marketization the process in which previously public services become increasingly like private businesses, facilitating competition between firms vying to attract consumers.

Marxism a political theory centred on the idea that socio-economic divisions within a society drive its evolution. Generally speaking, Marxists believe that all members of society should have access to the basic needs of life (e.g., food, water, medical care, housing, employment).

Material deprivation a lack of basic "materials," such as housing, food, and employment, needed for a certain standard of life.

Medical discourse society's conceptions of medical knowledge that influence our understanding of disease and its treatment. Medical discourse can vary among cultures.

Medical error (malpractice) physician error that breaches their legal contract with the patient. In such a circumstance, the physician is held culpable.

Medical gaze a term introduced by French scholar Michel Foucault. It describes a philosophy of health and illness that focuses on objective physical symptoms instead of patients' subjective experiences. Technologies such as the stethoscope contribute to the medical gaze by allowing doctors to observe such symptoms without any patient input, "bypassing" the patient.

Medical pluralism the existence of a diversity of medical perspectives.

Medical tourism international travel for the sake of acquiring medical treatment.

Medicalization the process in which conditions and behaviours that were previously considered a normal part of life come to be understood as medical problems (e.g., the conceptualization of inattention and hyperactivity as ADHD).

Mind–body dualism a theory by Rene Descartes (seventeenth-century philosopher) stating that the mind and the body are two separate, discrete entities.

Molecular gaze observing health at a microscopic, molecular level.

Moral hazard problem arises when insured patients heavily utilize available health care resources. As a result, they drive up the cost of insurance for everyone involved.

Morbidity the prevalence and incidence of a disease in a given population.

Mortality rate of deaths in a population over a period of time.

Multidisciplinarity an approach to an issue that uses the knowledge of various disciplines with little overlap or communication between them. In this approach, people with different areas of expertise work in parallel to reach discrete conclusions on a common issue (see Table 2.1 in Chapter Two).

Neoliberalism a theory of political economy derived from liberalism. Emphasizes capitalism, individual wealth, and private property. For neoliberals, markets are inherently good, self regulating, and necessary. Government interventions, such as taxes or redistributive processes for wealth, are not encouraged.

One Health an updated version of One Medicine. Stresses the importance of maintaining the health of all species and our overall ecosystem in an increasingly globalized society.

One Medicine an attempt to unite human and veterinary medicine as a result of the discovery that humans and animals are interrelated.

Paradigm a widely excepted explanation or framework for understanding a given issue.

Patriarchal relating to a patriarch, the male head of a society. In the context of this textbook, "patriarchal" refers to a male-dominated society.

Physical reductionism the act of analyzing a physical entity in light of its smallest parts. An example of this could be analyzing diseases on a microbiological level or studying the immunology of human blood types.

Placebo effect noticeable effects of treatment that occur when participant is given a placebo (for example, an inert sugar pill) and told it will be effective.

Political economy the relationship between an interdependent government system and economy. Political economists inquire into the relationship between the state and the market at a given moment in time.

Popular health sector individuals' personal experiences with health or illness. Members of the general population can consult one another, individually and as a group, to obtain health-related information, identify and diagnose their symptoms, or share their own health-related experiences.

Population health originally, an approach to health that stresses the importance of ensuring the health of the broader population and the social determinants of health. It aims to reduce income inequality to improve everyone's quality of life and, in turn, decrease the government's health care budget. The concept of population health changes with context.

Premium the fee charged for insurance coverage for a given period of time.

Primary care physicians medical doctors who function as the first point of contact for a patient.

Principal–agent relationship a relationship in which the principal contracts an agent to work in the principal's best interest. Such a relationship involves an element of trust. Economists use this term to describe the relationship between a patient and health care practitioner.

Professional domains the knowledge and practice of specific trained professions (e.g., nursing, social work).

Professional health sector encompasses health care workers who have been licensed and regulated. Examples include nurses and doctors.

Professionalization the process through which practitioners adhere to a set of legal requirements to create a uniformly regulated standard of quality. This allows professions to assert their legitimacy and competence amid other vocations.

Psycho-social stress stress related to one's position in society. For example, living with a low socio-economic status may introduce the added stress of securing housing and feeding one's family.

Quackery giving the false, unfounded impression of using a scientific method and rationale.

Qualitative information that cannot be quantified (measured in numbers). Qualitative analysis utilizes interviews, observations, and other non-numerical data. Qualitative data addresses *how* something is over *how much* of it there is.

Quantitative relating to numbers and measurable phenomena. Quantitative analysis deals with statistics, measurements, and other numerical data.

Race and ethnicity Contested terms. Some may use these terms to refer to genetic linkage and biological characteristics (e.g., skin and eye colour) but social scientists emphasize that these categories are socially constructed with little true biological meaning.

Randomized controlled trials A research method that divides participants, at random, into two groups. Researchers will conduct some form of research on one group (for example, exposing them to a new drug) while the other group will be a "control" group (and therefore will not receive any new treatments or interventions). These trials are an intrinsic part of evidence-based medicine as they help determine the effect, if any, of a medical treatment.

Rawlsian theory of social justice the political philosophy of John Rawls (1971). Centres on the concept of a "social contract" in which individuals define their own concept of a just society. Ideally this society would distribute wealth and power equally among all of its citizens.

Regimen and control a basic tenet of biomedicine, stating that all illnesses and diseases can be prevented through a closely monitored, controlled, and regimented healthy lifestyle.

Secularization the process in which society has become increasingly detached from religious influence.

Single-payer model how health insurance works in Canada. The government pays all health care providers directly for their services.

Social capital Refers to the strength of a society's social fabric. This includes levels of trust, civic engagement, and a sense of belonging. These traits can have a positive influence on health.

Social constructionism A theory that holds that knowledge, definitions, and social roles are not fixed or inherent but are a dynamic product of society. For example, gender roles are a social construct.

Social essentialism a sociological perspective stating that the characteristics of an object are determined by social perception and society as a whole. For technology, this means that we as humans determine the moral value of technology in how we use it.

Social gradient ranking in society based on socio-economic status and one's relative position in a market economy.

Social identity our sense of self in relation to society as a whole and its broader social structures. While the definition of this term is not widely agreed upon, some components of social identity can include one's gender, race, and age.

Social movements groups of individuals mobilized around a common cause.

Socio-environmental model considers the impact of society and how its structures affect an individual's health. It also takes into account how social structures affect our behaviour and therefore our health.

Specific etiology from –*aita*, the Greek word for "cause." Specific etiology suggests that illnesses have a unique, identifiable cause.

Structures of identification societal structures (e.g., gender, sexuality, class) that shape our individual experience and our identity, though our experiences are inherently different from anyone else's.

Surveillance gaze observing the entire population medically to dictate what constitutes normal health, and categorizing individuals accordingly.

Technogovernance the notion that technology shapes the entirety of the patient–carer relationship.

Technological determinism a sociological perspective on technology. Views technology as a dominant, independent, uncontrollable force in society, with its own free will and logic.

Technology the material artifacts we use to improve our everyday lives or the world around us.

Technology-in-practice a sociological perspective on technology, arguing that technology's moral value comes from its context. Technology in the health care field, for example, is only one aspect of a broader network of the health care system, and its value comes in the value of its position in this framework.

Technomedicine the practice of medicine that is heavily dependent on technological devices and advancements.

The sick role how society views sick people and how societies expect sick people should behave.

Third-payer relationship the process through which an insurance company, or another third party, pays the health care provider on behalf of a patient.

Transdisciplinarity an approach to an issue in which a researcher moves across various disciplines, looking at their intersections and how they relate to the overarching concept at hand. In such an approach, researchers tend to work beyond their usual disciplines (see Table 2.1 in Chapter Two).

Universal coverage health insurance that covers an entire demographic or population. Universal coverage is mandatory: citizens must enrol and cannot opt out.

Vitalism the concept that human life is a result of a universal or spiritual energy force.

Voluntary coverage health insurance that individuals can opt to buy of their own volition. Such coverage is generally organized through private companies and is therefore competitive.

Wellbeing being healthy and content with one's life, having one's basic needs met. More than just the absence of disease.

Index